CANCER INCIDENCE IN FIVE CONTINENTS

ISBN 978-3-540-03475-9   ISBN 978-3-642-85849-9 (eBook)
DOI 10.1007/978-3-642-85849-9

UNION INTERNATIONALE CONTRE LE CANCER
INTERNATIONAL UNION AGAINST CANCER

Cancer Incidence in Five Continents

A Technical Report

Edited by:

Richard DOLL - Peter PAYNE - John WATERHOUSE

Distributed for the

INTERNATIONAL UNION AGAINST CANCER

by

SPRINGER-VERLAG BERLIN - HEIDELBERG - NEW YORK

CONTRIBUTORS

Dr. G. Batten
: Hawaii Tumor Registry,
Cancer Commission of Hawaii Medical Association,
P.O. Box 3378,
Honolulu, Hawaii 96801, U.S.A.

Dr. O. Bjarnason
: Cancer Registration,
Iceland Cancer Society,
Suourgata 22,
P.O. Box 150, Reykjavik, Iceland.

Professor G. Bras
: Department of Pathology,
University of the West Indies Medical School,
Kingston 7, Jamaica, W.I.

Dr. W.S. Burnett
: Bureau of Cancer Control,
Division of Chronic Disease Services,
Department of Health,
State of New York,
84, Holland Avenue,
Albany, New York 12208, U.S.A.

* Dr. J. Clemmesen
: Danish Cancer Registry,
Strandboulevarden 49,
Copenhagen Ø, Denmark.

* Professor P. Correa
: Department of Pathology,
Faculty of Medicine,
Universidad del Valle,
Cali, Colombia.

Professor J.N.P. Davies
: Department of Pathology,
Albany Medical College,
Albany, New York, U.S.A.

* Dr. R. Doll
: M.R.C. Statistical Research Unit,
University College Hospital Medical School,
115, Gower Street,
London, W.C. 1, England.

Professor G.M. Edington
: Department of Pathology,
University of Ibadan,
Ibadan, Nigeria.

* Dr. H. Eisenberg
: Cancer Registry,
Connecticut State Department of Health,
Chronic Disease Control Section,
79, Elm Street,
Hartford, Connecticut, U.S.A.

* Dr. W. Haenszel
: Biometry Branch,
National Cancer Institute - NIH,
Bethesda, Maryland 20014, U.S.A.

Dr. M. Hakama
: Finnish Cancer Registry,
Liisankatu, 21 B,
Helsinki, Finland.

Dr. V.H. Handy
: Bureau of Cancer Control,
Division of Chronic Disease Services,
Department of Health,
State of New York,
84, Holland Avenue,
Albany, New York 12208, U.S.A.

Dr. W. Heinsohn

Statistisches Landesamt der Freien und
                          Hansestadt Hamburg,
Steckelhörn 12,
2 Hamburg 11, W. Germany.

* Dr. J. Higginson

International Agency for Research on Cancer,
c/o World Health Organization,
Avenue Appia,
1211, Geneva, Switzerland.

Dr. R. A. Kenney

Faculty of Medicine,
University of Singapore,
Sepoy Lines, Singapore, 3.

* Dr. J. Kmet

Institute of Oncology,
Vrazov trg št. 4,
Ljubljana, Yugoslavia.

* Professor J. Knowelden

Department of Preventive Medicine and Public
                          Health,
The University,
Sheffield 10, England.

Dr. G. Llanos

Department of Pathology,
Faculty of Medicine,
Universidad del Valle,
Cali, Colombia.

Dr. C. M. U. Maclean

M. R. C. Unit for Research on the
                         Epidemiology of Mental Illness,
Royal Edinburgh Hospital,
Edinburgh 10, Scotland.

Dr. V. A. Marcial

Radiotherapy and Cancer Division,
Puerto Rico Nuclear Center,
Caparra Heights Station,
San Juan, Puerto Rico 00935.

Dr. I. Martinez

Central Cancer Registry,
Division of Cancer Control,
Department of Health,
Puerto Rico.

Dr. L. Meinsma

Centrale Kanker Registratie,
De Lairessestraat 33,
Amsterdam, The Netherlands.

Professor J. Moroder

División del Cáncer y Enfermedades Crónicas,
Servicio Nacional de Salud,
Agustinas 715, Santiago, Chile.

Dr. C. S. Muir

Department of Pathology,
Faculty of Medicine,
University of Singapore,
Sepoy Lines, Singapore, 3.

* Dr. A. G. Oettlé

South African Institute for Medical Research,
Cancer Research Unit,
Hospital Street,
Johannesburg, South Africa.

* Mr. P. M. Payne

South Metropolitan Cancer Registry,
Clifton Avenue,
Belmont,
Sutton, Surrey, England.

* Dr. E. Pedersen

The Norwegian Cancer Registry,
The Norwegian Radium Hospital,
Oslo, Norway.

CONTRIBUTING ORGANIZATIONS

Cancer Commission of the Hawaiian Medical Association.

The Cancer Registry of Norway.

Central Cancer Registry, National Organization of the Netherlands against
Cancer.

Connecticut State Department of Health.

The Danish Cancer Registry, National Anti-Cancer League.

The Department of Health, Puerto Rico.

England and Wales
    Regional Cancer Registry, Birmingham

    Regional Cancer Registry, Liverpool

    The South Metropolitan Cancer Registry

    South Western Regional Cancer Records Bureau

The Finnish Cancer Registry

The Icelandic Cancer Registry, Iceland Cancer Society

The Institute of Oncology, Slovenia

The Israel Cancer Registry

The Jamaica Cancer Registry

National Cancer Institute of Canada
    Alberta Tumour Registry

    Manitoba Tumour Registry

    New Brunswick Tumour Registry

    Newfoundland Tumour Registry

    Saskatchewan Tumour Registry

National Health Service, Chile

New York State Department of Health

The New Zealand Cancer Registry

Regional Office of Statistics, City of Hamburg

The Swedish Cancer Registry

CONTENTS

PREFACE

The suggestion that cancer incidence rates for different parts of the world should be brought together in a single volume arose in discussion among members of the Geographical Pathology Committee of the International Union Against Cancer during a symposium in Mexico in 1964. That there was a need for such a volume rapidly became apparent when the directors of cancer registries were asked for their opinion. Of those approached, all but one responded enthusiastically and immediately agreed to contribute. In the event, data have been collected from 32 cancer registries in 24 countries, and 39 scientists have contributed personally by describing the character of their registry and by collecting and submitting figures in a standard way.

The form in which the book appears was suggested by a committee of 15 members, which met at the Ciba Foundation in London in May, 1965, and the editors have been guided in their work by the results of the discussions that took place at that meeting. In a few instances, it has not been possible to follow the Committee's advice, for reasons of finance, and the text which was written by the editors may, in some places, have inadvertently misrepresented the Committee's views. The editors, therefore, take full personal responsibility for all defects in both style and scientific presentation.

It is a pleasure to acknowledge the help that has been given in the collection of information about individual registries by the Cancer Unit of the World Health Organization, and particularly by Dr. A. Tuyns who took part in the meeting of the Editorial Committee. We are most grateful also to the Ciba Foundation, whose hospitality enabled the Committee to meet in London under such pleasant conditions, and to the British Empire Cancer Campaign for a generous contribution to the expenses of the meeting.

Finally, it is our sad duty to report the death of two contributors, Professor Moroder and Professor Prates. Their energy and scientific competence made itself felt, not only in Chile and Mozambique, but throughout the world, and we hope that this volume may be regarded as being in part a memorial to them.

Richard Doll,
Peter Payne,
John Waterhouse.

Chapter I
INTRODUCTION

In the development of knowledge about the cause of a disease, the first and most difficult stage is the search for clues on which hypotheses can be based. In this search, no road can be guaranteed to lead to success, but if past experience is any guide, one of the most rewarding is likely to be that which leads to a comparison of the frequency with which the disease occurs in different communities in different areas and at different times.

Attempts to use this approach in relation to cancer have been made from the time when Percival Pott described the peculiar liability of chimney sweeps to the development of cancer of the scrotum. Such attempts were, at first, limited in scope and confined to a few types of cancer and a few localities, and it was not until this century that Bashford (1905, 1908) and Hoffman (1915) set out to examine the distribution of the different types of cancer on a worldwide scale. These early studies contributed some notable observations - particularly, but not exclusively, in relation to occupational hazards. Most attempts were, however, abortive and little factual knowledge was gained. In retrospect, this is hardly surprising, since the medical services had not yet been developed sufficiently for accurate records to be made of the frequency of diseases which were as rare and as difficult to diagnose as most of the cancers.

In the last 30 years, however, the situation has changed dramatically. Medical services have been expanded, diagnosis has been improved and better statistical techniques have been employed. A mass of useful information has consequently been collected and it is now becoming possible to piece together a realistic picture of the distribution of cancer over a large part of the inhabited world. This information was at first limited to mortality rates and to accounts of clinical and pathological series in which the numbers of one type of cancer were expressed as a proportion of all cancers or, for example, of all hospital admissions. Both these types of information provide only an indirect estimate of incidence, but they have their use. In some circumstances they may be sufficient; in others they may be all that is practicable to obtain.

Mortality rates are adequate for studies of comparative incidence in countries where the accuracy of death certification is high, and for cancers which have a high fatality rate. Clinical and pathological series are more difficult to assess. At best they can provide evidence only of proportional incidence and this will necessarily be affected by the frequency of occurrence of conditions other than the cancer under special study. They are, however, often the only type of information that can be obtained from areas where the provision of medical services is far below the optimum level, and in these circumstances they may provide useful, though necessarily uncertain, pointers to the fact that a particular cancer is almost unknown, or moderately or very common.

The most valuable data are, undoubtedly, the rates obtained by recording the occurrence of every case of cancer in a defined community over a specified period. Such incidence rates are never easy to obtain and it is only recently that they have become available on at all a large scale. They are now being collected regularly in some countries, while in others they have been collected only for a limited period as a specific research project. Some of the results are published routinely in detailed annual reports. Others have not been published at all or have been reported in only an abbreviated form in one of the medical journals. Even when the results have been reported in full, comparisons have not always been easy to make. For one thing, the reports in which the data appear are not all widely available; for another, registries have not all used the same break down of age groups and they have commonly combined the rarer types of cancer in groups in different ways.

The object of this book is, therefore, to bring together the available cancer incidence data in one place and to present them all in the same way, so that the research worker can make whatever comparison between them he chooses. Since incidence varies with time, it is clearly desirable to compare data for different communities collected over the same period. Whenever possible, therefore, the rates in chapters IV and V refer to the years 1960-62. If, however, rates were available only for some other period, they have been included, so long as it was between 1950 and 1965. Sometimes, also, the population covered by the cancer registry is small (for example, in Iceland) and, in these circumstances, it has been thought better to include data for a longer period, to reduce the amount of random error in the rates due to the small number of cases. Apart from Connecticut, New York State and Denmark, registries have not operated for long enough to allow comparisons to be made at different times. No attempt has, therefore, been made to include more than one set of data for each registry, and any study of trends in cancer incidence on a worldwide scale must await the collection of more data.

The registries that have co-operated in producing this book do not include all the registries now active. Some have been omitted because the country in which they operate is already adequately represented. Others, because there was doubt about the completeness with which registration was effected. Cancer registration is undertaken in different countries for different purposes, and research is not always the principal objective. In some countries it serves primarily for cancer control and less stress may then be laid on completeness of registration, than on completeness of follow-up. For research purposes, however - and particularly for the present purpose of enabling incidence to be compared at different ages, in different places and at different times - completeness of registration is vital. Registries were, therefore, invited to participate only when there was reason to believe that registration was practically complete and, in particular, when it was known that all deaths attributed to cancer were automatically reported to the registry by the national or local authorities responsible for the registration of deaths. Exceptions were made only when the registration data referred to communities for which reliable mortality rates were lacking. In this situation even incomplete data have value. They can, for example, provide clear evidence for an unusually high incidence of a particular cancer (as is provided by the rates for naso-pharyngeal cancer among the Chinese in Singapore) and for this reason it was thought that it would be useful to include them. The extent to which complete data have been collected by each registry is described in the introductory text before each set of Tables and the reader should always consult this before making use of the reported rates. Detailed evidence of the reliability of the figures could not, unfortunately, be obtained for every registry in the time available. Such figures as could be obtained for the proportion of cases diagnosed histologically and for the proportion registered as a result of death certification alone are summarized in the Appendix.

In addition to the incidence data and the basic facts relating to the character of each registry, needed for interpretation of the data, we have included a variable amount of information describing, in a more detailed way, the work of some of the registries and the results they have obtained. In one instance, we had the opportunity of including a full-length article and as it contained much that was new and concerned a country of major international interest (Iceland) we have published it in extenso.

For information about populations not included in these Tables, the reader is referred to the annual publications of the World Health Organization (1965a and 1965b) and to the mortality rates brought together in a series of books by Professor Segi and his colleagues in Japan (Segi, 1960; Segi and Kurihara, 1962, 1963 and 1964). The history of cancer registration has been fully described by Stocks (1959) and by Clemmesen (1965), and it is unnecessary to repeat it here. References to earlier publications on incidence are also given by Clemmesen (1965) and, in chapter IV of this book, in the sections referring to the work of individual registries.

Chapter II
REGISTRATION

DEFINITION

Cancer registration is a procedure whereby selected information about all cancer patients occurring in a precisely defined population is brought together centrally as soon as possible after diagnosis.

Unfortunately, some rather vague terms have had to be used in this definition as well as others which, while not in themselves vague, require elaboration.

First, there is the use of the word "all" in the phrase "all cancer patients". This is not vague but it idealizes the definition to an extent that makes it impossible to realize in practice. For reasons that will be examined later, no registry can be sure that it has registered every cancer patient nor that it has not included a few patients who do not have cancer.

Secondly, the word "cancer" (and all its synonyms) is vague since no universally acceptable definition of it has been presented in the standard works on tumour pathology. A corollary of this is that cancer registries, while in general agreement as to the kinds of diseases that they record, may differ in their handling of a number of pre-invasive groups and of histogenic categories containing tumours of low lethality.

Thirdly, the phrase "in a presisely defined population" must also be explained. The population which a cancer registry considers is usually, though not necessarily, geographical. If it is geographical, it may be national (for example, Norway, Sweden, Israel or Chile), or it may be sub-national : that is, it may relate to states or provinces (for example, Connecticut or Alberta), to municipalities (for example, Hamburg) or to areas defined for the purpose of hospital administration (for example, the Birmingham region in England). Cancer registration that is not related primarily to geographical populations may still need to be circumscribed geographically; for example.

> all rubber workers in England and Wales,
> all twin siblings of cancer patients in Denmark,
> or   all Bantu resident in Johannesburg.

Schemes that are not based solely on geographically defined populations seem not to be common except where they are being conducted on an ad hoc basis.

It is important that the population should be "precisely defined". The definition of the area itself in topographical terms is not difficult. What is more difficult is the maintenance of up-to-date information about the people living in the area. The most complete information of the kind required is that derived from periodic censuses. Unfortunately, these usually take place at long intervals and tables containing specialized information may not become available until several years after the enumeration. Some countries have now adopted sampling procedures to replace or supplement complete enumerations. In addition less detailed reports are published more frequently (usually annually) which give population estimates arrived at after allowance for registered births, deaths and migration. The first essential is that the population base used in the computation of morbidity rates should conform to the group of people who are liable to inclusion in the cancer registration scheme. It would not be satisfactory in a rapidly changing community, if population estimates from five years ago were applied to current cancer registrations. Nor would it be satisfactory if the population figures used contained large numbers of foreign nationals who were not subject to cancer registration within the area under consideration.

Fourthly, the phrase "as soon as possible after diagnosis" requires further explanation. While there are cancer registries which limit the collection of information to histologically verified disease, this is unusual. Most registries accept cases for registration diagnosed as cancer on the best evidence available at the time, even though this evidence may be only clinical. Clearly if this policy is not adopted a cancer registry can make only a limited contribution to epidemiological studies. A consequence of the policy is, however, that the figures for a particular period may never attain absolute stability. Diagnoses of cancer that were at one time accepted on clinical grounds may later be rejected on the basis of histological reports on an operation or autopsy specimen. Likewise, cancers may not be registered until long after patients first attend hospital with symptoms of their disease, simply because the diagnosis was not made originally. In some cases also, cancers may not be registered until after post mortem examination because the disease had not reached a sufficiently advanced stage to give rise to symptoms, or because the symptoms had been concealed.

Quite apart from difficulties of diagnosis there are other, administrative, reasons why the registration of cancer information may be delayed for a longer period than would normally be desirable. In some hospitals, for instance, it may be necessary for those concerned with cancer registration to wait until other departments whose requirements are deemed more urgent have completed their work on the case records. With the more lethal cancers, a high proportion of deaths may occur during this period of delay, and it is thus impossible to attain a situation in which all cancer patients are registered while still alive.

PURPOSES

The purposes of cancer registration are several and vary from one registry to another. The most important, and the one with which all are concerned, is the collection of statistical data to enable the incidence of each type of cancer to be determined by sex and by age. Such data are used both for planning the development of hospital services and in the study of aetiology, by allowing comparisons of cancer incidence to be made between different areas. As an extension of this, registries that are established on a longterms basis can provide evidence of trends in incidence with time - information which is again of value for both administrative and research purposes.

Some registries place special emphasis on research; and, in these, efforts may be made to obtain information about differences in incidence in different sections of the population. The type of information that can be obtained is usually limited by the information that is available about the population from census data. Sometimes, however, cancer registries can, themselves, add to this by collecting the relevant data at an ad hoc census or from a suitably chosen sample. Sometimes also a special population may be defined by others who depend on the registry's co-operation for the detection of cases.

A quite distinct purpose is the collection of follow-up data and the calculation of survival rates following different types of treatment and in different centres. Such information is of interest to the participating hospitals as a guide to the efficacy of their treatment and to the national health authorities for purposes of cancer control. The use of such data in the evaluation of new methods of treatment is, however, not without danger and the clinical and follow-up data collected by cancer registries should not normally be regarded as an adequate replacement for controlled clinical trials.

6

Finally, the archives of a registry provide an invaluable source of material for clinical and other research workers who need access to more cases of a particular type of cancer than they would normally achieve. This is of particular value in the study of rare cancers - for example, the cancers of childhood - but it may also be of value when the number of cases that has to be studied is unusually large.

OPERATION OF CANCER REGISTRIES

There has been no international agreement, and little in the way of recommendations, as to how cancer registries should carry out their functions. Even within such countries as the United Kingdom and the U.S.A. the regional or state registries operate independently and in a variety of ways. These differences show themselves at every level from underlying purposes and policies to the finer details of day to day routine. Some of these differences have no noticeable effect on global comparisons and international co-operation, but others obviously do.

Permanent and Temporary Schemes

The first point of variation is the permanence or otherwise of the registry. Most registries have been established with the intention that they should continue indefinitely. But others (for example, the registry of cancer cases in the Johannesburg Bantu) were created solely for a limited objective, such as the determination of cancer incidence in the population in a defined period.

Statutory and Voluntary Schemes

Most cancer registries are able to function only if they can convince participating hospitals of the value of the work they are doing and if they undertake to provide reciprocal statistical services. Statutes making cancer a notifiable disease do exist (for example, in New York State); but they are not common. There is an obvious disinclination to frame laws regarding a disease that is lacking in precise definition and which can easily be ignored without causing any obvious dislocation to the medical services.

Incentives

Where cancer registration is voluntary it is a common practice to offer special incentives to the participating hospitals or to the staff who undertake the necessary work. First, is the return of useful information - and this may mean that a registry has to register all patients who seek investigation or treatment in hospitals within the area, irrespective of whether they reside in the registry's defined population. It would not impress the staff of a hospital if the services provided by the registry were limited to patients living in one area when, in fact, a high proportion of the hospital's patients came from another.

Secondly, financial incentives may be given. Varying sums may be paid to the registering hospital or doctor providing the information, depending on whether it consists of an initial registration, or a follow-up or necropsy report (as by the Danish Cancer Registry). Alternatively, a fixed sum of money may be apportioned between the contributing hospitals at the end of each year, on the basis of the kinds and quantities of information they have each submitted (as in Connecticut). The latter method, while requiring more book-keeping, probably makes for better budgetary control.

Responsibility for Abstracting Information

Some advantage might be derived if the medical history and the results of the clinical examination of cancer patients were recorded on special forms at the time of the patient's first examination. Unfortunately this kind of arrangement is difficult to achieve, since most clinics do not deal exclusively with cancer patients. In any event the history and clinical assessment are only a part of the record; other items, such as details of treatment, the results of radiographic and other special investigations and pathological reports, are not available until later. It has, therefore, become general for the abstracting process to be done when the initial investigations and treatment have been completed and usually when a firm diagnosis has been made. Much superfluous paper-work is thereby avoided.

There is, however, some difference of opinion about who should abstract the data. It is often maintained that only medically qualified personnel should do this and that if lay staff do it, errors will arise from their inability to interpret the records properly and from their failure to look for important annotations in particular situations. In many countries, however, doctors are already burdened with much paper-work and they resist any further impositions of this kind, especially when the benefit accruing to individual patients is not obvious. If, in these circumstances, doctors are required to do the work, they may in fact be less accurate than lay staff and certainly much more liable to allow arrears to accumulate. Unless there is definite willingness on the part of doctors to co-operate, it is probably better to rely on lay staff and to ask medical staff merely to operate a system that will ensure that : (a) all registerable cases are readily identifiable; and (b) all the required information is present in the case records in a form which makes interpretation by lay staff relatively simple. The latter objective is most easily achieved by arranging that case records should, as far as possible, take the form of a series of questionnaires.

The use of lay clerks for abstracting cancer information is, however, not without its difficulties. At all but the largest hospitals, there may not be enough work for full-time employment and troubles often arise when responsibilities are divided between several jobs. If clerical labour is short, either because of inability to attract staff, or because of budgetary limitations, hospital administrators will have a natural inclination to assign their staff to work that directly serves the ends of the hospital rather than the needs of an outside organization; and this is particularly likely to be so when the organization lacks statutory support.

Some registries for example, the South Metropolitan Cancer Registry in England - have tried to overcome these problems through the use of peripatetic clerks on their own staff. The advantages of this system are that :

1. Preliminary training by the registry makes for greater uniformity of standards;

2. The clerks are subject to the discipline of the registry in a way that hospital clerks cannot be; and

3. The clerks can specialize absolutely in the work of cancer registration and can, therefore, become highly efficient.

The main disadvantage is that a substantial amount of time and money must be spent in travelling, and thought must be given to the arrangement of itineraries so as to minimize the average cost of each registration.

Registerable diseases

It has already been noted that cancer registries may vary in regard to the classes of disease that they register. For the vast majority of cancers, the nature of which is obvious, there is complete agreement. The differences occur mainly in certain borderline groups. These are considered in detail in chapter III.

Other sources of variation are that some registries concern themselves only with histologically verified cancers, or only with patients who have at some time attended hospital for investigation or treatment.

Some registries limit themselves to recording patients and ignore further tumours that may occur in a patient who has had one previously. Most, however, concern themselves with tumours rather than patients, and a patient with a second primary tumour should appear in the records twice. This makes it important to distinguish between bilateral primary tumours in paired organs and a single primary tumour with extension or metastasis into the contralateral organ. Obviously, however, it would be very difficult to extend this principle to the recognition and registration of multiple tumours at the same site, and this has not been attempted.

Information recorded at the time of registration

The phrase "at the time of registration" is intended here to exclude information which is normally derived as part of the follow-up procedure or which is normally gleaned from death certificates or necropsy reports. It has been the custom in some areas for hospitals to use a simple provisional form of registration containing a minimum of information about suspected cancer cases and to follow this later with a detailed confirmatory registration or with an account of why registration is not being pursued. We assume here that registration is carried out as a single process.

The amount and type of information which is sought must depend on :

(a) the quality and quantity of staff available in the contributing hospitals and at the registry;

(b) the amount of detail needed for the provision of reports and services;

(c) the reliability of the proposed items of information and indeed whether they are likely to have been elicited from patients at all; and

(d) the equipment that is available for data processing and analysis.

A list of the items that a well-staffed and well-equipped registry might include are set out in the following Table. A smaller registry without mechanical or electronic data processing equipment would probably attempt only the more essential items. The Table includes a column of remarks regarding the difficulty of obtaining the information and its reliability.

A proportion of patients will already have died at the time of registration and details of death would in this case be included on the registration form. These details are, however, considered later under the general heading of follow-up information.

Items of information that may be included in the initial registration

Item No.	Nature of Item	Remarks
	BASIC PERSONAL INFORMATION	
1	Full name of patient	
2	Address	
3	Sex	
4	Date of birth and/or age	If age alone is recorded it should be age last birthday.
5	Marital state	Often not available for males.

6	Occupation (s)	Often not available for females and retired persons; often ambiguous (labourer, process worker, etc.).
	HOSPITAL ATTENDANCES	
7	Hospitals attented	
8	Hospital case No.　(at each hospital)	
9	Consultant　(at each hospital)	
10	Date first attented　(at each hospital)	
11	Method of reference　(to each hospital)	From family doctor, special clinic, other hospital, etc.
	HISTORY & SYMPTOMATOLOGY	
12	Previous major illnesses including other malignancies	
13	Possible predisposing factors	Often elicited only by clinicians with special interests.
14	Family history	Often elicited only by clinicians with special interests.
15	First symptom	Symptoms are usually well recorded but it is often difficult to identify which was the first.
16	Other symptoms	
17	Date of onset of first symptom and/or duration of symptoms	Unreliable if symptoms are un-dramatic or of gradual onset.
18	Number of pregnancies or live births (females only)	"Pregnancies" probably more useful but cannot be recorded as reliably as live births.
	CLINICAL ASSESSMENT	
19	General condition of patient	Possibly under various systemic headings.

20	Size and degree of infiltration of primary tumour	Items 20, 21 and 22 are, for many cancer sites, conveyed by the so-called TNM system of staging promulgated by the International Union Against Cancer.
21	Palpability and mobility of regional lymph nodes	
22	Sites of clinically detectable distant metastases	
23	Overall clinical stage	One of four categories (I - IV).
24	Other special clinical signs	
25	Concomittant diseases	Especially conditions likely to affect prognosis of choice of treatment; may include pregnancy and lactation.
	INVESTIGATIONS	
		It may be recorded merely that these investigations were or were not done, or dates and results may also be included.
26	Radiography	Including special techniques (tomography, ventriculography, etc.).
27	Endoscopy and other purely exploratory operations	
28	Various biochemical tests	
29	Haematology	
30	Radio-isotope studies	
31	Histological examinations with nature of specimen	
32	Other investigations	
33	DIAGNOSIS	Anatomical and histological.
34	SUMMARY OF INITIAL TREATMENT	In broad terms.
	INITIAL SURGICAL TREATMENT	
35	Nature of operation	
36	Where done?	

37	By whom?	
38	Date on which done	
39	Details of anaesthetic	
40	Immediate result (complications, etc.)	

EXTERNAL RADIOTHERAPY

41	Type of apparatus	Voltage or, in case of telecurie therapy, the nature of the source.
42	Dose in roentgens or rads	Possibly several measurements, e.g. maximum and minimum tumour dose, skin dose, gland dose, etc.
43	Area(s) irradiated	
44	Number and arrangement of fields	
45	Special techniques	Rotation methods, hyperbaric oxygen, etc.
46	Duration of course in days	
47	Radiotherapist	

OTHER RADIOTHERAPY

48	Nature of radioactive material used	
49	Mode of administration or application	
50	Site of administration or application	
51	Number of sources used (where applicable)	
52	Number of administration or applications	
53	Date of first administration or application	
54	Duration of administration or application	Including "permanent"
55	Radiotherapist (and surgeon if applicable)	

HORMONE TREATMENT

56	General method	By drugs, surgery, or radiation ablation, (If by surgery or radiation details required would be similar to those given above.)

	If by drugs :	
57	Nature of drugs(s)	
58	Mode of administration	
59	Regime	
60	Result including side effects	
61	Physician	
	CHEMOTHERAPY	
62-66	As for 57-61 above	
67	IMMEDIATE ASSESSMENT OF TREATMENT	Radical, palliative, incomplete, or untreated.

The form or record card on to which all or some of this information is abstracted should be designed to make the task as simple as possible. The design must in fact be related to the methods that are intended for subsequent recording and analysis (punched cards, data tape, etc.). It is important to stress that the acquisition of information on such a comprehensive list of items would be necessary only at a registry which was set up to provide a very wide range of services. Moreover, such a registry would have to be very well staffed and equipped. A registry with more limited functions, for example simple epidemiological studies, could manage very well with records containing only a few of these items.

Indexing

One of the features that registries are most likely to have in common is that of maintaining an up-to-date index of all registered cases. This is kept principally to verify that each registration is new. The index is usually maintained on small cards or on strips, with each card or strip carrying the minimum of information for identification. In countries or regions where the inhabitants are uniquely indentified by some code number (such as might be assigned for social security or health service purposes), it may be possible to use this as the key for filing the index cards. This cannot be done, however, if the number sometimes fails to be recorded in hospital case records. For this reason index cards are usually filed by surname and forenames in alphabetical order. In checking new registrations against the index, other useful secondary items are the address, the date of birth and the diagnosis. The maiden name of married women may also be essential. One of the problems of maintaining an index in name order in this way is that the same patient may be registered from two hospitals for the same disease, and his name may be spelt in two different ways. In such a case, duplication can easily arise. This difficulty can sometimes be overcome by introducing phonetic principles into the filing system - for example, by using the Soundex system; at other times, it may be necessary to utilize background information like place of birth.

When a registration has been established as new, it is assigned a registry serial number distinct from any case numbers that may have been assigned to the patient at hospitals he has visited. This number is entered on the registration documents and also on the new index card which must be created and filed for each tumour as soon as possible.

Coding

When, as is usually the case, the registered information must ultimately be stored on punched cards or some similar medium, the translation of the information into coded form is a major operation. It is a process involving a high proportion of the staff and requiring great care and an intimate understanding of the data on which it is being performed.

One economy derives from the fact that questions requiring only one or more of a few alternative answers can be dealt with by ringing or ticking the appropriate alternatives. If these alternatives are each associated with a code number or character, those indicated can be punched directly without any additional coding. Moreover, data which are essentially numerical can be punched directly in the same way.

The main problems of coding are, therefore, those concerned with questions to which the possible answers are non-quantitative and numerous. Such items are the diagnosis, histology, occupation, municipal area of residence, hospitals, consultants and so on. Invariably this type of information must be coded by reference to a manual of some kind. Some of the necessary codes will obviously be designed to suit local needs (hospitals, consultants and municipal areas); others may be widely used and have national or international status. Some of the most useful of the latter relate to the nomenclature and classification of diseases (World Health Organization, 1957; American Medical Association, 1961), tumours (World Health Organization, 1957; American Cancer Society, 1953), operations (American Medical Association, 1961, General Register Office, 1966a), and occupations (General Register Office, 1966b).

Follow-up procedures

Follow-up is usually thought of as providing the means of carrying out evaluations of treatment and of ensuring that patients remain under regular medical supervision, but it also has some importance in epidemiological studies. For example, it provides a means of verifying at regular intervals whether the original diagnosis is maintained and whether the patient has suffered any new malignancies. Both of these pieces of knowledge serve to improve the quality of the data for epidemiological purposes. Some registries, however, have concentrated on the registration process and have hardly concerned themselves with follow-up at all. Among those that do engage in follow-up there are many ways in which their practice varies. These include :

(a) Certain types of cancer (for example, skin cancer) may not be followed at all, or may be followed for less than the maximum period.

(b) The maximum period may vary as may the intervals between successive follow-up reports. Annual intervals are usual, but they may be made longer after, say, five or ten years.

(c) Follow-up information may be sought exclusively from hospitals or also from general practitioners. In the last resort, follow-up may be obtained from patients themselves, but this is unusual.

(d) Sometimes registries send hospitals lists of patients due for follow-up. The hospital then completes a questionnaire for each listed patient and returns it. An alternative is for the registry to prepare pre-headed questionnaires, one for each patient, and send them to the appropriate hospitals or doctors for completion. Punched card tabulators or computers can be used to prepare these lists or pre-headed questionnaires. A simpler procedure is to have a panel for recording periodic follow-up information on the card that was used for the purpose of initial registration. These cards are then sent back and forth between registry and hospital when follow-up becomes due.

(e) The actual information asked for in a follow-up request may vary widely. The most important single fact is whether the patient has survived. If the patient is alive, it may further be necessary to know whether or not he has any clinical or other evidence of disease, the nature of any recurrence or persistence of the disease since the last report and how and where this was treated. If he has died the date and cause of death will be needed, the distribution of the disease at the time of death and whether this information was derived from from necropsy examination.

The use of death certificates

A great many registries now benefit from arrangements whereby the appropriate government department or local health authority makes available copies of certificates relating to recent cancer deaths in the area. This has a twofold value.

(a) it helps towards the achievement of full registration; and

(b) it makes possible the provision of a death notification service to hospitals by registries.

When death certificates are received at the registry they are checked against the master index and divided into those relating to cases already registered and others.

If the subject is not already registered but has died in a hospital, action can be taken to obtain a registration from that hospital. If, however, he died at home, the certificate was presumably signed by a general practitioner who must first be written to, to find out which hospitals the patient attended and when. If the patient never attended hospital, the practitioner may be asked to answer a few questions regarding the patient's symptoms and their duration, and what treatment was given. The answers to these questions can then be used by the registry to provide the basis for a simple form of registration. The cases registered in this way constitute a special group; they concern for the most part rather old patients and, since they have never been investigated in hospital, the diagnosis may often be suspect.

The effect of using death certificates to secure registration in the manner described above has to be carefully considered. If the procedure is used by a registry whose more formal processes of registration are incomplete, the consequences will be that highly lethal cancers will be more adequately registered than the others. If, however, death certificates are not used, morbidity rates may be recorded for the highly lethal cancers that are lower than the mortality rates.

Data processing

For the smaller cancer registration schemes nothing more complicated than hand-sorted edge punched cards or feature cards is required. As the a-amount of material and the number of items of information in each record increases, these methods tend to become inadequate and the need for access to a punched card installation is increasingly felt, not only as an aid to statistical analysis, but also as a means of mechanizing dull, repetitive clerical operations. Even punched card installations tend to be inadequate as the number of records increases, especially when the number of items in each record are so numerous that they cannot be contained on a single punched card. This would certainly be the situation if all the information referred to previously were required for each record. It would then be necessary to consider the use of a computer, since records of virtually any length can be buitt up on magnetic tape or magnetic cards, using ordinary punched cards or punched paper tape as the input medium. Apart from their much greater speed, computers have many other advantages. For example :

(a) Conventional punched cards machines can produce only raw statistical tables. Much additional work using desk calculating machines may be necessary before tables and statistics derived from them are ready for publication. Computers, on the other hand, can proceed directly from the raw data to the finished tables and statistics.

(b) The computer can be programmed to carry out a large number of consistency checks on the information in each record, and to print out lists of definite or probable errors for further investigation.

(c) New items of information can be derived by the computer from the original items and these can be included in the record and stored on magnetic tape. Thus, if the patient's date of birth is given, the age need not be calculated by the coding clerk; it can, instead, be derived and stored by the computer. The same is true of the various possible intervals, such as survival time, which are derived by subtracting one date from another.

(d) Statistical diagrams can be prepared by using digital plotters or cathode ray display devices connected to the computer.

(e) One important possibility is the partial or total elimination of coding and punching by proceeding directly from the original document to the punched medium using mechanical or electronic devices. This has long been possible through the use of mark sense punching machines, but these require that the original document is in the form of a punched card. More recently it has been possible to translate marked documents of varying sizes into punched paper tape.

FUTURE OF CANCER REGISTRATION

Sources of Further Information

With the passing of time, it must be expected that more permanent cancer registries will be established in many different parts of the world. This will represent an advance, not only for the areas in which they are established, but also to the registries already in existence; for the value of each individual registry is enhanced by the establishment of others.

It would, of course, be wrong to seek international agreement which would limit the freedom of individual registries in regard to the kind of information they record; but it would be very helpful if each registry could conform to certain basic requirements in regard to such simple matters as the age groups utilized in analysis, the categories of disease which should be registered and the degree of sub-division which should be available within these categories.

Collaboration between cancer registries will also be helped by any growth there may be in mutual understanding among those who work in medicine. Doctors who use the same words do not always mean the same thing and any trend towards unity in terminology must inevitably benefit work concerned with international comparisons such as we are presenting here. Internationally agreed systems of classification are of such value that it is worthwhile to set aside long cherished personal notions in order to make use of them. This is perhaps nowhere more true today than in the clinical staging of tumours - a field in which the International Union Against Cancer has made intensive efforts in recent years.

Ultimately medical records may be standardized and computorized at the national level to such an extent that there is no need for cancer regustration as a distinct activity. Information about cancer patients may then be selected out from the records covering all diseases and be available on a very large scale. This development would be welcome, provided that the service to research and administration was at least as good as that provided by separate cancer registries as at present.

For further information about the value of cancer registries and their method of organization the reader is referred to the publications of indivual cancer registries, listed in chapter IV, to the World Health Organization's reports (World Health Organization, 1959, 1962, 1964, and 1966) and to articles by Payne (1961 and 1965) and Stocks (1959). The use of mechanised aids is discussed in detail by Casey and Perry (1958) and Hogben and Cross (1960)

Chapter III
CLASSIFICATION

METHOD

The international classification recommended by the World Health Organization (1957) has been used, with minor modifications, by all cancer registries and we have adopted it as the basis of our classification. We have, however, not used all the categories separately, as the numbers of cases recorded in some categories are small and the distinction between others is not always easy to make. We have, therefore, grouped together some of the three digit numbers and, at the same time, retained the subdivisions of others whenever this seemed both practicable and helpful :- for example, we have grouped together the international list numbers 202 and 205 (reticuloses other than lymphosarcoma, reticulosarcoma and Hodgkin's disease and mycosis fungoides) and retained separately numbers 155.0 and other subdivisions of 155 (primary malignant tumours of the liver and malignant tumours of the gall bladder, extrahepatic bile ducts and "multiple sites" within the liver).

Detailed definitions of the international list numbers are given at the end of this chapter together with an account of the modifications that have been adopted. These modifications arise partly from practical difficulties in determining the criteria for the use of the international classification, and partly from the fact that some three digit categories include different types of tumours with, in all probability, different causes. The use of a single system of classification does not, however, eliminate all diffidulties. Many factors affect its application in practice, and the results obtained by different registries are not always comparable.

SPECIAL DIFFICULTIES

Tumours of the central nervous system present the special difficulty that benign and malignant tumours may have a similar clinical course. Even grossly malignant tumours seldom metastasize and both may produce death by pressure on vital centres in the brain. Since surgery is not always carried out, a substantial proportion of these tumours are not examined histologically and they are commonly diagnosed as cerebral tumours, without sepcification of their malignant or benign character. The proportion of cases diagnosed histologically ᴸ or clinically by a sufficiently descriptive diagnosis - varies greatly from place to place and, within one place, from time to time. The best procedure is, therefore, to register all tumours of the central nervous system under one head and, if desired, to specify those known to be malignant histologically in a subheading. All contributors were asked to do this, but registration practice varies and it was not always possible.

Tumours of the urinary bladder present a somewhat different problem in that there are neither clinical nor pathological criteria which allow a clear and uniform distinction to be made between papillomas that will behave like benign tumours and those that will eventually manifest malignancy. As these papillomas form a substantial proportion of all bladder tumours, and as progression can be prevented by thorough treatment, the incidence of malignant tumours will clearly be affected by differences in the efficiency of the medical services. The best solution is to register both papillomas and carcinomas of

19

the bladder under one rubric. This, however, has not yet become standard practice and differences in procedure in this respect will affect comparison of the incidence of bladder "cancer" reported by different registries.

Tumours of the salivary glands present a similar difficulty. Recurrence without metastasis is common and it is difficult to forecast the clinical course on histological grounds alone. Criteria for classification of these tumours differ, and the character of the data recorded by each registry needs to be considered before incidence rates are compared.

Another and extremely difficult problem has been introduced by the recognition and treatment of pre-invasive lesions of the cervix uteri. The relationship between "carcinoma-in-situ" and classical invasive cancer has not been established with complete clarity, but it seems probable that the incidence of invasive cancer can be appreciably reduced by routine examination of cervical smears and the treatment of women whose smears show the presence of apparently neoplastic cells. Such routine examinations are now being carried out on a large scale in some countries and the question arises whether pre-invasive lesions should be included in the figures for cancer incidence. If they are not included, the cervix cancer incidence will probably be reduced - which will be satisfactory from a public health point of view, but will mislead anyone wanting to use the figures for the study of aetiology. If they are included, the apparent incidence of cervix cancer will be increased. The age distribution of the two types of lesion is, moreover, grossly different. The incidence of "carcinoma-in-situ" is maximal at ages 20-29 years and falls off rapidly as age increases, whereas the incidence of invasive cancer does not reach a maximum until after the age of 45 years. Data which include both types of lesion will, therefore, show a different age distribution from data derived from cases of invasive cancer alone. Since a small-scale screening programme can provide enough cases of carcinoma-in-situ to affect appreciably the incidence rates for the combined lesions at young ages, figures for "carcinoma-in-situ" have usually been excluded. Even so, comparisons between the recorded rates for the different registries can be assessed properly only when the extent of routine cytological screening programmes is also known. Pre-invasive lesions may also be diagnosed occasionally in other sites. The number of such cases is, however, small and differences in their classification are unlikely to introduce any serious bias into the comparison of current rates.

With some other cancers, the principal difficulty is the lack of adequate criteria for determining the organ of origin. This is most apparent with cancers of the colon and rectum. The anatomical definition of the upper end of the rectum is not easy to recognize clinically and cancers at the recto-sigmoid junction - which should be classified, according to the international classification, with cancer of the rectum - may easily be classed with cancer of the colon. This would not matter if the recto-sigmoid region was not a common site for cancer, but in many countries it is. The incidence of cancer of the colon and cancer of the rectum should, therefore, always be examined together to see whether differences in the incidence of one or other disease could be accounted for by differences in the level at which they are normally separated.

Similar difficulties are met with in separating cancers of different parts of the pharynx (here mostly grouped together) and in distinguishing cancer of the pharynx form cancer the larynx. Less confusion might occur if cancer of the intrinsic larynx were considered alone, but this was not possible with the present data as it not given a separate code number in the relevant international list (World Health Organization, 1957).

With one exception no attempt has been made to show separately figures for different histological types. This is unavoidable at present, as there is neither sufficient agreement about the appropriate classifications to use, nor is the proportion of cases examined histologically sufficiently large or suf-

20

ficiently constant. This is a defect of the present data (and of nearly all other cancer incidence data) as many of the different histological types have different causes. Certainly sarcomas and carcinomas, and myeloid and lymphatic leukaemias have different causes; and so may some of the different types of carcinoma (for example, squamous carcinoma and adenocarcinoma of the bronchus). If these differences could be taken into account, the incidence rates of some types of cancer would, in all probability, differ by much more than they do now when all histological types are classed together.

A difficulty of an entirely different type is that some registries intentionally abandon part of the classification, omitting some cancers and including conditions that are not uniformly regarded as neoplastic. The most important of these discrepancies is the failure to register cancer of the skin - as in Norway and New Zealand. The reason for omitting this type of cancer is that the condition is common and easily treatable; and interest in it is not always sufficient to justifiy the large amount of work required to obtain a high standard of registration. When skin cancer is omitted, the incidence recorded for all cancers is, of course, substantially reduced. It is, however, better to omit skin cancers altogether than to try and include them, but succeed in registering only a small proportion of the total.

In contrast, polycythaemia vera is sometimes included, though it is officially classified as a disease of the blood. It is always a relatively rare disease and its inclusion has no appreciable effect on the total rate for all cancers.

CLASSIFICATION BY SITE OF ORIGIN

The definition of the international list numbers recommended by the World Health Organization (1957) and used, with minor modifications, in the present text is as follows :

International List Number	Type of Tumour	Modification in Present Text
140	Malignant neoplasm of lip	
141	Malignant neoplasm of tongue	
142	Malignant neoplasm of salivary gland	
143	Malignant neoplasm of floor of mouth	) 143 and 144
144	Malignant neoplasm of other parts of mouth, and of mouth unspecified	)) grouped together)
145	Malignant neoplasm of oral nasopharynx	see 147
146	Malignant neoplasm of nasopharynx	
147	Malignant neoplasm of hypopharynx	) 145, 147 and 148)
148	Malignant neoplasm of pharynx, unspecified	) grouped together
150	Malignant neoplasm of oesophagus	
151	Malignant neoplasm of stomach	
152	Malignant neoplasm of small intestine, including duodenum	
153	Malignant neoplasm of large intestine, except rectum	
154	Malignant neoplasm of rectum, including recto-sigmoid junction, excluding anus	
155	Malignant neoplasm of biliary passages, and of liver (stated to be primary site)	

155.0	Malignant neoplasm of liver (primary site)	includes also cases classifiable under 155.8
155.1	Malignant neoplasm of gall-bladder and extrahepatic bile ducts including ampulla of vater	not used; see 155.1
155.8	Malignant neoplasm of multiple sites classifiable to both 155.0 and 155.1	
156	Malignant neoplasm of liver (secondary and unspecified)	sometimes grouped with "other neoplasms"
157	Malignant neoplasm of pancreas	
158	Malignant neoplasm of peritoneum	grouped with "other neoplasms"
159	Malignant neoplasm of unspecified digestive organs	grouped with "other neoplasms"
160	Malignant neoplasm of nose, nasal cavities, middle ear, and accessory sinuses	
161	Malignant neoplasm of larynx	
162	Malignant neoplasm of bronchus and trachea, and of lung specified as primary	))) 162 and 163) grouped together))
163	Malignant neoplasm of lung, unspecified as to whether primary or secondary	
164	Malignant neoplasm of mediastinum	grouped with "other neoplasms"
165	Malignant neoplasm of thoracic organs (secondary)	grouped with "other neoplasms"
170	Malignant neoplasm of breast	
171	Malignant neoplasm of cervix uteri	
172	Malignant neoplasm of corpus uteri	
173	Malignant neoplasm of other parts of the uterus, including chorion-epithelioma	
174	Malignant neoplasm of uterus (unspecified)	
175	Malignant neoplasm of ovary, fallopian tube, and broad ligament	
176	Malignant neoplasm of other and unspecified female genital organs	
177	Malignant neoplasm of prostate	
178	Malignant neoplasm of testis	
179	Malignant neoplasm of other and unspecified male genital organs	
179.0	Malignant neoplasm of penis	
Other sub-divisions of 179	Malignant neoplasm of other specified, unspecified, and multiple sites	not used; grouped with "other neoplasms", when 179.0 is shown separately
180	Malignant neoplasm of kidney	
181	Malignant neoplasm of bladder and other urinary organs	
181.0	Malignant neoplasm of bladder	

181.7, 181.8	Malignant neoplasm of other urinary organs, and multiple sites	not used; grouped with "other neoplasms", when 181.0 is shown separately
190	Malignant melanoma of skin	
191	Other malignant neoplasm of skin	
192	Malignant neoplasm of eye	
193	Malignant neoplasm of brain and other parts of nervous system	includes number 223 and 237, unless otherwise specified
194	Malignant neoplasm of thyroid gland	
195	Malignant neoplasm of other endocrine glands	
196	Malignant neoplasm of bone	
197	Malignant neoplasm of connective tissue	
198	Secondary and unspecified neoplasm of lymph nodes	grouped with "other neoplasms"
199	Malignant neoplasm of other and unspecified sites	grouped with "other neoplasms"
200	Lymphosarcoma and reticulosarcoma	
201	Hodgkin's disease	
202	Other forms of lymphoma (reticulosis)	202 and 205 grouped together
203	Multiple myeloma (plasmocytoma)	
204	Leukaemia and aleukaemia	
205	Mycosis fungoides	see 202
223	Benign neoplasm of brain and other parts of nervous system	see 193
237	Neoplasm of unspecified nature of brain and other parts of nervous system	see 193

CLASSIFICATION BY HISTOLOGICAL TYPE

The following types of neoplasm are coded as malignant unless specified as benign (World Health Organization, 1957) :

Acanthoma

Adamantinocarcinoma

Adamantinoma

Adeno-acanthoma

Adeno-angiosarcoma

Adenocancroid

Adenocarcinoma

Adenomyosarcoma

Adenosarcoma

Angiofibrosarcoma

Angiosarcoma

Astroblastoma

Astrocytoma

Astroglioma

Basal cell carcinoma

Blastocytoma

Blastoma

Bowen's epithelioma

Cancer, any type

Cancerous, any condition so qualified

Cancroid

Carcinoma, any type

Carcinomatous, any condition so qualified

Carcinosarcoma

Chondro-endothelioma

Chondromyxosarcoma

Chondrosarcoma

23

Chordoma
Chorionepithelioma
Cystadenocarcinoma
Cystosarcoma, except
   phyllodes
Dysgerminoma
Embryoma
Encephaloid (tumour)
Endothelioma
Ependymoblastoma
Ependymoma
Epithelial tumour
Epithelioma
Ewing's tumour
Fibroblastoma
Fibrocarcinoma
Fibrochondrosarcoma
Fibro-endothelioma
Fibroliposarcoma
Fibromyxosarcoma
Fibrosarcoma
Glioblastoma
Glioma
Glioneuroma
Gliosarcoma
Grawitz's tumour
Haemangioblastoma
Haemangiosarcoma
Hepatoma
Hypernephroma
Krukenberg's tumour
Leiomyosarcoma
Lipomyosarcoma
Lipomyxosarcoma
Liposarcoma

Lymphangiosarcoma
Lymphepithelioma
Lympho-epithelioma
Medulloblastoma
Medullo-epithelioma
Melanoblastoma
Melanocarcinoma
Melano-epithelioma
Melanoma
Melanosarcoma
Melanotic tumour
Mixed cell tumour
Myosarcoma
Myxochondrosarcoma
Myxofibrosarcoma
Myxosarcoma
Naevocarcinoma
Nephroma
Neuroblastoma
Neurocytoma
Neuro-epithelioma
Neurofibrosarcoma
Neuroglioma
Neurosarcoma
Nevocarcinoma
Oligodendroblastoma
Oligodendroglioma
Oligodendroma
Osteoblastoma
Osteocarcinoma
Osteochondro-
   carcinosarcoma
Osteochondro-
   myxosarcoma
Osteochondrosarcoma

Osteofibrosarcoma
Osteosarcoma
Paget's disease of
   breast, nipple,
   or skin
Pancoast's syndrome
   or tumour
Papillo-
   adenocarcinoma
Papillocarcinoma
Peri-endothelioma
Perithelioma
Pinealoblastoma
Psammocarcinoma
Retinoblastoma
Rhabdomyosarcoma
Rhabdosarcoma
Rodent ulcer, except
   of cornea
Sarcocarcinoma
Sarcoma
Sarcomatous, any
   condition so qualified
Scirrhus
Seminoma
Spermatoblastoma
Spongioblastoma
Spongiocytoma
Sympathoblastoma
Sympathogonioma
Syncytioma
Syringocarcinoma
Teratoma (cystic)
   of testis
Wilms' tumour
Xanthosarcoma

All these tumours are classified together when they originate in the same organ. Melanoma is an exception, as it is always separated from other tumours when it arises in the skin. Many registries maintain independent records for sarcomas and some other special tumours, but there is not as yet sufficient experience to justify comparing them internationally in the present volume.

Chapter IV
INCIDENCE

TABULATION OF DATA

The figures reported by each registry are set out in identical form. Each set of data is given in 3 Tables, Table A showing the relevant population and Table B and C the age-specific incidence rates for males and for females.

Populations are given in units of 100,000 so that 0.4430 indicates 44,300 persons. Figures are given separately for each sex and for each 5-year age group from 0-4 years to 80-84 years, and for 85 years and over. In some few instances, however, the oldest age groups have had to be combined, because of lack of information.

The total number of cases recorded and the number occurring in subjects of unknown age are shown separately for each type of cancer for males (Table B) and for females (Table C). The numbers occurring at each age have been omitted, to save space. They can be derived quickly, however, by dividing the age-specific incidence rates at each site by the corresponding figures in the last row of the Table - that is, by the rates that would have been observed if only one case had occurred in that age group over the whole period - and rounding off to the nearest integer. The accuracy of the calculation can be checked by multiplying the incidence rates by the population in the corresponding sex and age groups and by the number of years for which cancers were registered.

All incidence rates are given as rates per 100,000 persons per year, the male rates in Table B and the female rates in Table C. A crude rate is given for each type of cancer at all ages and age-specific rates are given in 5-year age groups. In many instances the number of cases recorded for a particular type of cancer is very small and the age-specific incidence rate is correspondingly unreliable. We have preferred, however, to give the rates for each site and for every registry in a standard way, rather than to alter the age grouping for smaller registries or for rarer types of cancer. It is always possible to obtain more reliable rates by combining the results into larger groups, but it would not have been possible to obtain figures for small groups from larger ones.

In the calculation of the age-specific rates, no allowance has been made for the cases occurring in subjects of unknown age. These cases are, however, included in the crude rate for all ages.

Age-standardized rates for each type of cancer for each registry are brought together for ease of comparison in Chapter V.

DESCRIPTION OF REGISTRIES

The incidence data reported by each registry are preceded by a brief account of the registry and of the population served by it set out in note form in a standard way. For many of the registries these notes are preceded and amplified by a more detailed text, which has been prepared by the contributors personally concerned in the work of the registry.

On aspect of the registry population which was particularly difficult to describe in a standard way was their occupational structure. When available, this is useful information as it indicates an important element in the economic and social characteristics of the population and may be relevant to any local peculiarities in the distribution of tumours of different sites.

The subject was discussed exhaustively at the meeting of the editorial committee. It was clear that only very general categories could be used if it was to apply equally throughout all of the wide range of areas included. The four groupings it was ultimately decided to use reveal clearly the major differences to be found between underdeveloped areas and those most highly developed. The categories are, however, so broad and general that they have presented considerable problems of classification to some of the registries which possessed very detailed occupational distributions. It is often difficult to decide between the categories of industry and commerce; and "personal service", which was included largely to accomodate some of the African areas, is capable of widely varying interpretations in more complex societies. Moreover, any one of several reference populations can be used as a base for expressing the occupational composition in proportional form: the whole population of both sexes, the male population only, or the employed population (of both sexes, or of one sex only). Wherever possible the nature of the reference population has been indicated. Where no further information is available no inferences have been attempted, but the data have been recorded as they were provided. Sometimes the occupational composition of the population was given in several forms: in such cases the employed male population has been selected for inclusion as the basis.

MOZAMBIQUE, LOURENÇO MARQUES

Registry Title and Address : Lourenço Marques Cancer Survey, Department of Pathology, Hospital Central Miguel Bombarda, Lourenço Marques, Mozambique. Commenced 1st May, 1956 and terminated 30th April, 1961. Supported financially by the Portugese Government and the National Cancer Association of South Africa.

Registration. Cases are registered by medical staff from hospital in-patients and out-patients, radiotherapy departments, pathology departments, death certificates and doctors attending cases at home. Other registrations come from the Mortuary, the Department of Statistics, two Mission hospitals, three private nursing homes, twelve state or municipal or company outpatient clinics, from the Medical Officer of Health for Lourenço Marques and from the port Health Authority. Registration is more than 90 % complete.

Follow-up. All patients with tumours reported from the Pathology Department of the Central Hospital of Lourenço Marques have been followed up since May 1961.

Physical Description. The Registry covers the area of the city of Lourenço Marques with a clearly defined area of 56 square kilometres and a peri-urban area of 60 square kilometres. The city lies in flat sandy country on the estuary Espirito Santo where the Umbeluzi River reaches the Indian Ocean. Its boundary line is 5 kilometres from the city limits. The city lies at latitude 26º South and longitude 33º East, and the total registration area is 116 square kilometres.

Demographic Description. Total population of area under survey 99,030. The population comprises 60 % Thonga (Ronga) Shangana group, 30 % Bitonga and Chope people, 10 % other tribes including Chuabos and Macuas. The religious groups are 51 % Catholic, 23 % Protestant, 4 % Moslem, and 22 % have other religions (African) or no religion. The main occupational composition is industry 4.5 %, commerce 0.7 % agriculture 76 % and personal service 3.8 %.

Medical Services. Total number of hospital beds of all kinds 1,266. Total number of doctors in practice in registration area 105. Tribal customs and religious beliefs might cause 5 % or more of the population to abstain from, or unduly to delay seeking medical advice. Cancer causes approximately 18.2 % of all deaths.

Publications. Flegg and Lutz(1959); Prates and Torres (1959).

TABLE 1 A
MOZAMBIQUE, LOURENCO MARQUES :
POPULATION (100, 000s), MEAN 1956 - 61

AGE (In years)	MALES		FEMALES	
	No.	Per Cent	No.	Per Cent
0 –	0.0720	13.39	0.0770	17.01
5 –	0.0540	10.04	0.0561	12.40
10 –	0.0470	8.74	0.0340	7.51
15 –	0.1010	18.78	0.0369	8.15
20 –	0.0540	10.04	0.0504	11.14
25 –	0.0540	10.04	0.0514	11.36
30 –	0.0320	5.95	0.0325	7.18
35 –	0.0280	5.21	0.0309	6.83
40 –	0.0250	4.65	0.0270	5.97
45 –	0.0240	4.46	0.0154	3.40
50 –	0.0175	3.25	0.0119	2.63
55 –	0.0110	2.05	0.0106	2.34
60 – and over	0.0182	3.38	0.0185	4.09
–	–	–	–	–
–	–	–	–	–
–	–	–	–	–
–	–	–	–	–
TOTAL	0.5377	100.00	0.4526	100.00

NOTES

TO TABLES 1 A, B and C

(I)   Period of registration 1. 5. 56 to 30. 4. 61.

(II)   No cases recorded under I. L. numbers 145, 147-8, 156, 173-5, 178, 190, 201-2, 203 or 205.

(III) I. L. number 193 excludes benign and unspecified tumours of the central nervous system.

(IV)   Carcinoma in situ excluded.

TABLE 1 B
MOZAMBIQUE, LOURENCO MARQUES :
MALE INCIDENCE RATES, 1956 - 60.

INTER-NATIONAL LIST No.	AVERAGE ANNUAL INCIDENCE PER 100,000 AGE IN YEARS																		ALL AGES	No. OF CASES IN WHOLE PERIOD		INTER-NATIONAL LIST No.
	0-	5-	10-	15-	20-	25-	30-	35-	40-	45-	50-	55-	60-	65-	70-	75-	80-	85- AND OVER		AGE UN-KNOWN	ALL AGES	
140	0.0	0.0	0.0	0.0	0.0	0.0	0.0	0.0	0.0	0.0	0.0	0.0	0.0						0.0	0	0	140
141	0.0	0.0	0.0	0.0	0.0	0.0	0.0	0.0	0.0	0.0	0.0	0.0	0.0						0.0	0	0	141
142	0.0	0.0	0.0	0.0	0.0	0.0	0.0	0.0	0.0	0.0	0.0	0.0	0.0						0.0	0	0	142
143-4	0.0	0.0	0.0	2.0	3.7	0.0	0.0	0.0	0.0	0.0	0.0	54.5	11.0						2.2	0	6	143-4
146	0.0	0.0	0.0	0.0	0.0	0.0	0.0	7.1	0.0	0.0	11.4	18.2	11.0						1.1	0	3	146
150	0.0	0.0	0.0	0.0	0.0	0.0	0.0	14.3	8.0	0.0	22.9	0.0	22.0						2.6	0	7	150
151	0.0	0.0	0.0	0.0	0.0	0.0	0.0	0.0	0.0	0.0	11.4	0.0	0.0						1.1	0	3	151
152	0.0	0.0	0.0	0.0	0.0	0.0	0.0	0.0	0.0	0.0	0.0	0.0	0.0						0.0	0	0	152
153	0.0	0.0	0.0	0.0	0.0	3.7	0.0	7.1	8.0	0.0	0.0	18.2	0.0						1.5	0	4	153
154	0.0	0.0	0.0	0.0	0.0	0.0	0.0	0.0	0.0	0.0	0.0	0.0	0.0						0.0	0	0	154
155.0	0.0	3.7	51.1	77.2	181.5	151.9	162.5	192.9	264.0	116.7	80.0	90.9	87.9						98.2	2	264	155.0
155.1	0.0	0.0	0.0	0.0	0.0	0.0	0.0	0.0	0.0	0.0	0.0	0.0	0.0						0.0	0	0	155.1
157	0.0	0.0	0.0	0.0	0.0	3.7	0.0	0.0	0.0	0.0	0.0	0.0	11.0						0.7	0	2	157
160	0.0	0.0	0.0	0.0	0.0	0.0	0.0	0.0	0.0	0.0	0.0	0.0	0.0						0.0	0	0	160
161	0.0	0.0	0.0	0.0	0.0	0.0	0.0	0.0	8.0	0.0	0.0	18.2	0.0						0.7	0	2	161
162-3	0.0	0.0	0.0	2.0	0.0	0.0	0.0	0.0	8.0	8.3	11.4	0.0	22.0						2.2	0	6	162-3
170	0.0	0.0	0.0	0.0	0.0	0.0	0.0	0.0	0.0	0.0	0.0	0.0	0.0						0.0	0	0	170
177	0.0	0.0	0.0	0.0	0.0	0.0	0.0	7.1	0.0	0.0	11.4	54.5	54.9						3.7	0	10	177
179.0	0.0	0.0	0.0	0.0	0.0	0.0	6.3	0.0	8.0	8.3	11.4	18.2	0.0						1.9	0	5	179.0
180	0.0	0.0	0.0	0.0	0.0	0.0	0.0	0.0	0.0	0.0	0.0	0.0	22.0						0.7	0	2	180
181.0	0.0	0.0	0.0	0.0	3.7	3.7	12.5	7.1	24.0	16.7	22.9	90.9	76.9						8.9	0	24	181.0
191	0.0	0.0	0.0	0.0	3.7	0.0	18.8	0.0	0.0	16.7	0.0	0.0	22.0						4.8	0	13	191
192	0.0	0.0	0.0	0.0	0.0	0.0	12.5	14.3	0.0	0.0	0.0	54.5	0.0						1.5	0	4	192
193	5.6	0.0	0.0	5.9	0.0	11.1	0.0	0.0	0.0	0.0	0.0	0.0	11.0						2.2	0	6	193
194	0.0	0.0	0.0	0.0	0.0	0.0	0.0	0.0	0.0	0.0	11.4	0.0	11.0						0.7	0	2	194
195	0.0	0.0	0.0	0.0	0.0	0.0	0.0	0.0	0.0	0.0	0.0	0.0	0.0						0.0	0	0	195
196	0.0	0.0	4.3	2.0	0.0	0.0	12.5	0.0	8.0	8.3	0.0	18.2	11.0						1.9	0	5	196
197	0.0	3.7	8.5	4.0	3.7	3.7	6.3	0.0	0.0	0.0	0.0	0.0	11.0						3.3	0	9	197
200	0.0	3.7	0.0	11.9	18.5	7.4	0.0	7.1	0.0	0.0	0.0	0.0	22.0						6.7	0	18	200
204	2.8	0.0	0.0	4.0	0.0	3.7	0.0	7.1	0.0	0.0	0.0	18.2	0.0						2.6	0	7	204
OTHER	0.0	0.0	0.0	0.0	0.0	0.0	0.0	0.0	0.0	0.0	0.0	18.2	0.0						0.4	0	1	OTHER
140-205	8.3	11.1	63.8	108.9	214.8	188.9	231.3	264.3	336.0	175.0	194.3	454.5	406.6						149.9	2	403	140-205
RATE PER CASE IN PERIOD	2.78	3.70	4.26	1.98	3.70	3.70	6.25	7.14	8.00	8.33	11.43	18.18	10.99						0.37	-	-	RATE PER CASE IN PERIOD

TABLE 1 C
MOZAMBIQUE, LOURENCO MARQUES :
FEMALE INCIDENCE RATES, 1956 - 60.

AVERAGE ANNUAL INCIDENCE PER 100,000

INTER-NATIONAL LIST No.	0–	5–	10–	15–	20–	25–	30–	35–	40–	45–	50–	55–	60–	65–	70–	75–	80–	85– AND OVER	ALL AGES	No. of cases AGE UNKNOWN	No. of cases ALL AGES	INTER-NATIONAL LIST No.
140	0.0	0.0	0.0	0.0	0.0	0.0	0.0	0.0	0.0	0.0	0.0	0.0	0.0						0.0	0	0	140
141	0.0	0.0	0.0	0.0	0.0	0.0	0.0	0.0	0.0	0.0	0.0	0.0	0.0						0.0	0	0	141
142	0.0	0.0	0.0	0.0	0.0	7.8	0.0	0.0	0.0	0.0	16.8	0.0	21.6						2.2	0	5	142
143-4	0.0	0.0	0.0	10.8	0.0	0.0	0.0	0.0	7.4	0.0	33.6	0.0	0.0						2.2	0	5	143-4
146	0.0	0.0	0.0	0.0	0.0	0.0	0.0	0.0	0.0	0.0	0.0	0.0	0.0						0.0	0	0	146
150	0.0	0.0	0.0	0.0	0.0	0.0	0.0	0.0	0.0	0.0	0.0	0.0	0.0						0.0	0	0	150
151	0.0	0.0	0.0	0.0	0.0	0.0	0.0	0.0	0.0	0.0	0.0	0.0	21.6						0.9	0	2	151
152	0.0	0.0	0.0	0.0	0.0	0.0	0.0	0.0	0.0	0.0	0.0	0.0	0.0						0.0	0	0	152
153	0.0	0.0	0.0	0.0	0.0	0.0	0.0	0.0	0.0	0.0	0.0	18.9	10.8						0.9	0	2	153
154	0.0	0.0	0.0	0.0	0.0	0.0	0.0	0.0	0.0	0.0	0.0	0.0	0.0						0.0	0	0	154
155.0	0.0	0.0	17.6	10.8	47.6	35.0	36.9	25.9	81.5	51.9	16.8	75.5	54.1						27.0	0	61	155.0
155.1	0.0	0.0	0.0	0.0	0.0	0.0	0.0	0.0	0.0	0.0	0.0	0.0	0.0						0.0	0	0	155.1
157	0.0	0.0	0.0	5.4	0.0	0.0	0.0	0.0	0.0	0.0	0.0	18.9	10.8						0.9	0	2	157
160	0.0	0.0	0.0	0.0	0.0	0.0	0.0	0.0	0.0	0.0	0.0	0.0	0.0						0.0	0	0	160
161	0.0	0.0	0.0	0.0	0.0	0.0	0.0	0.0	0.0	26.0	0.0	0.0	0.0						0.9	0	2	161
162-3	0.0	0.0	0.0	0.0	0.0	0.0	0.0	6.5	0.0	0.0	0.0	0.0	10.8						0.9	0	2	162-3
170	0.0	0.0	0.0	0.0	0.0	0.0	0.0	0.0	14.8	0.0	0.0	56.6	0.0						2.2	0	5	170
171	0.0	0.0	0.0	0.0	7.9	7.8	6.2	45.3	66.7	26.0	84.0	75.5	97.3						18.6	1	42	171
172	0.0	0.0	0.0	0.0	0.0	0.0	12.3	6.5	0.0	0.0	0.0	0.0	10.8						1.8	0	4	172
176	0.0	0.0	0.0	0.0	0.0	0.0	0.0	0.0	0.0	0.0	0.0	0.0	21.6						1.3	0	3	176
180	2.6	0.0	0.0	0.0	0.0	3.9	0.0	0.0	0.0	0.0	0.0	0.0	0.0						0.9	0	2	180
181.0	0.0	0.0	0.0	0.0	4.0	11.7	12.3	0.0	14.8	39.0	33.6	94.3	32.4						9.3	0	21	181.0
191	2.6	0.0	0.0	0.0	0.0	0.0	0.0	6.5	0.0	13.0	0.0	37.7	43.2						4.0	0	9	191
192	5.2	0.0	0.0	0.0	0.0	3.9	0.0	6.5	0.0	13.0	16.8	0.0	0.0						2.7	0	6	192
193	2.6	0.0	0.0	5.4	4.0	7.8	0.0	0.0	0.0	0.0	0.0	0.0	0.0						1.8	0	4	193
194	0.0	0.0	0.0	0.0	0.0	0.0	0.0	0.0	0.0	0.0	16.8	0.0	10.8						1.3	0	3	194
195	0.0	0.0	0.0	0.0	0.0	0.0	0.0	0.0	0.0	0.0	0.0	0.0	0.0						0.0	0	0	195
196	0.0	0.0	5.9	0.0	0.0	3.9	0.0	0.0	0.0	0.0	16.8	0.0	0.0						1.3	0	3	196
197	0.0	0.0	0.0	0.0	0.0	3.9	6.2	6.5	0.0	0.0	0.0	0.0	0.0						1.3	0	3	197
200	2.6	3.6	0.0	5.4	0.0	0.0	6.2	6.5	0.0	0.0	0.0	18.9	0.0						2.7	0	6	200
204	0.0	0.0	0.0	0.0	4.0	0.0	6.2	6.5	0.0	13.0	0.0	0.0	10.8						1.8	0	4	204
OTHER	0.0	0.0	0.0	0.0	0.0	0.0	0.0	0.0	0.0	13.0	0.0	0.0	0.0						0.4	0	1	OTHER
140-205	15.6	3.6	23.5	37.9	67.5	85.6	86.2	116.5	185.2	181.8	235.3	396.2	356.8						87.1	1	197	140-205
RATE PER CASE IN PERIOD	2.60	3.57	5.88	5.42	3.97	3.89	6.15	6.47	7.41	12.99	16.81	18.87	10.81						0.44	–	–	RATE PER CASE IN PERIOD

Note: Figures in column 60– relate to the years 60 and over.

NIGERIA, IBADAN

A Cancer Registry was established at the University College Hospital, Ibadan, Nigeria, in 1960, with the aid of a generous grant from the British Empire Cancer Campaign, with the object of assessing the incidence of malignant disease in the population. The staff consisted of a full-time senior research assistant, a copy typist and an interpreter.

Ibadan, the capital city of the Western Region of Nigeria, appeared most suitable for such an investigation. The population was thought to be in the region of 500,000 and a census was to be held in 1961 - later postponed until 1962. The 1962 census unfortunately was never published but a provisional population figure of 479,000 was obtained for Ibadan. A further census has since been taken, and the original figure should be accepted with some reserve, although it is doubtful if a more accurate figure will be obtained in the near future. The breakdown of this figure of 479,000 into age and sex groups was obtained from the results of a W.H.O. sample survey of the population undertaken in 1962; and we are indebted to Dr. Hahn of the W.H.O. for making these figures available (Edington and Mordean, 1965).

The medical facilities in Ibadan consisted of the University College Hospital, a 500-bedded teaching hospital including all the major specialties, a 225-bedded government hospital with a medical staff of between 15 and 20, a small Catholic Mission Hospital with two doctors, and approximately 10 general practitioners in the town itself. A Cancer Research Committee was formed of interested consultants in the two main hospitals, and all practising physicians in Ibadan were approached and requested to notify every case of suspected malignant disease to the Registry. It was found that the mission hospital and private practitioners tended to refer possible cases of malignant disease to the specialist hospital clinics whence they were notified to the Registry. All wards and outpatient departments were visited and the records of the Medical Records Department, the Radiology Department, the Pathology Department and theatre lists of the two hospitals concerned were examined regularly.

By this means it was thought that most patients suffering from malignant disease attending either private practitioners or hospitals would be detected. A survey of the Ibadan population showed that over 90 per cent of the population would attend hospital if sick.

Patients were classified by age and sex and were included in the Ibadan population group if resident in Ibadan for at least one year; cases occurring in other patients were included in the general register which also included malignant conditions seen in material received for histopathological diagnosis from outstations. From the general register, which also included Ibadan cases, relative ratio frequencies were calculated. Only Ibadan patients were included in the rate study; when necessary the residence qualification (one year) was confirmed by house visiting, since patients who were anxious to obtain admission to hospital occasionally gave a false Ibadan address.

The estimation of age in the absence of vital statistics is difficult and if, on interview, the age was not known it was calculated from the patient's memory of local historical events listed in chronological order.

G.M. Edington,
C.M.U. MacLean.

Registry Title and Address : The Ibadan Cancer Registry, University College Hospital, Ibadan, Nigeria.
Commenced 1960. Supported financially by British Empire Cancer Campaign.

Registrations are made from hospital in-patients and out-patients, pathology departments and from doctors attending cases at home. Registration is thought to be less than 90 % complete for old people.

Follow-up. A small percentage of cases are followed up.

Physical Description. The Registry covers the city of Ibadan in the Western Region of Nigeria which is in the forest belt of West Africa. It lies at latitude 7^U 26' North and longitude 3^0 54' East. The total registration area is 18 square kilometres.

Demographic Description. Total population of area under survey 477,000. The population is comprised mainly of the Yoruba tribe, and the population is approximately 90 % agricultural. The entire registration population lives in Ibadan.

Medical Services. Total number of hospitals beds of all kinds 700. Total number of doctors in practice in registration area approximately 150. The use of native herbalists and medicines might unduly delay 5 % or more of the population seeking medical advice. It is not known what percentage of deaths is caused by cancer.

Publications. Annual reports in Annual Reports of the British Empire Cancer Campaign. Edington and MacLean (1965).

TABLE 2 A
NIGERIA, IBADAN :
POPULATION (100, 000s), 1962

AGE (In years)	MALES No.	MALES Per Cent	FEMALES No.	FEMALES Per Cent
0 –	0.4430	18.69	0.4260	17.75
5 –	0.3210	13.54	0.3630	15.13
10 –	0.2660	11.22	0.2450	10.21
15 –	0.2430	10.25	0.1600	6.67
20 –	0.2710	11.43	0.2770	11.54
25 –	0.2270	9.58	0.2770	11.54
30 –	0.1720	7.26	0.2030	8.46
35 –	0.1270	5.36	0.1490	6.21
40 –	0.0890	3.76	0.1070	4.46
45 –	0.0660	2.78	0.0750	3.13
50 –	0.0500	2.11	0.0430	1.79
55 –	0.0390	1.65	0.0320	1.33
60 –	0.0280	1.18	0.0210	0.88
65 –	0.0170	0.72	0.0110	0.46
70 – and over	0.0110	0.46	0.0110	0.46
–	–	–	–	–
–	–	–	–	–
–	–	–	–	–
TOTAL	2.3700	100.00	2.4000	100.00

NOTES

TO TABLES 2 A, B and C

(I) Period of registration 1.4.60 to 31.3.63.

(II) Population in 5-year age groups obtained by interpolation from data for 10-year age groups.

(III) I.L. number 142 includes "benign salivary glands".
" " 193 includes unspecified tumours of the central nervous system, but excludes benign tumours.
" " 196 includes adamantinomas.

(IV) Carcinoma in situ excluded.

TABLE 2 B
NIGERIA, IBADAN :
MALE INCIDENCE RATES, 1960 - 62.

AVERAGE ANNUAL INCIDENCE PER 100,000

INTER-NATIONAL LIST No.	0-	5-	10-	15-	20-	25-	30-	35-	40-	45-	50-	55-	60-	65-	70-	75-	80-	85- AND OVER	ALL AGES	AGE UNKNOWN	ALL AGES	INTER-NATIONAL LIST No.
140	0.0	0.0	0.0	0.0	0.0	0.0	0.0	0.0	0.0	0.0	0.0	0.0	11.9	0.0	0.0				0.1	0	1	140
141	0.0	0.0	0.0	0.0	0.0	0.0	0.0	0.0	0.0	0.0	0.0	8.5	0.0	0.0	0.0				0.1	0	1	141
142	0.0	0.0	0.0	0.0	0.0	0.0	0.0	0.0	3.7	10.1	0.0	0.0	23.8	0.0	0.0				0.7	0	5	142
143-4	0.0	0.0	0.0	0.0	0.0	0.0	1.9	2.6	3.7	0.0	0.0	0.0	0.0	19.6	0.0				0.6	0	4	143-4
146	0.0	0.0	0.0	0.0	0.0	0.0	0.0	0.0	3.7	0.0	0.0	0.0	0.0	19.6	0.0				0.3	0	2	146
145,147-8	0.0	0.0	0.0	0.0	0.0	0.0	0.0	0.0	0.0	0.0	0.0	0.0	0.0	0.0	0.0				0.0	1	0	145,147-8
150	0.0	0.0	0.0	0.0	0.0	0.0	0.0	0.0	0.0	0.0	6.7	0.0	11.9	0.0	0.0				0.4	0	3	150
151	0.0	0.0	0.0	0.0	1.2	1.5	0.0	2.6	15.0	30.3	20.0	25.6	47.6	78.4	30.3				3.9	0	28	151
152	0.0	0.0	0.0	0.0	0.0	0.0	0.0	0.0	3.7	0.0	0.0	0.0	0.0	0.0	0.0				0.6	0	4	152
153	0.0	0.0	0.0	0.0	0.0	0.0	1.9	0.0	3.7	5.1	0.0	8.5	0.0	0.0	0.0				0.6	0	4	153
154	0.0	0.0	1.3	0.0	0.0	0.0	3.9	0.0	0.0	10.1	0.0	8.5	0.0	0.0	0.0				0.8	0	6	154
155.0	0.0	0.0	0.0	2.7	3.7	5.9	7.8	18.4	30.0	15.2	13.3	25.6	59.5	0.0	0.0				5.9	1	42	155.0
155.1	0.0	0.0	0.0	0.0	0.0	0.0	0.0	0.0	0.0	0.0	0.0	0.0	0.0	0.0	0.0				0.0	0	0	155.1
156	0.0	0.0	0.0	0.0	1.2	0.0	0.0	2.6	0.0	0.0	6.7	0.0	0.0	19.6	0.0				0.3	0	2	156
157	0.0	0.0	0.0	0.0	1.2	1.5	1.9	5.2	3.7	5.1	6.7	0.0	0.0	0.0	0.0				1.1	0	8	157
160	0.8	0.0	0.0	0.0	0.0	0.0	1.9	2.6	3.7	10.1	6.7	8.5	0.0	0.0	0.0				1.1	0	8	160
161	0.0	0.0	0.0	0.0	0.0	0.0	0.0	0.0	0.0	0.0	6.7	0.0	11.9	0.0	0.0				0.6	0	4	161
162-3	0.0	0.0	0.0	0.0	1.2	0.0	1.9	2.6	0.0	0.0	6.7	0.0	11.9	0.0	0.0				0.7	0	5	162-3
170	0.0	0.0	0.0	0.0	0.0	0.0	0.0	0.0	0.0	0.0	0.0	0.0	0.0	0.0	0.0				0.0	0	0	170
177	0.0	0.0	0.0	0.0	2.5	0.0	0.0	0.0	0.0	5.1	13.3	34.2	47.6	78.4	90.9				2.5	1	18	177
178	0.0	0.0	0.0	0.0	0.0	0.0	0.0	0.0	0.0	0.0	0.0	0.0	0.0	0.0	0.0				0.4	0	3	178
179.0	0.0	0.0	0.0	1.4	0.0	0.0	0.0	0.0	0.0	0.0	6.7	0.0	0.0	0.0	0.0				0.1	0	1	179.0
180	1.5	1.0	0.0	0.0	0.0	0.0	0.0	0.0	0.0	0.0	6.7	0.0	0.0	0.0	0.0				0.6	0	4	180
181.0	0.0	0.0	0.0	0.0	0.0	0.0	0.0	0.0	11.2	0.0	6.7	0.0	47.6	19.6	30.3				1.4	0	10	181.0
190	0.0	0.0	0.0	0.0	1.2	0.0	0.0	2.6	0.0	0.0	0.0	0.0	0.0	19.6	0.0				0.4	0	3	190
191	0.0	0.0	0.0	0.0	1.2	1.5	1.9	0.0	0.0	5.1	0.0	0.0	11.9	0.0	0.0				1.0	2	7	191
192	2.3	1.0	0.0	0.0	0.0	0.0	0.0	0.0	0.0	0.0	0.0	0.0	0.0	0.0	0.0				0.6	0	4	192
193	0.8	2.1	0.0	1.4	0.0	0.0	0.0	0.0	0.0	0.0	0.0	0.0	19.6	0.0	0.0				0.7	0	5	193
194	0.0	0.0	0.0	0.0	2.5	0.0	0.0	2.6	7.5	0.0	0.0	0.0	0.0	0.0	0.0				0.7	0	5	194
195	0.0	0.0	0.0	0.0	0.0	0.0	0.0	0.0	0.0	0.0	0.0	0.0	0.0	0.0	0.0				0.0	0	0	195
196	0.0	0.0	0.0	0.0	1.2	5.9	0.0	0.0	3.7	5.1	0.0	0.0	0.0	0.0	0.0				1.0	0	7	196
197	1.5	0.0	0.0	2.7	0.0	2.9	0.0	0.0	0.0	5.1	0.0	17.1	0.0	0.0	0.0				1.1	1	8	197
200	3.0	19.7	13.8	2.7	4.9	1.5	7.8	7.9	11.2	5.1	26.7	0.0	0.0	19.6	0.0				8.3	0	59	200
201	0.0	0.0	2.5	2.7	2.5	1.5	1.9	0.0	7.5	5.1	6.7	0.0	0.0	19.6	0.0				1.8	0	13	201
203	0.0	0.0	0.0	0.0	0.0	0.0	0.0	2.6	0.0	0.0	0.0	0.0	0.0	0.0	0.0				0.1	0	1	203
204	0.8	1.0	6.3	2.7	0.0	0.0	5.8	13.1	0.0	20.2	0.0	8.5	11.9	19.6	0.0				3.4	0	24	204
OTHER	0.0	1.0	0.0	0.0	0.0	1.5	3.9	0.0	18.7	10.1	26.7	0.0	35.7	58.8	0.0				3.2	2	23	OTHER
140-205	10.5	26.0	23.8	15.1	24.6	23.5	42.6	65.6	131.1	146.5	160.0	145.3	333.3	392.2	151.5				44.7	8	318	140-205
RATE PER CASE IN PERIOD	0.75	1.04	1.25	1.37	1.23	1.47	1.94	2.62	3.75	5.05	6.67	8.55	11.90	19.61	30.30				0.14	-	-	RATE PER CASE IN PERIOD

TABLE 2 C

NIGERIA, IBADAN :

FEMALE INCIDENCE RATES, 1960 - 62.

INTERNATIONAL LIST No.	0-	5-	10-	15-	20-	25-	30-	35-	40-	45-	50-	55-	60-	65-	70-	75-	80-	85- AND OVER	ALL AGES	No. of cases AGE UNKNOWN	No. of cases ALL AGES
140	0.0	0.0	0.0	0.0	0.0	0.0	0.0	0.0	0.0	0.0	0.0	0.0	0.0	0.0	0.0				0.0	0	0
141	0.0	0.0	0.0	0.0	0.0	0.0	0.0	0.0	0.0	0.0	0.0	0.0	0.0	0.0	0.0				0.0	0	0
142	0.0	0.0	0.0	0.0	0.0	0.0	0.0	0.0	9.3	0.0	0.0	0.0	0.0	0.0	0.0				0.4	0	3
143-4	0.0	0.0	0.0	0.0	0.0	0.0	0.0	0.0	0.0	0.0	0.0	0.0	0.0	0.0	0.0				0.0	0	0
146	0.0	0.0	0.0	0.0	0.0	0.0	0.0	0.0	0.0	0.0	0.0	0.0	0.0	0.0	0.0				0.0	0	0
145,147-8	0.0	0.0	0.0	0.0	0.0	0.0	0.0	0.0	0.0	0.0	0.0	0.0	0.0	0.0	0.0				0.0	0	0
150	0.0	0.0	0.0	0.0	0.0	0.0	0.0	0.0	0.0	0.0	0.0	0.0	0.0	0.0	0.0				0.1	1	1
151	0.0	0.0	0.0	0.0	0.0	0.0	3.3	2.2	6.2	13.3	7.8	10.4	31.7	30.3	0.0				1.9	0	14
152	0.0	0.0	0.0	0.0	0.0	0.0	0.0	0.0	0.0	0.0	0.0	0.0	0.0	0.0	0.0				0.0	0	0
153	0.0	0.0	0.0	0.0	0.0	0.0	0.0	0.0	3.1	4.4	7.8	0.0	0.0	0.0	30.3				0.6	0	4
154	0.0	0.0	0.0	0.0	0.0	0.0	0.0	2.2	3.1	8.9	0.0	0.0	0.0	0.0	0.0				0.6	0	4
155.0	0.0	0.0	0.0	0.0	0.0	0.0	0.0	4.5	0.0	13.3	0.0	31.3	0.0	0.0	0.0				1.1	0	8
155.1	0.0	0.0	0.0	0.0	0.0	0.0	0.0	0.0	0.0	0.0	0.0	10.4	0.0	0.0	0.0				0.1	0	1
156	0.0	0.0	0.0	0.0	0.0	0.0	0.0	0.0	0.0	0.0	23.3	0.0	0.0	0.0	0.0				0.6	0	4
157	0.0	0.0	0.0	0.0	0.0	0.0	0.0	2.2	0.0	8.9	7.8	10.4	0.0	0.0	0.0				0.7	0	5
160	0.0	0.0	0.0	0.0	0.0	0.0	0.0	0.0	0.0	0.0	0.0	0.0	0.0	0.0	0.0				0.0	0	0
161	0.0	0.0	0.0	0.0	0.0	0.0	0.0	0.0	0.0	0.0	0.0	0.0	0.0	0.0	0.0				0.0	0	0
162-3	0.0	0.0	0.0	0.0	0.0	0.0	0.0	4.5	0.0	8.9	0.0	0.0	15.9	0.0	0.0				0.7	1	5
170	0.0	0.0	0.0	0.0	0.0	4.8	6.6	24.6	21.8	17.8	108.5	41.7	47.6	90.9	0.0				7.6	1	55
171	0.0	0.0	0.0	0.0	0.0	0.0	0.0	17.9	24.9	57.8	100.8	83.3	47.6	90.9	60.6				8.2	1	59
172	0.0	0.0	0.0	0.0	0.0	0.0	0.0	0.0	0.0	0.0	0.0	0.0	0.0	0.0	0.0				0.0	0	0
173	0.0	0.0	0.0	2.1	3.6	2.4	2.3	8.9	9.3	0.0	0.0	0.0	0.0	0.0	0.0				2.1	0	15
174	0.0	0.0	0.0	0.0	0.0	0.0	0.0	0.0	0.0	0.0	0.0	0.0	0.0	0.0	0.0				0.0	0	0
175	0.0	0.9	0.0	0.0	0.0	6.0	6.6	4.5	12.5	4.4	46.5	41.7	31.7	30.3	0.0				4.3	0	31
176	0.0	0.0	0.0	0.0	0.0	0.0	0.0	0.0	0.0	0.0	15.5	0.0	0.0	0.0	0.0				0.3	0	2
180	0.8	0.0	0.0	0.0	0.0	0.0	0.0	2.2	0.0	0.0	0.0	0.0	0.0	0.0	0.0				0.3	0	2
181.0	0.0	0.0	0.0	2.1	0.0	0.0	0.0	0.0	0.0	4.4	15.5	10.4	0.0	0.0	0.0				0.7	0	5
190	0.0	0.0	0.0	0.0	0.0	0.0	0.0	0.0	0.0	4.4	7.8	0.0	15.9	0.0	0.0				0.4	0	3
191	0.8	0.0	0.0	0.0	1.2	0.0	0.0	0.0	0.0	0.0	0.0	0.0	0.0	0.0	0.0				0.4	0	3
192	0.8	0.0	0.0	0.0	0.0	0.0	0.0	0.0	0.0	0.0	0.0	0.0	0.0	0.0	0.0				0.1	0	1
193	1.6	0.0	0.0	0.0	0.0	0.0	0.0	0.0	0.0	0.0	0.0	0.0	0.0	30.3	0.0				0.3	0	2
194	0.0	0.0	1.4	0.0	0.0	1.2	0.0	2.2	3.1	0.0	23.3	0.0	0.0	30.3	0.0				1.5	0	11
195	0.0	0.0	0.0	0.0	1.2	1.2	0.0	0.0	0.0	0.0	0.0	0.0	0.0	0.0	0.0				0.4	2	3
196	0.0	0.0	0.0	2.1	1.2	0.0	0.0	0.0	0.0	0.0	0.0	0.0	0.0	0.0	0.0				0.4	0	3
197	0.0	0.0	0.0	0.0	0.0	0.0	0.0	2.2	0.0	0.0	7.8	0.0	0.0	30.3	0.0				0.8	0	6
200	0.8	9.2	9.5	4.2	3.6	6.0	1.6	4.5	12.5	8.9	38.8	20.8	15.9	0.0	0.0				6.4	1	46
201	0.0	0.0	0.0	0.0	0.0	0.0	0.0	0.0	0.0	4.4	0.0	10.4	0.0	0.0	0.0				0.3	0	2
203	0.0	0.0	0.0	0.0	0.0	0.0	0.0	0.0	0.0	0.0	0.0	0.0	0.0	0.0	0.0				0.0	0	0
204	0.0	1.8	0.0	0.0	0.0	4.8	1.6	0.0	3.1	8.9	23.3	0.0	47.6	0.0	0.0				2.2	0	16
OTHER	0.0	0.0	0.0	0.0	0.0	1.2	3.3	4.5	15.6	4.4	23.3	10.4	31.7	30.3	0.0				2.6	1	19
140-205	3.9	12.9	10.9	12.5	13.2	27.7	26.3	87.2	127.7	177.8	457.4	281.3	285.7	363.6	90.9				45.8	8	330
RATE PER CASE IN PERIOD	0.78	0.92	1.36	2.08	1.20	1.20	1.64	2.24	3.12	4.44	7.75	10.42	15.87	30.30	30.30				0.14	-	-

AVERAGE ANNUAL INCIDENCE PER 100,000 — AGE IN YEARS

Note : Figures in column 70— relate to the years 70 and over.

SOUTH AFRICA, JOHANNESBURG (BANTU)

Registry Title and Address : The Johannesburg Cancer Survey, 1953-1955, The South African Institute for Medical Research, Hospital Street, Johannesburg, South Africa. Commenced 1st January, 1953 and terminated 31st December, 1955. Principal sources of financial support were Research Grant (C - 1716) from the National Cancer Institute, National Institutes of Health, United States Public Health Service; a grant from the Department of Education, Arts and Sciences of the Union Government; the National Cancer Association of South Africa; and the South African Institute for Medical Research.

Registration. Cases were registered by medical staff from hospital in-patients, but in addition it was found necessary to screen all case histories. This was done by the authors. Hospital out-patients were not registered except for a single large clinic at Alexandra Township where registrations were made by doctors. Records from radiotherapy and pathology departments and death certificates were screened by the authors. Doctors attending cases at home were paid for each registration made. Pathologists in medico-legal departments also registered cases which were screened by the authors. Registration is likely to be less than 90 % complete for Zionist religious groups and old people.

Follow-up. No cases are followed up.

Physical Description. The Registry covers the metropolitan area of Johannesburg, consisting of the municipal area, and the peri-urban Bantu Townships, notably Alexandra township in the north-east and a cluster of townships in the south west. Johannesburg, in the southern Transvaal, is the largest city in South Africa, having a total population at the time of the survey of 800,000. It is situated at the northern limit of the Highveld inland plateau at a mean altitude of 5,850 feet. Although only 3⁰ from the Tropic of Capricorn it has an excellent temperate climate with an average duration of sunlight of 8.7 hours (73 %). The amount of cosmic and ultraviolet irradiation is high. It lies at the centre of the Witwatersrand Goldfields on the watershed of the Vaal River to the south, running westwards into the Atlantic; and to the north into the Jukskei and Crocodile rivers, running into the Limpopo and eastwards into the Indian Ocean. It is 300 miles from the Indian Ocean coast. Johannesburg lies at latitude 26⁰ 11' South and longitude 28⁰ 4' East. The municipal area has a maximum diameter of 11.5 miles (18.5 kilometres) but there are outlying native townships which extended at the time of the survey up to 12 miles (19 kilometres) from the centre of the city. The total registration area comprised the municipal area of 94 square mile (243 square kilometres) with another 26.5 square miles (69 square kilometres) of Bantu housing of which approximately one half had been settled by the time of this survey. The total populated area surveyed was 108 square miles, or 280 square kilometres.

Demographic Description. Total Bantu population of area under survey 478,464 (shown in Table 3A as 477,200 after excluding 1,245 persons of unknown age and rounding off). The main occupational composition of the economically active registered population is : industry 5 %, commerce 54 %, agriculture 3 % and personal service 38 %. The entire registration population lives in a conurbation of more than 100,000.

Medical Services. Total number of hospital beds of all kinds 2,570. Total number of doctors in practice in registration area 160 full-time staff, with additional part-time staff; 385 doctors in private practice treated Bantu and Coloured patients. Religious beliefs, chiefly of the Zionist Christian group, prevent about 5 % of the population from calling in medical advice until the subject is moribund. Tribal customs and adherence to the tribal medical men cause delay, in that a proportion (30 %) will attend the tribal practitioner first. Only 2 % stated that they would use the traditional doctor alone. One person only (0.2 % of the sample) stated that he would leave the city if he fell ill. Ignorance of the early signs of cancer led to delay so that a large proportion were advanced cases on first seeing a doctor. Cancer caused approximately 1 % of all deaths certified.

Publications. Higginson and Oettlé (1957a, 1957b, 1958a, 1958b, 1960 and 1966); Oettlé (1957, 1960 and 1964); Oettlé and Higginson (1956).

TABLE 3 A
SOUTH AFRICA, JOHANNESBURG, BANTU :
POPULATION (100, 000s), 1954

AGE (In years)	MALES No.	MALES Per Cent	FEMALES No.	FEMALES Per Cent
0 –	0.2614	9.83	0.2761	13.07
5 –	0.1629	6.13	0.1889	8.94
10 –	0.1373	5.16	0.1643	7.78
15 –	0.2052	7.72	0.1736	8.22
20 –	0.2754	10.36	0.2727	12.91
25 –	0.3512	13.21	0.2724	12.89
30 –	0.3457	13.00	0.2483	11.75
35 –	0.3070	11.54	0.1732	8.20
40 –	0.2218	8.34	0.1163	5.50
45 –	0.1671	6.28	0.0830	3.93
50 –	0.1100	4.14	0.0551	2.61
55 –	0.0443	1.67	0.0270	1.28
60 –	0.0297	1.12	0.0216	1.02
65 –	0.0176	0.66	0.0150	0.71
70 –	0.0112	0.42	0.0118	0.56
75 – and over	0.0114	0.43	0.0135	0.64
–	–	–	–	–
TOTAL	2.6592	100.00	2.1128	100.00

NOTES

TO TAïBLES 3 A, B and C

(I) I.L. number 176 no case recorded.
   "   " 193 includes unspecified and some benign tumours of the central nervous system.

(II) One case of carcinoma in situ included (I.L. number 171).

TABLE 3 B

SOUTH AFRICA, JOHANNESBURG, BANTU :

MALE INCIDENCE RATES, 1953 - 55.

INTER-NATIONAL LIST No.	AVERAGE ANNUAL INCIDENCE PER 100,000 — AGE IN YEARS																		ALL AGES	No. OF CASES IN WHOLE PERIOD		INTER-NATIONAL LIST No.
	0-	5-	10-	15-	20-	25-	30-	35-	40-	45-	50-	55-	60-	65-	70-	75-	80-	85- and over		AGE UNKNOWN	ALL AGES	
140	0.0	0.0	0.0	0.0	0.0	0.0	0.0	1.1	0.0	0.0	3.0	0.0	0.0	0.0	0.0	0.0			0.3	0	2	140
141	0.0	0.0	0.0	0.0	0.0	0.0	0.0	2.2	1.5	0.0	6.1	0.0	11.2	18.9	29.8	0.0			1.0	0	8	141
142	0.0	2.0	0.0	0.0	0.0	0.0	1.0	1.1	0.0	0.0	0.0	0.0	0.0	0.0	0.0	0.0			0.4	0	3	142
143-4	0.0	0.0	0.0	0.0	0.0	0.0	1.0	0.0	0.0	2.0	3.0	7.5	22.4	37.9	0.0	29.2			1.0	0	8	143-4
146	0.0	0.0	0.0	1.6	1.2	0.9	1.0	0.0	1.5	0.0	0.0	0.0	11.2	0.0	0.0	0.0			0.8	0	6	146
145,147-8	0.0	0.0	0.0	0.0	0.0	0.0	1.0	0.0	0.0	0.0	0.0	0.0	0.0	0.0	0.0	0.0			0.1	0	1	145,147-8
150	0.0	0.0	0.0	0.0	0.0	0.0	0.0	6.5	9.0	14.0	54.5	22.6	33.7	37.9	0.0	233.9			6.8	1	54	150
151	0.0	0.0	0.0	0.0	1.2	0.0	1.0	5.4	6.0	16.0	18.2	30.1	56.1	56.8	59.5	58.5			5.1	0	41	151
152	0.0	0.0	0.0	0.0	0.0	0.0	0.0	0.0	0.0	0.0	3.0	0.0	0.0	0.0	0.0	0.0			0.1	0	1	152
153	0.0	0.0	0.0	0.0	0.0	0.0	0.0	0.0	1.5	4.0	3.0	7.5	11.2	18.9	0.0	0.0			0.9	0	7	153
154	0.0	0.0	0.0	0.0	0.0	0.9	0.0	0.0	0.0	0.0	0.0	7.5	11.2	0.0	29.8	29.2			0.6	0	5	154
155.0	0.0	0.0	2.4	1.6	2.4	9.5	11.6	19.5	24.0	35.9	39.4	52.7	33.7	113.6	119.0	58.5			14.2	0	113	155.0
155.1	0.0	0.0	0.0	0.0	0.0	0.0	0.0	0.0	0.0	0.0	0.0	0.0	0.0	0.0	0.0	0.0			0.0	0	0	155.1
156	0.0	0.0	0.0	0.0	0.0	0.0	1.0	0.0	0.0	0.0	0.0	0.0	0.0	18.9	0.0	0.0			0.1	0	1	156
157	0.0	0.0	0.0	0.0	0.0	1.9	1.0	1.1	0.0	4.0	9.1	7.5	22.4	0.0	0.0	29.2			1.3	0	10	157
160	0.0	0.0	0.0	0.0	0.0	0.0	0.0	0.0	3.0	0.0	0.0	0.0	0.0	18.9	29.8	0.0			1.0	0	8	160
161	0.0	0.0	0.0	0.0	0.0	0.0	0.0	0.0	0.0	6.0	6.1	0.0	11.2	18.9	29.8	0.0			1.0	0	8	161
162-3	0.0	0.0	0.0	0.0	0.0	0.0	1.9	2.2	7.5	19.9	36.4	37.6	11.2	18.9	29.8	29.2			5.0	0	40	162-3
170	0.0	0.0	0.0	0.0	0.0	0.0	0.0	0.0	1.5	2.0	0.0	0.0	0.0	0.0	29.8	0.0			0.4	0	3	170
177	0.0	0.0	0.0	0.0	0.0	0.0	0.0	0.0	0.0	0.0	9.1	30.1	33.7	94.7	89.3	87.7			2.6	0	21	177
178	0.0	0.0	0.0	0.0	0.0	0.0	1.0	2.2	0.0	0.0	0.0	7.5	0.0	0.0	0.0	29.2			0.3	0	2	178
179	0.0	0.0	0.0	0.0	0.0	0.0	0.0	0.0	1.5	0.0	6.1	7.5	0.0	18.9	0.0	0.0			1.0	0	8	179
180	0.0	0.0	0.0	0.0	0.0	0.0	0.0	2.2	0.0	2.0	3.0	7.5	11.2	0.0	0.0	0.0			0.6	0	5	180
181	0.0	0.0	0.0	0.0	1.2	0.9	1.0	2.2	1.5	4.0	12.1	7.5	22.4	0.0	0.0	0.0			2.1	1	17	181
190	0.0	0.0	0.0	0.0	0.0	0.0	1.0	0.0	1.5	0.0	3.0	0.0	0.0	18.9	0.0	0.0			0.6	1	5	190
191	0.0	0.0	0.0	0.0	0.0	0.0	2.9	2.2	0.0	2.0	3.0	7.5	0.0	18.9	0.0	0.0			1.1	0	9	191
192	2.6	0.0	0.0	0.0	0.0	0.9	0.0	0.0	1.5	0.0	6.1	0.0	0.0	0.0	0.0	0.0			0.6	0	5	192
193	1.3	2.0	2.4	1.6	2.4	0.0	2.9	4.3	0.0	0.0	0.0	0.0	0.0	0.0	0.0	0.0			1.8	0	14	193
194	0.0	0.0	0.0	0.0	0.0	0.0	0.0	0.0	1.5	0.0	0.0	0.0	0.0	0.0	0.0	0.0			0.1	0	1	194
195	0.0	0.0	2.4	1.6	0.0	0.0	0.0	0.0	0.0	0.0	0.0	0.0	0.0	0.0	0.0	0.0			0.3	0	2	195
196	0.0	0.0	0.0	0.0	0.0	0.9	1.0	0.0	0.0	0.0	6.1	0.0	0.0	0.0	0.0	0.0			0.4	0	3	196
197	0.0	2.0	2.4	0.0	1.2	2.8	0.0	3.3	0.0	2.0	3.0	15.0	0.0	0.0	59.5	0.0			1.9	0	15	197
200	1.3	2.0	0.0	4.9	0.0	0.9	0.0	2.2	0.0	0.0	0.0	7.5	0.0	0.0	0.0	0.0			0.8	0	6	200
201	0.0	0.0	0.0	0.0	1.2	1.9	0.0	1.1	1.5	4.0	0.0	0.0	0.0	0.0	0.0	0.0			1.3	0	10	201
203	0.0	2.0	2.4	3.2	0.0	0.0	1.0	3.3	0.0	2.0	3.0	7.5	0.0	0.0	0.0	0.0			0.8	0	6	203
204	2.6	0.0	0.0	1.6	0.0	2.8	1.0	1.1	3.0	2.0	0.0	7.5	0.0	18.9	0.0	0.0			2.3	0	18	204
202,205	0.0	0.0	0.0	0.0	0.0	0.9	1.0	1.1	0.0	0.0	0.0	0.0	0.0	0.0	0.0	0.0			0.6	0	5	202,205
OTHER	0.0	0.0	0.0	0.0	2.4	1.9	0.0	0.0	3.0	4.0	9.1	22.6	11.2	18.9	59.5	0.0			2.3	0	18	OTHER
140-205	7.7	10.2	12.1	16.2	13.3	27.5	29.9	63.0	72.1	127.7	245.5	308.5	314.3	587.1	565.5	584.8			61.3	2	489	140-205
RATE PER CASE IN PERIOD	1.28	2.05	2.43	1.62	1.21	0.95	0.96	1.09	1.50	1.99	3.03	7.52	11.22	18.94	29.76	29.24			0.13	-	-	RATE PER CASE IN PERIOD

TABLE 3 C
SOUTH AFRICA, JOHANNESBURG, BANTU :
FEMALE INCIDENCE RATES, 1953 - 55.

INTER-NATIONAL LIST No.	AVERAGE ANNUAL INCIDENCE PER 100,000 — AGE IN YEARS																		ALL AGES	No. OF CASES IN WHOLE PERIOD — AGE UNKNOWN	No. OF CASES IN WHOLE PERIOD — ALL AGES	INTER-NATIONAL LIST No.
	0-	5-	10-	15-	20-	25-	30-	35-	40-	45-	50-	55-	60-	65-	70-	75-	80-	85- AND OVER				
140	0.0	0.0	0.0	0.0	0.0	0.0	0.0	0.0	0.0	0.0	0.0	0.0	0.0	0.0	0.0	0.0			0.0	0	0	140
141	0.0	0.0	0.0	0.0	0.0	0.0	0.0	0.0	0.0	4.0	0.0	0.0	0.0	22.2	0.0	0.0			0.3	0	2	141
142	0.0	0.0	0.0	0.0	0.0	1.2	0.0	0.0	0.0	0.0	0.0	0.0	0.0	22.2	0.0	0.0			0.3	0	2	142
143-4	0.0	0.0	0.0	0.0	0.0	0.0	0.0	0.0	2.9	0.0	0.0	0.0	0.0	0.0	0.0	0.0			0.2	0	1	143-4
146	0.0	0.0	0.0	0.0	0.0	0.0	0.0	0.0	0.0	0.0	0.0	0.0	15.4	0.0	28.2	0.0			0.3	0	2	146
145,147-8	0.0	0.0	0.0	0.0	0.0	0.0	0.0	0.0	0.0	0.0	0.0	0.0	0.0	0.0	0.0	0.0			0.0	0	0	145,147-8
150	0.0	0.0	0.0	0.0	0.0	2.4	0.0	3.8	0.0	0.0	0.0	0.0	15.4	0.0	28.2	0.0			0.3	0	2	150
151	0.0	0.0	0.0	0.0	0.0	0.0	0.0	0.0	2.9	4.0	24.2	61.7	15.4	0.0	28.2	24.7			2.8	0	18	151
152	0.0	0.0	0.0	0.0	1.2	0.0	0.0	0.0	0.0	0.0	0.0	0.0	0.0	0.0	0.0	0.0			0.2	0	1	152
153	0.0	0.0	0.0	0.0	0.0	0.0	1.3	1.9	0.0	0.0	0.0	37.0	61.7	0.0	0.0	0.0			1.4	0	9	153
154	0.0	0.0	0.0	0.0	0.0	0.0	1.3	0.0	5.7	0.0	0.0	12.3	15.4	22.2	0.0	0.0			0.9	0	6	154
155.0	0.0	0.0	0.0	0.0	1.2	0.0	5.4	0.0	5.7	4.0	12.1	74.1	61.7	44.4	28.2	49.4			3.9	0	25	155.0
155.1	0.0	0.0	0.0	0.0	0.0	0.0	0.0	0.0	2.9	0.0	0.0	0.0	15.4	22.2	0.0	0.0			0.5	0	3	155.1
156	0.0	0.0	0.0	0.0	0.0	0.0	0.0	0.0	0.0	0.0	0.0	0.0	0.0	0.0	0.0	0.0			0.0	0	0	156
157	0.0	0.0	0.0	1.9	0.0	0.0	0.0	0.0	2.9	0.0	0.0	12.3	0.0	0.0	0.0	49.4			0.6	0	4	157
160	0.0	0.0	0.0	0.0	0.0	0.0	0.0	0.0	0.0	0.0	0.0	0.0	0.0	0.0	0.0	0.0			0.0	0	0	160
161	0.0	0.0	0.0	0.0	0.0	1.2	0.0	0.0	2.9	0.0	0.0	0.0	0.0	0.0	0.0	0.0			0.3	0	2	161
162-3	0.0	0.0	0.0	0.0	2.4	1.2	2.7	0.0	0.0	0.0	0.0	12.3	15.4	22.2	28.2	24.7			1.3	0	8	162-3
170	0.0	0.0	0.0	0.0	2.4	1.2	9.4	7.7	11.5	28.1	54.4	24.7	30.9	133.3	84.7	49.4			7.7	0	49	170
171	0.0	0.0	0.0	0.0	0.0	7.3	30.9	38.5	111.8	112.4	151.2	172.8	154.3	222.2	141.2	172.8			29.8	0	189	171
172	0.0	0.0	0.0	0.0	0.0	1.2	0.0	0.0	2.9	12.0	0.0	0.0	0.0	0.0	0.0	0.0			0.2	0	1	172
173	0.0	0.0	0.0	1.9	0.0	0.0	0.0	0.0	0.0	0.0	6.0	12.3	0.0	0.0	0.0	0.0			1.3	0	8	173
174	0.0	0.0	0.0	0.0	2.4	2.4	0.0	0.0	0.0	0.0	0.0	0.0	15.4	0.0	28.2	49.4			0.6	0	4	174
175	0.0	0.0	0.0	1.9	0.0	4.9	1.3	7.7	5.7	4.0	12.1	0.0	15.4	22.2	0.0	0.0			3.0	0	19	175
180	2.4	0.0	0.0	0.0	0.0	0.0	0.0	0.0	2.9	0.0	0.0	0.0	0.0	0.0	0.0	0.0			0.5	0	3	180
181	0.0	0.0	0.0	0.0	0.0	0.0	0.0	0.0	2.9	0.0	0.0	0.0	0.0	0.0	28.2	0.0			0.5	0	3	181
190	0.0	0.0	0.0	0.0	0.0	0.0	0.0	1.9	2.9	4.0	6.0	0.0	15.4	0.0	28.2	0.0			0.9	0	6	190
191	0.0	0.0	0.0	0.0	0.0	1.2	1.3	0.0	0.0	4.0	0.0	0.0	46.3	0.0	0.0	0.0			1.1	0	7	191
192	1.2	0.0	0.0	0.0	0.0	0.0	0.0	1.9	0.0	0.0	0.0	0.0	0.0	0.0	28.2	0.0			0.3	0	2	192
193	0.0	1.8	2.0	0.0	1.2	2.4	1.3	1.9	2.9	4.0	6.0	12.3	30.9	22.2	0.0	0.0			1.6	0	10	193
194	0.0	0.0	0.0	1.9	0.0	0.0	0.0	1.9	2.9	0.0	0.0	0.0	15.4	0.0	0.0	24.7			1.1	0	7	194
195	0.0	0.0	0.0	0.0	0.0	0.0	0.0	0.0	5.7	0.0	0.0	0.0	0.0	0.0	0.0	0.0			0.3	0	2	195
196	0.0	0.0	0.0	0.0	1.2	2.4	0.0	0.0	0.0	0.0	0.0	0.0	0.0	0.0	0.0	0.0			0.3	0	2	196
197	0.0	0.0	0.0	1.9	0.0	2.4	1.3	0.0	5.7	4.0	0.0	12.3	0.0	22.2	0.0	0.0			1.4	0	9	197
200	0.0	0.0	0.0	0.0	1.2	0.0	0.0	0.0	2.9	0.0	6.0	12.3	15.4	0.0	0.0	24.7			0.8	0	5	200
201	0.0	0.0	0.0	1.9	0.0	2.4	0.0	0.0	0.0	0.0	0.0	12.3	15.4	0.0	0.0	0.0			0.8	0	5	201
203	0.0	0.0	0.0	0.0	0.0	0.0	4.0	0.0	0.0	0.0	0.0	0.0	15.4	44.4	0.0	24.7			0.6	0	4	203
204	3.6	0.0	4.1	1.9	0.0	0.0	0.0	5.8	0.0	0.0	0.0	24.7	15.4	22.2	0.0	0.0			2.5	0	16	204
202,205	1.2	0.0	2.0	0.0	0.0	0.0	0.0	0.0	0.0	0.0	0.0	24.7	0.0	0.0	0.0	0.0			0.3	0	2	202,205
OTHER	1.2	0.0	0.0	0.0	1.2	0.0	1.3	1.9	0.0	4.0	12.1	24.7	30.9	0.0	56.5	0.0			2.1	0	13	OTHER
140-205	9.7	1.8	8.1	9.6	14.7	29.4	61.8	75.1	189.2	188.8	296.4	518.5	617.3	644.4	536.7	493.8			71.2	0	451	**140-205**
RATE PER CASE IN PERIOD	1.21	1.76	2.03	1.92	1.22	1.22	1.34	1.92	2.87	4.02	6.05	12.35	15.43	22.22	28.25	24.69			0.16	-	-	**RATE PER CASE IN PERIOD**

Note : Figures in column 75— relate to the years 75 and over.

UGANDA, KYADONDO

The registry was organised in the Department of Pathology of the Makerere College Medical School in 1951, because it was realised that the local pattern of types and sites of cancer differed considerably from that seen in Europe. A pilot survey revealed that very few cases seen in the outpatient departments of the various hospitals and ancillary diagnostic units were not forthwith admitted to the wards for further assessment when a cancerous condition was suspected. The aim was to register all cases of cancer seeking aid in the various medical units of the city. There were no private hospitals or nursing homes and few general practitioners and these chiefly looked after expatriate Asians and Europeans, (whose deaths alone were registered), and were dependent for all consultations on the hospitals or the diagnostic units. All the specialist medical services of Uganda were then concentrated in Kampala.

In 1952-1953 the registry operated on a retrospective basis by search of hospital records, with cards being filled in in out-patient departments for all cases not immediately admitted to the wards. All types of cancer (CD. Rubrics 140-205) were registered (Davies and Wilson, 1954). Analysis of the material showed that while few cases had apparently escaped registration essential details of age, sex or address were often missing. (Davies, Wilson and Knowelden, 1958). So in 1954 the registry was put on a current basis with the appointment of a cancer registrar and of an African social worker. The registrar regularly visited all wards and medical units recording details of all cases and these were subsequently visited by the social worker to check on the details. The following items of information were sought from all cases.

(1) Registration details : case number, hospital number, report numbers x-ray, biopsy, autopsy, operation, etc.
(2) Name, age, sex, tribe
(3) Address
(4) Site and type of tumour and major clinical details.

All available resources were devoted to obtaining these data and no attempt was made to accumulate other socio-economic or other data. As it was, numerous difficulties were encountered in obtaining the basic data; these and the steps taken to overcome them have been discussed elsewhere. (Davies, 1958 and 1963). Careful steps were taken to eliminate duplication of registrations and helpful in this respect was the keeping of a separate tumour site registry. Ages were obtained with fair accuracy, in part by the use of dated lists of local events appropriate to the area. Cases in which a histologic diagnosis was available were registered forthwith but cases without such a confirmation were individually considered by a broadly based cancer research committee. A master register was compiled of all cases and they were also recorded on specially printed "Key Sort" cards. All histologic slides were filed with the Registry. The histologic verification rate varied from 70-80 %.

The material collected in 1952-54 was analysed by Professor Knowelden and this revealed that the index of cancer reporting from the county of Kyadondo on a population basis was far higher than from any other area. This county included the Kampala conurbation and surrounding rural areas. The reasons for this higher reporting were carefully considered and it was concluded that it was due to the ready accessibility to the Kyadondo population of the Kampala hospitals. The local population had easy access, medical services were free, the population was receptive and readily sought aid from the hospitals in enormous numbers. While they may first consult some local healer (Gutkind and Southall, 1956) there is nothing to suggest that they would not seek help from the hospitals at least once in any serious illness. The older individuals appeared from the hospital records no less willing than the young to seek treatment, to submit to investigations and operations and to figure in the autopsy records.

It was decided in 1954 to continue to register all cases but to concentrate especially on those who gave addresses in Kyadondo. Much of the time of the social worker was devoted to visiting patient's homes and ascertaining that they were genuine residents of Kyadondo, these being defined as those who had lived in the county for at least one year prior to attending hospital with a neoplastic condition.

Thus from 1954-60 the Registry, which was financed by the British Empire Cancer Campaign, operated under uniform conditions and the material collected from the African population of the County of Kyadondo has been anlysed to obtain annual incidence rates. The Kyadondo population was known from a census taken in 1948 and though this was believed to be a very complete count the age distribution was only recorded in broad categories, 0-1: 1-4: 5-14: 15-45 and over 45 years, which were useless for comparative purposes. Various pilot surveys showed that more precise age groupings could be obtained and the Uganda authorities followed the total census in 1959 with a special sample census of 25 % of the population of Kyadondo to obtain more precise age groupings. The results agreed with those of the total census and provided adequate demographic data to permit the annual incidence rates for cancer to be calculated for the Kyadondo area. The total population in 1959 was over 200,000 and had increased by about 54 % over the 1948 total. About half the population of Kyadondo were members of the local Ganda tribe and the others were immigrants from a wide variety of tribes from many areas of Uganda and East Africa notably from Rwanda and Urundi. Comparisons were therefore possible between Ganda and Non-Ganda and these revealed some marked differences in the frequencies of certain cancers in these groups. (Davies, Knowelden and Wilson, 1965). These, and the obvious differences between the figures from Kyadondo and those from other African areas make it important to emphasise that the result of the Kyadondo region must only be taken as applying to this area and not necessarily to Uganda as a whole, and certainly not to other parts of Africa.

Two things are evident in Kyadondo, firstly that there is a deficiency of cancer in the older age groups as compared with European and American experience, a finding which took us by surprise (Davies, Wilson and Knowelden, 1962) and was certainly not anticipated; and secondly that the pattern of site and type differs markedly not merely from that of Europe and the U.S.A., but from that of other African areas. Due to the availability of adequate records extending back to 1897, a period before the population had come under westernising influences, it is possible to say (Davies et al., 1964) that the site and type pattern in Kampala has been present there, and remarkably stable, over at least six decades. Moreover, when details of the site and type of tumours are studied it is evident that in almost every case there are marked differences from the Europeans patterns which presumably reflect local environmental factors. The deficiencies in the older age groups certainly reflect in part these differences because some of the notable deficiencies are in those cancers which are particularly responsible for the rapid rise of the cancer rates with age in European communities. It is most unusual to find an occult cancer in an elderly African though this is a common finding in elderly Europeans.

The experience of the Kampala Cancer Registry would show that it is possible to obtain cancer rates in an underdeveloped country provided that there is full co-operation from the clinicians, that a carefully controlled registration net is built up and that a variety of procedures will enable adequate demographic data to be obtained.

J. N. P. Davies,
J. Knowelden.

Registry Title and Address : The Kampala Cancer Registry, Department of Pathology, Makerere College Medical School, Kampala, Uganda.
Commenced 1951. Supported financially by the British Empire Cancer Campaign.

Registration. Cases are registered by a cancer registrar and an African social worker from hospital in-patients, and by a member of the clinical staff from out-patients. The cancer registrar registers cases from pathology departments and also from death certificates of expatriate Europeans and Asians only. Registration is less than 90 % complete for the Muslim section of the population.

Follow-up. Only residents of Kyadondo are followed up but there is no specific cancer follow-up.

Physical description. Kyadondo includes the city of Kampala at the N.W. corner of Lake Victoria and the surrounding five urban and rural areas. The Registry is based on the Medical Units in Kampala, although cases are registered from all Uganda and neighbouring parts of Sudan, Congo, Burundi, Rwanda, Tanganyka and Kenya. Incidence rates have been calculated on Kyadondo County only. It lies between latitudes 0° $0'$ and 0° $1'$ and longitude is approximately 34° East. The total registration area is 1.914 square kilometres.

Demographic description. Total population of area under survey 203,970. The population is 100 % indigenous Africans, none of whom live in large conurbations.

Medical Services. Total number of hospital beds of all kinds approximately 1,500. Total number of doctors 120. 5 % or more of the population might delay seeking medical advice because of superstition and also because of the distance from the medical centres in Kampala. Autopsy statistics show cancer as approximately 11 % of all causes of death.

Publications. Davies (1958a, 1958b and 1963); Davies, Elmes, Hutt, Mtivalye, Owor and Shaper (1964); Davies, Knowelden and Wilson (1966); Davies and Wilson (1954); Davies, Wilson and Knowelden (1958, 1962); Guttkind and Southall (1956).

TABLE 4 A
UGANDA, KYADONDO :
POPULATION (100,000s), CENSUS 1959

AGE (in years)	MALES No.	MALES Per Cent	FEMALES No.	FEMALES Per Cent
0 –	0.1469	12.47	0.1411	16.38
5 –	0.1156	9.81	0.1094	12.70
10 –	0.0739	6.27	0.0596	6.92
15 –	0.1204	10.22	0.0902	10.47
20 –	0.1508	12.80	0.1134	13.16
25 –	0.1605	13.62	0.1030	11.95
30 –	0.1220	10.36	0.0675	7.83
35 –	0.0843	7.16	0.0463	5.37
40 –	0.0606	5.14	0.0358	4.16
45 –	0.0435	3.69	0.0264	3.06
50 –	0.0323	2.74	0.0192	2.23
55 –	0.0206	1.75	0.0140	1.62
60 –	0.0177	1.50	0.0148	1.72
65 –	0.0103	0.87	0.0080	0.93
70 –	0.0085	0.72	0.0060	0.70
75 –	0.0050	0.42	0.0034	0.39
80 –	0.0035	0.30	0.0024	0.28
85 – and over	0.0017	0.14	0.0011	0.13
TOTAL	1.1781	100.00	0.8616	100.00

NOTES
TO TABLES 4 A, B and C

(I)   I.L. number 193 excludes benign and unspecified tu-mours of the central nervous system.

(II)   Carcinoma in situ excluded.

TABLE 4 B
UGANDA, KYADONDO :
MALE INCIDENCE RATES, 1954 - 60.

AVERAGE ANNUAL INCIDENCE PER 100,000 — AGE IN YEARS

INTERNATIONAL LIST No.	No. of cases — Age Unknown	No. of cases — All Ages	All Ages (rate)	85– and over	80–	75–	70–	65–	60–	55–	50–	45–	40–	35–	30–	25–	20–	15–	10–	5–	0–
140	0	0	0.0	0.0	0.0	0.0	0.0	0.0	0.0	0.0	0.0	0.0	0.0	0.0	0.0	0.0	0.0	0.0	0.0	0.0	0.0
141	0	0	0.0	0.0	0.0	0.0	0.0	0.0	0.0	0.0	0.0	0.0	0.0	0.0	0.0	0.0	0.0	0.0	0.0	0.0	0.0
142	0	2	0.2	0.0	0.0	0.0	0.0	0.0	0.0	0.0	0.0	0.0	0.0	1.7	1.2	0.0	0.0	0.0	0.0	0.0	0.0
143-4	0	0	0.0	0.0	0.0	0.0	0.0	0.0	0.0	0.0	0.0	0.0	0.0	0.0	0.0	0.0	0.0	0.0	0.0	0.0	0.0
146	0	0	0.0	0.0	0.0	0.0	0.0	0.0	0.0	0.0	0.0	0.0	0.0	0.0	0.0	0.0	0.0	0.0	0.0	0.0	0.0
145,147-8	0	2	0.2	0.0	0.0	0.0	0.0	0.0	8.1	0.0	0.0	6.6	0.0	1.7	0.0	0.0	0.0	0.0	0.0	0.0	0.0
150	0	8	1.0	0.0	0.0	0.0	0.0	0.0	8.1	13.9	8.8	6.6	0.0	0.0	1.2	0.0	0.0	0.0	0.0	0.0	0.0
151	0	13	1.6	0.0	0.0	0.0	0.0	0.0	16.1	6.9	4.4	9.9	0.0	5.1	3.5	0.0	0.0	0.0	0.0	0.0	0.0
152	0	2	0.2	0.0	0.0	0.0	0.0	0.0	0.0	0.0	0.0	0.0	0.0	0.0	0.0	0.0	0.0	0.0	3.9	0.0	0.0
153	0	1	0.1	0.0	0.0	0.0	16.8	0.0	0.0	0.0	0.0	0.0	0.0	0.0	0.0	0.0	0.0	0.0	0.0	0.0	0.0
154	0	4	0.5	0.0	0.0	0.0	0.0	0.0	8.1	13.9	0.0	3.3	0.0	0.0	0.0	0.0	0.0	0.0	0.0	0.0	0.0
155.0	0	45	5.5	0.0	0.0	28.6	16.8	0.0	8.1	13.9	13.3	23.0	7.1	15.3	15.2	3.6	1.9	1.2	0.0	0.0	0.0
155.1	0	1	0.1	0.0	0.0	0.0	0.0	13.9	0.0	0.0	0.0	0.0	0.0	0.0	0.0	0.0	0.0	0.0	0.0	0.0	0.0
156	0	8	1.0	0.0	0.0	0.0	0.0	0.0	0.0	13.9	0.0	3.3	2.4	1.7	1.2	0.0	0.0	2.4	0.0	0.0	0.0
157	0	7	0.8	0.0	0.0	0.0	0.0	0.0	8.1	13.9	0.0	3.3	2.4	1.7	2.3	0.0	0.0	0.0	0.0	0.0	0.0
160	0	4	0.5	0.0	0.0	0.0	16.8	0.0	0.0	0.0	4.4	0.0	0.0	0.0	0.0	0.0	0.0	0.0	0.0	0.0	0.0
161	0	3	0.4	0.0	0.0	0.0	0.0	13.9	8.1	0.0	0.0	3.3	0.0	0.0	0.0	0.9	0.0	0.0	0.0	0.0	0.0
162-3	0	7	0.8	0.0	0.0	0.0	0.0	0.0	8.1	0.0	4.4	0.0	4.7	1.7	0.0	0.0	0.9	1.2	0.0	1.0	1.0
170	0	1	0.1	0.0	0.0	0.0	0.0	0.0	8.1	0.0	0.0	0.0	0.0	0.0	0.0	0.0	0.0	0.0	0.0	0.0	0.0
177	0	16	1.9	84.0	81.6	0.0	16.8	13.9	32.3	6.9	13.3	9.9	0.0	0.0	0.0	0.0	0.0	0.0	0.0	0.0	0.0
178	0	1	0.1	0.0	0.0	0.0	0.0	0.0	0.0	0.0	0.0	0.0	0.0	0.0	0.0	0.0	0.0	0.0	0.0	0.0	1.0
179	0	31	3.8	168.1	0.0	28.6	16.8	13.9	32.3	13.9	17.7	19.7	0.0	11.9	1.2	0.9	0.9	1.2	0.0	0.0	0.0
180	0	1	0.1	0.0	0.0	0.0	0.0	0.0	0.0	0.0	0.0	0.0	0.0	0.0	0.0	0.0	0.0	0.0	0.0	0.0	0.0
181.0	0	26	3.2	0.0	0.0	57.1	16.8	55.5	64.6	13.9	4.4	9.9	2.4	5.1	1.2	0.0	0.0	1.2	0.0	1.2	0.0
190	0	6	0.7	0.0	0.0	28.6	16.8	0.0	8.1	6.9	0.0	0.0	0.0	1.7	0.0	0.0	0.0	0.0	0.0	0.0	0.0
191	0	40	4.9	0.0	0.0	28.6	33.6	13.9	16.1	20.8	17.7	13.1	4.7	13.6	4.7	4.5	2.8	1.2	0.0	0.0	0.0
192	0	8	1.0	0.0	0.0	0.0	0.0	0.0	0.0	0.0	4.4	3.3	0.0	1.7	1.2	0.0	0.0	2.4	0.0	1.2	0.0
193	0	2	0.2	0.0	0.0	0.0	0.0	0.0	0.0	0.0	0.0	0.0	0.0	0.0	0.0	0.0	0.0	0.0	0.0	1.2	0.0
194	0	1	0.1	0.0	0.0	0.0	0.0	0.0	0.0	0.0	0.0	0.0	0.0	0.0	0.0	0.0	0.0	0.0	0.0	0.0	0.0
195	0	3	0.4	0.0	0.0	0.0	0.0	0.0	0.0	0.0	0.0	3.3	0.0	0.0	0.0	0.9	0.0	1.2	0.0	1.2	1.0
196	0	4	0.5	0.0	0.0	0.0	0.0	13.9	8.1	6.9	4.4	3.3	0.0	0.0	2.3	0.9	0.0	2.4	1.9	0.0	1.0
197	0	9	1.1	0.0	0.0	0.0	0.0	13.9	8.1	0.0	4.4	3.3	7.1	1.7	3.5	0.9	0.0	0.0	0.0	1.2	1.0
200	1	24	2.9	0.0	0.0	0.0	0.0	0.0	0.0	0.0	4.4	9.9	0.0	0.0	4.7	1.8	3.8	2.4	3.9	6.2	1.0
201	0	13	1.6	0.0	0.0	0.0	0.0	13.9	8.1	0.0	0.0	3.3	0.0	1.7	0.0	0.0	0.9	1.2	0.0	0.0	0.0
203	0	2	0.2	0.0	0.0	0.0	0.0	13.9	0.0	0.0	0.0	0.0	0.0	1.7	0.0	0.0	0.0	0.0	0.0	0.0	0.0
204	0	19	2.3	0.0	0.0	0.0	0.0	0.0	0.0	6.9	4.4	6.6	2.4	1.7	1.2	0.9	2.8	4.7	0.0	1.2	2.9
OTHER	0	11	1.3	0.0	40.8	0.0	0.0	13.9	0.0	13.9	8.8	3.3	0.0	1.7	2.3	0.9	0.0	0.0	0.0	0.0	0.0
140-205	1	325	39.4	252.1	122.4	171.4	151.3	180.3	234.1	152.6	115.0	137.9	33.0	71.2	46.8	16.9	13.3	20.2	9.7	13.6	8.8
RATE PER CASE IN PERIOD	–	–	0.12	84.03	40.82	28.57	16.81	13.87	8.07	6.93	4.42	3.28	2.36	1.69	1.17	0.89	0.95	1.19	1.93	1.24	0.97

TABLE 4 C
UGANDA, KYADONDO :
FEMALE INCIDENCE RATES, 1954 - 60.

AVERAGE ANNUAL INCIDENCE PER 100,000 — AGE IN YEARS

INTERNATIONAL LIST No.	0-	5-	10-	15-	20-	25-	30-	35-	40-	45-	50-	55-	60-	65-	70-	75-	80-	85- AND OVER	ALL AGES	AGE UNKNOWN	ALL AGES (cases)	INTERNATIONAL LIST No.
140	0.0	0.0	0.0	0.0	0.0	0.0	0.0	0.0	0.0	0.0	0.0	0.0	0.0	0.0	0.0	0.0	0.0	0.0	0.0	0	0	140
141	0.0	0.0	0.0	0.0	0.0	0.0	0.0	0.0	0.0	0.0	0.0	10.2	0.0	0.0	0.0	0.0	0.0	0.0	0.2	0	1	141
142	0.0	0.0	0.0	0.0	1.3	0.0	2.1	3.1	8.0	0.0	0.0	0.0	0.0	0.0	0.0	0.0	0.0	0.0	0.8	0	5	142
143	0.0	0.0	0.0	0.0	0.0	0.0	0.0	0.0	4.0	5.4	0.0	0.0	0.0	0.0	0.0	0.0	0.0	0.0	0.3	0	2	143-4
146	0.0	0.0	0.0	0.0	0.0	0.0	0.0	0.0	0.0	0.0	0.0	0.0	0.0	0.0	0.0	0.0	0.0	0.0	0.0	0	0	146
145,147-8	0.0	0.0	0.0	0.0	0.0	0.0	0.0	0.0	0.0	0.0	0.0	0.0	0.0	0.0	23.8	0.0	0.0	0.0	0.2	0	1	145,147-8
150	0.0	0.0	0.0	0.0	0.0	0.0	0.0	3.1	0.0	5.4	7.4	0.0	9.7	0.0	0.0	0.0	0.0	0.0	0.5	0	3	150
151	0.0	0.0	0.0	0.0	0.0	0.0	0.0	0.0	0.0	0.0	14.9	0.0	0.0	0.0	0.0	0.0	0.0	0.0	0.5	0	3	151
152	0.0	0.0	0.0	0.0	0.0	0.0	0.0	0.0	0.0	0.0	0.0	0.0	0.0	0.0	0.0	0.0	0.0	0.0	0.0	0	0	152
153	0.0	0.0	0.0	0.0	0.0	0.0	4.2	0.0	0.0	0.0	7.4	0.0	0.0	0.0	0.0	0.0	0.0	0.0	0.5	0	3	153
154	0.0	0.0	2.4	0.0	0.0	2.8	4.2	0.0	0.0	5.4	7.4	20.4	0.0	17.9	0.0	0.0	0.0	0.0	1.5	0	9	154
155.0	0.0	0.0	0.0	0.0	0.0	2.8	2.1	6.2	4.0	5.4	7.4	0.0	9.7	0.0	0.0	0.0	0.0	0.0	1.7	0	10	155.0
155.1	0.0	0.0	0.0	0.0	0.0	0.0	0.0	0.0	0.0	0.0	0.0	0.0	0.0	0.0	0.0	0.0	0.0	0.0	0.0	0	0	155.1
156	0.0	0.0	0.0	0.0	0.0	0.0	4.2	0.0	0.0	0.0	7.4	10.2	0.0	17.9	0.0	0.0	0.0	0.0	0.8	0	5	156
157	0.0	0.0	0.0	0.0	0.0	0.0	2.1	3.1	2.2	5.4	7.4	0.0	0.0	0.0	0.0	0.0	0.0	0.0	0.7	0	4	157
160	0.0	0.0	0.0	0.0	0.0	0.0	0.0	0.0	0.0	5.4	0.0	0.0	0.0	0.0	0.0	0.0	0.0	0.0	0.7	0	4	160
161	0.0	0.0	0.0	0.0	0.0	0.0	0.0	0.0	12.0	0.0	0.0	0.0	0.0	0.0	0.0	0.0	0.0	0.0	0.0	0	0	161
162-3	0.0	0.0	0.0	0.0	0.0	4.2	10.6	9.3	16.0	21.6	22.3	61.2	9.7	0.0	23.8	0.0	0.0	0.0	5.3	1	0	162-3
170	0.0	0.0	0.0	0.0	3.8	9.7	8.5	37.0	35.9	70.3	67.0	71.4	67.6	17.9	71.4	0.0	59.5	0.0	12.6	1	76	170
171	0.0	0.0	0.0	0.0	1.3	2.8	0.0	3.1	0.0	5.4	7.4	10.2	0.0	53.6	71.4	0.0	0.0	0.0	1.7	0	10	171
172	0.0	0.0	0.0	0.0	2.5	1.4	0.0	0.0	0.0	5.4	14.9	0.0	0.0	0.0	0.0	0.0	0.0	0.0	0.7	0	4	172
173-4	0.0	0.0	0.0	0.0	0.0	1.4	0.0	15.4	27.9	21.6	7.4	40.8	19.3	17.9	0.0	0.0	0.0	0.0	4.3	0	26	173-4
175	0.0	0.0	0.0	0.0	0.0	2.8	0.0	6.2	0.0	5.4	7.4	20.4	0.0	0.0	0.0	0.0	0.0	0.0	1.3	0	8	175
176	0.0	0.0	0.0	0.0	0.0	0.0	0.0	0.0	0.0	0.0	0.0	0.0	0.0	0.0	0.0	0.0	0.0	0.0	0.2	0	1	176
180	1.0	0.0	0.0	0.0	0.0	0.0	0.0	3.1	4.0	5.4	7.4	0.0	9.7	0.0	0.0	0.0	0.0	0.0	0.8	0	5	180
181.0	0.0	0.0	0.0	0.0	0.0	0.0	0.0	0.0	0.0	0.0	0.0	0.0	0.0	0.0	0.0	0.0	0.0	0.0	0.0	0	0	181.0
190	0.0	0.0	0.0	0.0	0.0	4.2	2.1	0.0	8.0	10.8	14.9	0.0	9.7	17.9	0.0	0.0	59.5	0.0	2.0	0	12	190
191	0.0	0.0	0.0	0.0	0.0	1.4	0.0	6.2	4.0	5.4	0.0	0.0	0.0	0.0	0.0	0.0	0.0	0.0	1.0	0	6	191
192	0.0	0.0	0.0	0.0	0.0	0.0	0.0	0.0	4.0	0.0	0.0	0.0	0.0	0.0	0.0	0.0	0.0	0.0	0.2	0	1	192
193	0.0	0.0	0.0	0.0	1.3	1.4	0.0	6.2	0.0	10.8	7.4	20.4	0.0	0.0	0.0	0.0	0.0	0.0	1.7	0	10	193
194	0.0	0.0	0.0	1.6	1.3	1.4	0.0	3.1	0.0	10.8	0.0	0.0	0.0	0.0	0.0	0.0	0.0	0.0	0.8	0	5	194
195	1.3	1.3	0.0	1.6	1.3	0.0	0.0	0.0	8.0	0.0	0.0	0.0	9.7	0.0	0.0	0.0	0.0	0.0	0.3	0	2	195
196	1.3	1.3	0.0	0.0	0.0	1.4	2.1	3.1	0.0	0.0	7.4	0.0	0.0	0.0	0.0	0.0	0.0	0.0	1.3	0	8	196
197	1.0	6.5	0.0	1.6	0.0	0.0	2.1	3.1	0.0	0.0	0.0	0.0	9.7	17.9	23.8	0.0	0.0	0.0	2.0	0	12	197
200	2.0	0.0	0.0	0.0	0.0	1.4	2.1	0.0	0.0	5.4	0.0	0.0	0.0	0.0	0.0	0.0	0.0	0.0	0.7	0	4	200
201	0.0	0.0	0.0	0.0	0.0	0.0	0.0	0.0	0.0	0.0	0.0	0.0	0.0	0.0	0.0	0.0	0.0	0.0	0.0	0	0	201
203	1.0	1.3	2.4	0.0	1.3	1.4	0.0	6.2	0.0	5.4	7.4	0.0	0.0	0.0	71.4	0.0	0.0	0.0	2.0	0	12	203
204	0.0	0.0	0.0	0.0	1.3	0.0	0.0	0.0	4.0	0.0	7.4	10.2	9.7	0.0	23.8	0.0	0.0	0.0	1.0	0	6	204
OTHER	0.0	0.0	0.0	0.0	1.3	0.0	0.0	0.0	4.0	0.0	7.4	10.2	9.7	0.0	23.8	0.0	0.0	0.0	1.0	0	6	OTHER
140-205	5.1	10.4	4.8	6.3	15.1	37.4	44.4	117.2	139.7	216.5	230.7	275.5	164.1	160.7	236.1	0.0	119.0	0.0	48.1	2	290	140-205
RATE PER CASE IN PERIOD	1.01	1.31	2.40	1.58	1.26	1.39	2.12	3.09	3.99	5.41	7.44	10.20	9.65	17.86	23.81	42.02	59.52	129.87	0.17	-	-	RATE PER CASE IN PERIOD

CANADA (5 PROVINCES)

Cancer registration in Canada is the responsibility of the provinces and there is no single national register. The National Cancer Institute, which is solely an administrative office, has, however, undertaken the co-ordination of the incidence material reported for this publication. Information about the various registries is given separately before the data for each province.

A. J. Phillips.

TABLE 5 A
CANADA (FIVE PROVINCES) :
POPULATION (100, 000s), 1961

AGE (In years)	MALES		FEMALES	
	No.	Per Cent	No.	Per Cent
0 –	2.8040	12.89	2.6710	12.97
5 –	2.5960	11.94	2.4800	12.04
10 –	2.2850	10.51	2.1940	10.65
15 –	1.7340	7.97	1.6660	8.09
20 –	1.3720	6.31	1.3560	6.58
25 –	1.3880	6.38	1.2990	6.31
30 –	1.4110	6.49	1.3340	6.48
35 –	1.3770	6.33	1.3660	6.63
40 –	1.2880	5.92	1.2490	6.06
45 –	1.1800	5.43	1.1160	5.42
50 –	1.0150	4.67	0.9140	4.44
55 –	0.8430	3.88	0.7400	3.59
60 –	0.6860	3.15	0.6240	3.03
65 –	0.5960	2.74	0.5440	2.64
70 –	0.5240	2.41	0.4580	2.22
75 –	0.3700	1.70	0.3190	1.55
80 –	0.1860	0.86	0.1710	0.83
85 – and over	0.0940	0.43	0.0970	0.47
TOTAL	21.7490	100.00	20.5980	100.00

NOTES

TO TABLES 5 A, B and C

(I)   Data for 5 provinces only.

(II)   Period registration 1960-62 inclusive for Alberta, Manitoba, Newfoundland and Saskatchewan and 1962-64 for New Brunswick.

(III)   I.L. number 156 based on data for 4 provinces only (excluding Manitoba).
       " "   174 " " " " " "   "
       " "   193 excludes benign and unspecified tumours of the central nervous system.

(IV)   Carcinoma in situ included.

TABLE 5 B
CANADA (FIVE PROVINCES) :
MALE INCIDENCE RATES, 1960 - 62.

INTER-NATIONAL LIST No.	No. of Cases — ALL AGES	No. of Cases — AGE UNKNOWN	ALL AGES	85- AND OVER	80-	75-	70-	65-	60-	55-	50-	45-	40-	35-	30-	25-	20-	15-	10-	5-	0-	INTER-NATIONAL LIST No.
140	1162	12	17.8	131.2	145.2	106.3	103.7	89.5	59.8	47.8	40.7	26.3	15.8	9.4	4.7	1.9	0.5	0.0	0.0	0.0	0.0	140
141	55	0	0.8	10.6	9.0	2.7	5.7	4.5	5.3	1.6	1.6	0.3	1.3	0.0	0.2	0.0	0.0	0.0	0.0	0.0	0.0	141
142	95	1	1.9	10.6	10.8	6.3	2.5	6.2	4.9	2.4	1.3	2.8	2.1	1.2	1.9	0.7	1.5	0.6	0.0	0.0	0.0	142
143-4	121	0	1.9	46.1	26.9	12.6	13.4	6.7	5.3	5.9	2.6	1.7	0.5	0.5	0.2	0.0	0.0	0.0	0.1	0.0	0.0	143-4
146	32	0	0.5	0.0	0.0	2.7	0.0	2.2	2.9	2.4	1.0	1.1	0.8	0.2	0.0	0.0	0.2	0.2	0.0	0.0	0.0	146
145,147-8	47	1	0.7	0.0	7.2	7.2	3.8	5.0	3.9	0.8	1.0	0.8	0.5	0.0	0.2	0.0	0.0	0.0	0.0	0.0	0.0	145,147-8
150	163	5	2.5	31.9	28.7	33.3	15.3	11.7	11.2	4.3	3.9	1.4	1.3	0.0	2.8	1.0	0.2	0.2	0.0	0.0	0.0	150
151	1502	0	23.0	223.4	258.1	216.2	179.4	119.1	87.5	59.7	31.9	18.9	7.5	3.1	2.8	1.0	0.2	0.2	0.0	0.0	0.0	151
152	45	0	0.7	3.5	7.2	9.0	5.1	2.2	3.4	0.4	0.7	1.4	0.3	0.2	0.0	0.0	0.0	0.0	0.0	0.0	0.0	152
153	1165	9	17.9	191.5	195.3	166.7	136.8	87.8	69.0	36.8	23.0	15.5	9.1	4.1	3.8	1.4	0.5	0.0	0.0	0.0	0.0	153
154	734	1	11.2	117.0	114.7	112.6	81.4	62.6	34.0	27.7	19.0	11.9	4.1	1.9	0.9	0.7	0.0	0.0	0.0	0.0	0.0	154
155.0	67	0	1.0	10.6	7.2	8.1	5.7	4.5	5.8	2.8	2.0	1.1	0.3	0.0	0.2	0.0	0.0	0.0	0.1	0.0	0.2	155.0
155.1	112	0	1.7	21.3	12.5	18.9	13.4	10.6	3.4	4.3	4.3	1.1	0.5	0.0	0.0	0.2	0.0	0.0	0.0	0.0	0.0	155.1
156	51	0	0.8	0.0	5.4	5.4	7.0	3.9	3.4	0.8	1.3	1.1	1.0	0.0	0.0	0.2	0.0	0.0	0.0	0.1	0.2	156
157	482	3	7.4	74.5	73.5	64.0	59.2	41.5	29.6	21.0	10.5	5.1	1.8	1.0	0.2	0.2	0.0	0.4	0.1	0.0	0.0	157
160	44	0	0.7	3.5	3.6	2.7	3.8	5.0	3.9	2.8	0.3	0.8	0.5	0.5	0.0	0.0	0.0	0.0	0.0	0.0	0.0	160
161	145	0	2.2	7.1	10.8	18.9	12.7	14.5	9.2	6.7	4.9	3.4	1.0	0.0	0.5	0.0	0.0	0.2	0.0	0.0	0.0	161
162-3	1686	1	25.8	117.0	125.4	140.5	183.2	181.8	132.7	85.0	48.9	25.7	11.9	5.6	2.6	0.5	0.7	0.0	0.0	0.0	0.0	162-3
170	24	0	0.4	0.0	3.6	3.6	3.2	3.9	0.5	0.8	0.7	0.3	0.0	0.0	0.0	0.0	0.0	0.0	0.0	0.0	0.1	170
177	2019	1	30.9	673.8	569.9	434.2	309.8	160.5	77.3	22.1	8.9	2.8	0.0	0.0	0.0	0.2	0.0	0.0	0.0	0.0	0.6	177
178	153	1	2.3	0.0	1.8	1.8	1.9	2.2	1.9	2.4	2.0	3.7	3.9	7.5	5.9	6.0	1.5	1.0	0.1	0.0	0.0	178
179.0	59	1	0.9	14.2	12.5	9.0	3.8	4.5	1.5	1.6	0.7	2.5	0.8	0.0	0.0	0.5	0.0	0.0	0.0	0.0	0.0	179.0
180	378	3	5.8	39.0	30.5	42.3	28.0	21.3	19.0	18.6	14.4	9.6	4.7	1.2	1.9	0.2	0.0	0.4	0.1	0.4	1.9	180
181.0	837	6	12.8	180.9	147.0	123.4	89.7	76.1	52.5	26.1	15.8	6.8	3.4	4.4	1.4	0.2	0.0	0.0	0.0	0.0	0.0	181.0
190	130	1	2.0	10.6	10.8	13.5	8.9	10.6	6.8	3.2	2.6	4.0	2.3	1.2	1.4	0.7	0.5	0.6	0.3	0.9	0.0	190
191	3723	32	56.8	734.0	630.8	499.1	383.0	274.0	183.2	137.6	87.4	53.7	36.5	18.2	9.4	5.3	0.5	0.6	0.3	0.1	1.1	191
192	84	0	1.3	7.1	10.8	4.5	5.1	2.2	1.0	1.2	1.3	9.0	0.8	0.7	0.2	0.0	0.2	0.0	0.3	0.1	1.1	192
193	338	0	5.2	7.1	0.0	3.6	10.2	11.2	17.0	12.7	10.2	10.5	7.2	5.1	4.3	2.6	1.9	2.3	1.3	2.7	3.9	193
194	56	2	0.9	3.5	5.4	1.8	5.1	3.9	4.9	2.0	0.7	1.1	0.8	1.2	0.2	0.5	0.0	0.2	0.4	0.0	0.0	194
195	21	1	0.3	0.0	0.0	0.9	1.9	0.0	1.0	0.4	0.0	0.6	0.8	0.2	0.0	0.0	0.2	0.6	0.0	0.1	0.2	195
196	75	0	1.1	3.5	3.6	2.7	4.5	2.2	2.9	1.6	2.0	0.3	0.5	0.5	0.7	1.4	1.0	1.5	1.3	0.8	0.1	196
197	149	1	2.3	3.5	16.1	8.1	8.9	8.9	5.8	4.7	2.3	3.4	1.6	2.9	0.5	1.4	1.5	1.3	0.3	0.9	1.0	197
200	278	1	4.3	17.7	26.9	23.4	23.5	14.0	15.5	7.9	8.2	3.1	3.6	1.7	1.9	2.9	1.7	1.7	1.6	0.9	1.0	200
201	176	0	2.7	7.1	9.0	7.2	5.7	5.2	5.8	5.9	3.3	4.8	2.3	2.4	4.3	3.1	4.9	0.0	0.4	0.5	0.4	201
203	142	0	2.2	17.7	16.1	14.4	12.7	11.2	13.6	7.5	3.9	0.8	1.0	1.5	0.0	0.0	0.0	0.0	0.0	0.0	0.0	203
204	485	1	7.4	42.6	52.0	53.2	40.7	29.6	20.4	16.2	10.5	3.7	3.6	3.6	3.3	0.7	1.5	2.1	1.8	3.3	4.5	204
202,205	52	0	0.8	3.5	12.5	6.3	2.5	2.2	2.4	1.6	1.0	0.8	1.3	0.5	0.7	0.0	0.0	0.2	0.3	0.0	0.1	202,205
OTHER	300	1	4.6	60.3	41.2	29.7	30.5	21.8	15.1	9.9	10.2	4.2	3.1	1.2	0.9	0.2	0.2	0.6	0.0	0.4	1.0	OTHER
140-205	17167	85	263.1	2826.2	2641.6	2217.1	1811.7	1325.5	923.2	597.1	384.9	246.3	138.5	81.8	55.8	33.1	19.2	15.6	7.9	10.3	16.3	140-205
RATE PER CASE IN PERIOD	-	-	0.02	3.55	1.79	0.90	0.64	0.56	0.49	0.40	0.33	0.28	0.26	0.24	0.24	0.24	0.24	0.19	0.15	0.13	0.12	RATE PER CASE IN PERIOD

TABLE 5 C
CANADA (FIVE PROVINCES) :
FEMALE INCIDENCE RATES, 1960 - 62.

Columns 0- through 85- AND OVER and the first ALL AGES column give AVERAGE ANNUAL INCIDENCE PER 100,000 (AGE IN YEARS). The AGE UNKNOWN and final ALL AGES columns give NO. OF CASES IN WHOLE PERIOD.

INTERNATIONAL LIST No.	0-	5-	10-	15-	20-	25-	30-	35-	40-	45-	50-	55-	60-	65-	70-	75-	80-	85- AND OVER	ALL AGES (rate)	AGE UNKNOWN	ALL AGES (cases)	INTERNATIONAL LIST No.
140	0.0	0.0	0.0	0.0	0.2	0.5	0.0	0.2	0.0	1.2	1.5	3.2	3.2	4.9	8.7	7.3	5.8	17.2	1.0	0	60	140
141	0.0	0.0	0.0	0.0	0.0	0.5	0.0	0.0	0.3	0.6	2.2	1.4	1.2	1.2	4.4	3.1	11.7	3.4	0.6	0	37	141
142	0.0	0.0	0.6	0.0	0.5	1.5	2.0	2.2	2.7	2.1	2.9	2.7	6.4	4.3	4.4	5.2	1.9	10.3	1.5	0	94	142
143-4	0.0	0.0	0.0	0.0	0.0	0.0	0.5	0.2	0.0	1.2	0.7	0.9	2.1	1.2	7.3	10.4	7.8	10.3	0.7	0	44	143-4
146	0.1	0.1	0.0	0.0	0.0	0.0	0.0	0.2	0.5	0.6	0.4	0.9	0.5	1.2	3.6	1.0	0.0	0.0	0.3	0	18	146
145,147-8	0.0	0.0	0.0	0.2	0.5	0.0	0.0	0.0	0.3	1.2	0.4	1.4	1.6	3.1	3.6	1.0	3.9	3.4	0.4	0	27	145,147-8
150	0.0	0.0	0.0	0.0	0.5	0.8	0.5	0.0	0.3	1.5	1.8	5.3	5.3	5.5	11.6	10.4	13.6	6.9	1.1	0	70	150
151	0.0	0.1	0.0	0.0	0.5	0.3	1.5	3.4	5.1	6.9	10.2	31.1	40.1	65.6	69.9	104.5	132.6	123.7	10.5	5	651	151
152	0.0	0.0	0.0	0.2	0.0	0.3	0.2	0.2	0.8	0.3	1.8	2.3	2.7	6.1	2.9	2.1	1.9	6.9	0.7	0	42	152
153	0.0	0.0	0.2	0.0	1.2	1.0	4.7	5.4	9.3	25.1	35.0	47.3	75.9	104.2	135.4	164.1	171.5	209.6	19.2	8	1184	153
154	0.0	0.0	0.0	0.0	0.2	0.5	1.2	2.7	5.1	10.2	13.9	23.4	32.1	39.8	56.8	62.7	74.1	61.9	7.8	3	484	154
155.0	0.0	0.1	0.0	0.0	0.0	0.0	0.2	0.2	1.3	0.3	0.4	0.9	0.5	3.1	2.9	8.4	9.7	6.9	0.6	0	37	155.0
155.1	0.0	0.0	0.0	0.0	0.0	0.0	0.2	0.2	0.3	1.2	5.5	7.2	11.2	23.9	30.6	40.8	48.7	34.4	3.5	0	214	155.1
156	0.0	0.0	0.0	0.0	0.0	0.0	0.0	0.5	0.3	0.9	0.7	0.9	2.1	6.7	4.4	6.3	3.9	10.3	0.7	0	43	156
157	0.0	0.0	0.0	0.0	0.0	0.3	0.7	0.0	1.9	3.0	5.8	16.7	17.6	22.7	42.2	44.9	68.2	72.2	4.9	0	301	157
160	0.0	0.0	0.2	0.0	0.0	0.3	0.2	0.2	0.5	1.2	1.5	0.9	1.6	1.8	0.0	6.3	3.9	10.3	0.5	0	33	160
161	0.0	0.0	0.0	0.0	0.0	0.3	0.0	0.0	0.0	1.2	0.4	0.0	1.1	0.0	3.6	3.1	5.8	6.9	0.3	0	20	161
162-3	0.0	0.0	0.0	0.2	0.0	0.0	1.5	0.7	2.4	5.4	11.3	18.9	18.2	19.6	26.9	31.3	19.5	24.1	4.2	0	261	162-3
170	0.0	0.0	0.0	0.0	1.7	6.2	19.7	47.6	108.6	142.5	146.6	144.6	160.3	173.4	188.5	241.4	237.8	233.7	51.5	5	3181	170
171	0.0	0.0	0.0	0.0	3.4	16.4	37.7	67.6	61.4	66.3	59.8	48.2	43.8	43.5	42.9	35.5	42.9	24.1	24.4	5	1509	171
172	0.0	0.0	0.2	0.0	0.0	0.0	3.2	8.3	12.8	28.1	37.2	50.9	59.3	57.6	41.5	29.3	35.1	24.1	11.7	0	720	172
173	0.0	0.0	0.0	0.0	0.7	0.3	0.7	0.2	0.0	1.2	0.7	0.9	2.7	3.7	1.5	0.0	0.0	0.5	0.5	2	32	173
174	0.0	0.0	0.0	0.0	0.0	0.0	0.0	0.2	0.0	0.0	1.5	1.4	1.1	1.8	3.6	3.1	1.9	0.0	0.4	1	23	174
175	0.1	0.0	0.3	1.8	2.5	1.8	3.5	8.8	11.5	22.7	33.9	34.2	42.7	40.4	33.5	51.2	52.6	20.6	10.4	2	642	175
176	0.1	0.0	0.0	0.0	0.0	0.3	0.5	2.0	1.3	1.5	4.4	6.3	7.5	9.8	13.1	17.8	29.3	24.1	2.2	0	135	176
180	1.2	0.8	0.2	1.4	0.0	0.3	1.0	0.5	2.4	4.8	8.4	9.9	12.8	16.5	11.6	18.8	17.5	17.2	3.2	0	195	180
181.0	0.0	0.0	0.0	0.0	0.0	0.0	0.0	0.0	0.8	2.4	4.4	6.3	5.9	15.3	11.6	18.8	48.7	41.2	3.1	0	190	181.0
190	0.1	0.1	0.2	0.6	0.7	2.3	3.5	2.9	3.5	2.4	2.6	5.9	5.3	4.9	7.3	9.4	9.7	10.3	2.1	2	131	190
191	1.1	0.1	0.2	0.2	2.5	4.6	10.5	13.9	28.8	42.1	64.2	73.4	110.0	172.8	220.5	336.5	430.8	474.2	35.9	26	2217	191
192	2.5	2.8	1.5	1.4	0.7	0.5	0.0	0.2	0.3	0.9	0.7	2.7	2.1	0.6	2.9	1.0	5.8	0.0	0.6	0	39	192
193	0.0	0.1	0.9	1.2	1.5	2.1	2.5	3.9	5.9	7.5	9.8	9.0	10.7	8.0	6.6	5.2	5.8	0.0	3.9	0	242	193
194	0.5	0.1	0.2	0.4	1.2	2.6	2.0	3.7	3.7	4.8	3.3	6.3	2.1	6.7	7.3	10.4	3.9	6.9	2.4	3	150	194
195	0.2	0.8	1.7	2.6	0.0	0.0	0.0	0.0	0.5	0.3	1.1	1.8	0.0	0.0	0.0	0.0	0.0	0.0	0.3	0	18	195
196	0.5	0.3	0.8	0.8	1.0	0.5	0.2	0.2	0.0	0.6	1.1	0.0	1.1	1.2	2.9	2.1	0.0	3.4	0.9	1	57	196
197	0.1	0.3	0.2	1.4	1.7	1.5	1.7	1.0	2.1	2.1	2.9	5.9	3.7	4.3	8.0	8.4	7.8	3.4	1.8	0	113	197
200	0.2	0.3	0.0	2.0	0.7	0.0	2.0	1.7	2.9	3.9	3.3	8.6	4.3	15.9	11.6	16.7	21.4	17.2	2.6	0	158	200
201	0.0	0.3	0.0	1.8	2.7	3.8	2.0	1.5	1.9	2.7	0.4	3.2	3.7	3.7	8.7	1.0	0.0	0.0	1.7	0	104	201
203	0.0	0.0	1.7	0.0	0.0	0.0	0.0	0.2	1.3	0.6	2.2	4.1	6.4	8.6	9.5	10.4	3.9	3.4	1.2	0	75	203
204	4.0	2.2	0.0	1.8	1.2	1.8	3.7	2.4	3.5	3.9	2.9	7.7	12.8	15.3	20.4	39.7	19.5	24.1	4.7	0	288	204
202,205	0.1	0.0	0.0	0.0	0.0	0.3	0.5	0.5	1.1	0.6	1.5	1.8	3.7	2.5	3.6	3.1	1.9	0.0	0.6	0	40	202,205
OTHER	0.2	0.0	0.2	0.0	0.0	1.5	1.5	1.5	3.7	6.3	6.6	9.0	15.0	23.9	24.0	53.3	42.9	58.4	4.6	2	286	OTHER
140-205	11.4	8.3	8.8	15.2	24.6	52.6	110.2	186.7	289.3	411.9	495.6	602.3	742.0	945.5	1117.2	1444.1	1604.3	1604.8	229.2	69	14165	140-205
RATE PER CASE IN PERIOD	0.12	0.13	0.15	0.20	0.25	0.26	0.25	0.24	0.27	0.30	0.36	0.45	0.53	0.61	0.73	1.04	1.95	3.44	0.2	-	-	RATE PER CASE IN PERIOD

CANADA, ALBERTA

There are three cancer clinics in the province of Alberta, the major one being in the capital city of Edmonton. A record of a case of cancer occurring anywhere in the province is submitted to the clinic in Edmonton where the data are transferred to punch cards. Since the payment of professional fees is based upon the submission of these reports, it is doubtful if many cases are missed.

Registry Title and Address : Alberta Provincial Cancer Registry, Edmonton Cancer Clinic, 11250 - 84th Avenue, Edmonton, Alberta, Canada. Supported financially by Provincial Government.

Registration. Registrations are made by doctors from hospital in-patients and out-patients, and from radiotherapy and pathology departments; from death certificates by Provincial Registrars; and also by doctors attending cases at home.

Follow-up. All registrations are followed up for life.

Physical Description. The Registry covers the province of Alberta, which is situated in western Canada between British Columbia on the west and Saskatchewan on the east. It lies between latitudes 49° and 60° north and longitudes 102° and 110° west. Total registration area is 661, 188 square kilometres.

Demographic Description. Total population of area under survey 1, 332, 000. Fifty per cent of the population live in conurbations of more than 100, 000.

Medical Services. Total number of hospital beds of all kinds 11,678. Total number of doctors in practice in registration area 1, 513. Cancer causes approximately 17 % of all deaths.

Publications. Registry Report included in Annual Report of Department of Health of Alberta.

TABLE 6 A
CANADA, ALBERTA :
POPULATION (100,000s), 1961

AGE (in years)	MALES		FEMALES	
	No.	Per Cent	No.	Per Cent
0-	0.9220	13.37	0.8770	13.65
5-	0.8160	11.84	0.7740	12.04
10-	0.6670	9.68	0.6370	9.91
15-	0.5030	7.30	0.4870	7.58
20-	0.4440	6.44	0.4480	6.97
25-	0.4970	7.21	0.4600	7.16
30-	0.5070	7.35	0.4610	7.17
35-	0.4630	6.72	0.4540	7.07
40-	0.4130	5.99	0.3970	6.18
45-	0.3640	5.28	0.3390	5.28
50-	0.3090	4.48	0.2740	4.26
55-	0.2690	3.90	0.2200	3.42
60-	0.2120	3.08	0.1760	2.74
65-	0.1720	2.49	0.1450	2.26
70-	0.1540	2.23	0.1240	1.93
75-	0.1060	1.54	0.0850	1.32
80-	0.0520	0.75	0.0440	0.68
85- and over	0.0240	0.35	0.0240	0.37
TOTAL	6.8940	100.00	6.4260	100.00

NOTES

TO TABLES 6 A, B and C

(I)   I.L. number 193 excludes benign and unspecified tumours of the central nervous system.

(II)   Carcinoma in situ included.

TABLE 6 B
CANADA, ALBERTA :
MALE INCIDENCE RATES, 1960 - 62.

INTER-NATIONAL LIST No.	0-	5-	10-	15-	20-	25-	30-	35-	40-	45-	50-	55-	60-	65-	70-	75-	80-	85- and over	ALL AGES	AGE UN-KNOWN	ALL AGES	INTER-NATIONAL LIST No.
						AVERAGE ANNUAL INCIDENCE PER 100,000 — AGE IN YEARS															No. OF CASES IN WHOLE PERIOD		
140	0.0	0.0	0.0	0.0	0.8	0.7	4.6	10.8	17.8	24.7	37.8	53.3	62.9	79.5	69.3	100.6	89.7	83.3	15.3	0	316	140
141	0.0	0.0	0.0	0.0	0.0	0.0	0.7	0.0	1.6	0.0	2.2	1.2	9.4	1.9	6.5	3.1	12.8	13.9	1.0	0	20	141
142	0.0	0.0	0.0	0.7	0.0	0.0	0.7	0.0	0.0	2.7	0.0	1.2	3.1	7.8	2.2	3.1	6.4	0.0	0.7	0	15	142
143-4	0.0	0.0	0.0	0.0	0.0	0.0	0.0	0.7	1.6	0.9	2.2	5.0	6.3	3.9	17.3	9.4	25.6	13.9	1.5	0	32	143-4
146	0.0	0.0	0.0	0.0	0.8	0.0	0.0	0.0	0.8	1.8	1.1	1.2	1.6	1.9	0.0	6.3	0.0	0.0	0.5	0	10	146
145,147-8	0.0	0.0	0.0	0.0	0.0	0.0	0.7	0.0	0.8	0.9	0.0	1.2	3.1	7.8	6.5	3.1	6.4	0.0	0.7	0	15	145,147-8
150	0.0	0.0	0.0	0.0	0.0	0.0	0.0	0.0	2.4	0.9	4.3	3.7	3.1	11.6	8.7	25.2	19.2	13.2	1.7	0	35	150
151	0.0	0.0	0.0	0.0	0.0	0.0	0.0	1.4	5.6	13.7	21.6	54.5	77.0	112.4	138.5	138.4	109.0	180.6	16.1	0	333	151
152	0.0	0.0	0.0	0.0	0.0	0.0	0.0	0.7	0.8	1.8	0.0	0.7	0.0	1.9	4.3	3.1	6.4	0.0	0.4	0	9	152
153	0.0	0.0	0.0	0.7	0.0	0.7	4.6	2.9	7.3	14.7	28.0	29.7	55.0	95.0	149.4	125.8	224.4	83.3	15.5	0	321	153
154	0.0	0.0	0.0	0.0	0.0	0.7	1.3	2.2	3.2	11.9	18.3	16.1	31.4	54.3	71.4	113.2	76.0	97.2	9.1	0	189	154
155.0	0.0	0.0	0.0	0.0	0.0	0.0	0.0	0.0	0.0	0.0	0.0	0.0	3.1	1.9	6.5	3.1	0.0	13.9	0.4	0	8	155.0
155.1	0.0	0.0	0.0	0.0	0.0	0.0	0.0	0.0	1.6	1.8	3.2	2.5	6.3	7.8	17.3	18.9	6.4	0.0	1.5	0	31	155.1
156	0.7	0.0	0.0	0.0	0.0	0.7	0.0	0.7	1.6	1.8	1.1	1.2	6.3	5.8	2.2	3.1	6.4	0.0	0.9	0	19	156
157	0.0	0.0	0.0	0.0	0.0	0.0	0.0	0.7	2.4	4.6	5.4	9.9	25.2	38.8	32.5	34.6	38.5	69.4	4.6	0	95	157
160	0.0	0.0	0.0	0.0	0.0	0.0	0.0	0.7	0.0	0.0	1.1	3.7	6.3	6.3	0.0	0.0	0.0	0.0	0.4	0	9	160
161	0.0	0.0	0.0	0.0	0.0	0.7	0.7	0.0	0.8	2.7	3.2	8.7	3.1	17.4	6.5	22.0	0.0	13.9	1.8	0	37	161
162-3	0.0	0.0	0.0	0.0	0.8	0.7	2.0	1.4	5.6	14.7	57.2	84.3	110.1	170.5	149.4	122.6	57.7	27.8	20.7	0	428	162-3
170	0.0	0.0	0.0	0.0	0.0	0.0	0.0	0.0	0.0	0.9	2.2	1.2	0.0	0.0	4.3	6.3	6.4	0.0	0.4	0	9	170
177	0.0	0.0	0.0	0.0	0.0	0.0	0.0	0.0	0.0	2.7	5.4	19.8	61.3	149.2	218.6	349.1	423.1	625.0	22.4	0	463	177
178	1.1	0.0	0.0	0.0	2.3	6.7	6.6	8.6	5.6	5.5	3.2	0.0	0.0	5.8	2.2	3.1	0.0	0.0	2.9	0	61	178
179.0	0.0	0.8	0.0	1.3	0.0	0.0	0.0	0.0	0.8	2.7	0.0	0.0	1.6	1.9	2.2	6.3	12.8	27.8	0.6	0	13	179.0
180	2.2	0.0	0.0	0.0	0.0	0.0	2.0	1.4	2.4	10.1	16.2	16.1	25.2	9.7	32.5	31.4	19.2	0.0	5.0	0	104	180
181.0	0.0	0.0	0.0	0.7	0.0	0.7	0.0	2.9	1.6	5.5	8.6	21.1	39.3	75.6	80.1	100.6	115.6	111.1	9.6	0	198	181.0
190	0.0	0.0	0.0	1.3	0.0	1.3	0.0	2.2	4.0	4.6	4.3	5.0	4.7	13.6	8.7	18.9	12.8	0.0	2.2	0	46	190
191	1.4	0.0	0.0	1.3	0.0	4.0	10.5	20.9	28.2	47.6	84.1	119.0	157.2	217.1	326.8	399.4	467.9	472.2	44.0	0	911	191
192	0.0	0.0	0.0	0.7	3.0	0.0	3.9	0.7	0.0	0.9	0.0	0.0	0.0	0.0	0.0	0.0	12.8	13.9	0.4	0	9	192
193	3.6	1.6	0.5	0.7	0.0	2.0	0.0	6.5	5.6	6.4	8.6	13.6	15.7	9.7	10.8	3.1	12.8	0.0	4.4	0	92	193
194	0.0	0.0	0.0	0.7	0.6	0.7	0.0	2.2	0.0	0.0	1.1	2.5	3.1	0.0	6.5	0.0	0.0	0.0	0.6	0	12	194
195	0.0	0.0	0.0	0.7	0.8	0.0	0.0	0.0	0.0	0.0	0.0	1.2	1.6	0.0	2.2	0.0	0.0	0.0	0.2	0	5	195
196	0.0	1.2	2.0	1.3	0.0	1.3	0.7	0.0	0.8	1.8	2.2	1.2	3.1	1.9	6.5	3.1	6.4	0.0	1.1	0	23	196
197	0.7	0.8	0.5	1.3	1.5	2.7	0.7	2.9	0.8	1.8	2.2	5.0	4.7	13.6	8.7	12.6	25.6	13.9	2.4	0	50	197
200	1.4	1.6	1.5	1.3	2.3	4.0	1.3	1.4	3.2	2.7	5.4	6.2	11.0	5.8	21.6	9.4	19.2	13.9	3.4	0	70	200
201	0.7	0.8	0.5	2.7	0.0	2.0	5.9	2.2	2.4	3.7	4.3	8.7	3.1	0.0	4.3	0.0	6.4	0.0	2.3	0	47	201
203	0.0	0.0	0.0	0.0	0.0	0.0	0.0	1.4	1.6	1.8	4.3	9.9	7.9	1.9	13.0	6.3	19.2	0.0	1.7	0	35	203
204	3.6	1.6	1.5	2.0	0.0	0.0	3.9	3.6	3.2	2.7	7.6	11.2	17.3	27.1	26.0	34.6	32.1	13.9	5.2	0	108	204
202,205	0.0	0.0	0.5	0.0	0.0	0.0	0.0	0.7	1.6	0.9	1.1	1.2	0.0	0.0	0.0	6.3	32.1	0.0	0.7	0	14	202,205
OTHER	0.4	0.0	0.0	0.7	0.8	0.0	2.0	1.4	2.4	2.7	7.6	11.2	9.4	15.5	19.5	22.0	12.8	27.8	3.1	0	64	OTHER
140-205	15.9	8.6	7.0	14.6	12.8	28.8	53.3	80.6	117.8	203.3	354.9	531.6	779.9	1168.6	1482.7	1748.4	1903.8	1930.6	205.8	0	4256	140-205
RATE PER CASE IN PERIOD	0.36	0.41	0.50	0.66	0.75	0.67	0.66	0.72	0.81	0.92	1.08	1.24	1.57	1.94	2.16	3.14	6.41	13.89	0.05	-	-	RATE PER CASE IN PERIOD

TABLE 6 C
CANADA, ALBERTA :
FEMALE INCIDENCE RATES, 1960 - 62.

AVERAGE ANNUAL INCIDENCE PER 100,000 — AGE IN YEARS

INTER-NATIONAL LIST No.	0–	5–	10–	15–	20–	25–	30–	35–	40–	45–	50–	55–	60–	65–	70–	75–	80–	85– AND OVER	ALL AGES	AGE UNKNOWN	NO. OF CASES ALL AGES	INTER-NATIONAL LIST No.
140	0.0	0.0	0.0	0.0	0.0	1.4	0.0	0.7	0.0	1.0	2.4	6.1	3.8	6.9	18.8	23.5	7.6	27.8	1.6	0	31	140
141	0.0	0.0	0.0	0.0	0.0	0.0	0.0	0.0	0.0	0.0	2.4	1.5	3.8	0.0	2.7	0.0	0.0	0.0	0.3	0	6	141
142	0.0	0.0	1.0	0.0	0.0	0.0	2.2	0.7	1.7	2.0	0.0	3.0	7.6	6.9	5.4	0.0	0.0	0.0	1.1	0	21	142
143–4	0.0	0.0	0.0	0.0	0.0	0.0	0.0	0.7	0.0	1.0	1.2	0.0	0.0	0.0	5.4	11.8	7.6	0.0	0.5	0	9	143–4
146	0.0	0.0	0.0	0.0	0.0	0.0	0.0	0.0	0.8	0.0	1.2	1.5	0.0	2.3	2.7	0.0	0.0	0.0	0.2	0	3	146
145,147–8	0.0	0.0	0.0	0.7	0.0	0.0	0.0	0.0	0.0	0.0	0.0	1.5	5.7	9.2	10.8	15.7	0.0	13.9	0.3	0	5	145,147–8
150	0.0	0.0	0.0	0.0	0.7	0.7	0.0	2.2	5.0	5.9	0.0	0.0	0.0	0.0	0.0	0.0	7.6	0.0	0.9	0	18	150
151	0.0	0.0	0.0	0.0	0.0	0.0	0.7	0.0	0.8	0.0	13.4	18.2	24.6	48.3	43.0	90.2	60.6	27.8	6.4	0	124	151
152	0.0	0.0	0.0	0.0	0.0	0.0	0.0	4.4	7.6	0.0	0.0	1.5	3.8	0.0	0.0	0.0	7.6	0.0	0.3	0	5	152
153	0.0	0.0	0.0	0.0	0.0	0.0	2.9	0.7	3.4	19.7	25.5	33.3	89.0	92.0	110.2	164.7	136.4	111.1	14.4	0	278	153
154	0.0	0.0	0.0	0.0	0.0	0.0	1.4	0.0	0.0	11.8	10.9	16.7	15.2	34.5	51.1	58.8	45.5	0.0	5.3	0	102	154
155.0	0.0	0.0	0.0	0.0	0.0	0.0	0.0	0.0	0.8	0.0	0.0	0.0	0.0	0.0	0.0	3.9	7.6	0.0	0.1	0	2	155.0
155.1	0.0	0.0	0.0	0.0	0.0	0.0	0.0	0.7	0.8	0.0	6.1	9.1	17.0	20.7	32.3	47.1	22.7	0.0	3.0	0	57	155.1
156	0.0	0.0	0.0	0.0	0.0	0.0	0.0	0.0	1.7	0.0	0.0	0.0	1.9	11.5	8.1	7.8	0.0	0.0	0.7	0	13	156
157	0.0	0.0	0.0	0.0	0.0	0.0	1.4	0.0	0.0	3.9	4.9	18.2	15.2	20.7	34.9	11.8	53.0	13.9	3.4	0	65	157
160	0.0	0.0	0.0	0.0	0.0	0.7	0.0	0.0	0.0	1.0	0.0	0.0	0.0	0.0	0.0	15.7	7.6	0.0	0.4	0	7	160
161	0.0	0.0	0.0	0.0	0.0	0.0	1.4	0.7	0.0	0.0	1.2	0.0	0.0	0.0	0.0	3.9	0.0	0.0	0.1	0	2	161
162–3	0.0	0.0	0.0	0.7	0.0	0.0	1.4	0.7	4.2	6.9	12.2	19.7	18.9	23.0	29.6	27.5	0.0	27.8	4.0	0	78	162–3
170	0.0	0.0	0.0	0.0	0.7	5.8	13.0	51.4	110.0	133.7	153.3	139.4	149.6	158.6	190.9	231.4	257.6	138.9	46.9	0	905	170
171	0.0	0.0	0.0	0.0	0.7	13.0	24.6	46.3	41.1	63.9	59.6	50.0	45.5	39.1	43.0	35.3	45.5	13.9	20.0	0	385	171
172	0.0	0.0	0.0	0.0	0.0	0.0	1.4	8.1	9.2	26.5	35.3	51.5	72.0	59.8	43.0	31.4	7.6	13.9	10.6	0	204	172
173	0.0	0.0	0.0	0.0	0.0	0.0	0.7	0.0	0.0	0.0	0.0	0.0	0.0	0.0	0.0	0.0	0.0	0.0	0.1	0	1	173
174	0.0	0.0	0.0	0.0	0.0	0.0	0.0	0.0	0.0	0.0	0.0	0.0	0.0	0.0	0.0	0.0	0.0	0.0	0.0	0	0	174
175	0.0	0.0	0.5	3.4	1.5	0.7	4.3	3.7	12.6	15.7	30.4	19.7	43.6	39.1	24.2	54.9	30.3	27.8	8.2	0	158	175
176	0.4	0.0	0.0	0.0	0.0	0.7	0.0	2.9	2.5	0.0	2.4	6.1	5.7	11.5	18.8	11.8	22.7	27.8	2.0	0	38	176
180	1.1	0.9	0.0	0.0	0.0	0.0	0.0	1.5	1.7	3.9	15.8	9.1	13.3	16.1	13.4	31.4	7.6	0.0	3.1	0	60	180
181.0	0.0	0.0	0.0	0.7	0.0	0.7	0.0	0.0	0.8	2.0	3.6	6.1	7.6	11.5	18.8	47.1	30.3	41.7	2.4	0	46	181.0
190	0.0	0.0	0.5	0.7	0.0	2.9	4.3	6.6	4.2	2.9	3.6	12.1	3.8	6.9	10.8	0.0	7.6	0.0	2.6	0	50	190
191	0.8	0.0	0.0	0.7	1.5	3.6	9.4	13.2	23.5	41.3	69.3	71.2	117.4	156.3	174.7	298.0	378.8	375.0	29.1	0	561	191
192	2.3	0.0	0.5	0.0	0.0	1.4	0.0	0.0	0.0	0.0	2.4	1.5	1.9	2.3	5.4	0.0	15.2	0.0	0.6	0	11	192
193	0.0	2.6	0.0	2.7	1.5	1.4	0.7	5.1	7.6	4.9	4.9	6.1	5.7	2.3	8.1	3.9	7.6	0.0	3.1	0	60	193
194	0.0	0.0	0.0	0.0	1.5	4.3	3.6	4.4	1.7	4.9	2.4	3.0	1.9	11.5	2.7	3.9	0.0	0.0	2.1	0	40	194
195	0.0	0.0	0.0	0.0	0.0	0.0	0.0	0.0	0.0	1.0	1.2	4.5	0.0	0.0	0.0	0.0	0.0	0.0	0.3	0	5	195
196	0.4	1.7	2.1	4.8	1.5	0.7	0.0	0.0	0.0	0.0	1.2	0.0	1.9	0.0	5.4	3.9	0.0	0.0	1.1	0	22	196
197	0.0	0.4	0.0	0.0	2.2	0.7	2.9	0.7	3.4	2.9	3.6	7.6	7.6	9.2	5.4	3.9	15.2	0.0	2.0	0	39	197
200	0.4	0.0	0.0	1.4	0.7	0.0	0.7	2.2	0.8	1.0	0.0	9.1	5.7	9.2	5.4	23.5	15.2	0.0	1.7	0	32	200
201	0.0	0.0	0.0	2.1	2.2	5.8	0.7	0.0	1.7	1.0	0.0	3.0	13.3	2.3	13.4	0.0	0.0	0.0	1.4	0	27	201
203	0.0	0.0	0.0	0.0	0.0	0.0	0.0	3.7	0.8	2.0	2.4	4.5	2.7	0.0	2.7	7.8	7.6	0.0	1.0	0	19	203
204	3.4	0.9	2.1	2.7	0.0	0.7	2.2	3.7	0.8	2.0	3.6	7.6	9.5	16.1	10.8	15.7	7.6	13.9	3.2	0	61	204
202,205	0.4	0.0	0.0	0.0	0.0	0.7	0.7	0.7	0.0	0.0	0.0	1.5	5.7	0.0	0.0	0.0	7.6	0.0	0.5	0	9	202,205
OTHER	0.4	0.0	0.0	0.0	0.0	0.7	0.7	1.5	3.4	3.9	6.1	9.1	22.7	27.6	13.4	51.0	30.3	41.7	3.8	0	73	OTHER
140–205	9.5	6.5	7.3	20.5	14.9	45.7	80.3	163.7	252.7	367.7	484.2	553.0	738.6	855.2	965.1	1333.3	1257.6	916.7	188.4	0	3632	140–205
RATE PER CASE IN PERIOD	0.38	0.43	0.52	0.68	0.74	0.72	0.72	0.73	0.84	0.98	1.22	1.52	1.89	2.30	2.69	3.92	7.58	13.89	0.05	–	–	RATE PER CASE IN PERIOD

CANADA, MANITOBA

In this province, a special committee undertook to study the incidence of cancer and the recorded annual rate has increased steadily since the beginning of this effort in 1956. This is one of two provinces where cancer is a reportable disease by law, but a check of this statute showed that it was less than 50 % effective. The efficiency of the data now recorded for Manitoba is directly dependent upon willing cooperation. All pathologists submit copies of malignant diagnoses and there is good indication that doctors are reporting cases which are not biopsied. The data can be regarded as complete.

Registry Title and Address : Manitoba Provincial Cancer Registry, c/o Manitoba Cancer Foundation, 700 Bannatyne Avenue, Winnipeg, Manitoba. Supported financially by the Provincial Government.

Registration. Cases are registered by doctors from hospital in-patients and out-patients, from radiotherapy and pathology departments; by Provincial Registrar from death certificates; and by doctors attending cases at home.

Follow-up. All registrations are followed up for life.

Physical Description. The Registry covers the province of Manitoba which lies between Saskatchewan on the west and Ontario on the east. It lies between latitudes 49⁰ and 60⁰ north and between longitudes 102⁰ and 95⁰ west. The total registration area is 650,000 square kilometres.

Demographic Description. Total population of area under survey 921,700. Fifty per cent of the population live in conurbations of more than 100,000.

Medical Services. Total number of hospital beds of all kinds 6,906. Total number of doctors in practice in registration area is 1,085. Cancer causes approximately 18 % of all deaths.

Publications. Annual Report of Manitoba Cancer Foundation.

TABLE 7 A
CANADA, MANITOBA :
POPULATION (100,000s), 1961

AGE (in years)	MALES No.	MALES Per Cent	FEMALES No.	FEMALES Per Cent
0-	0.5510	11.76	0.5250	11.58
5-	0.5190	11.08	0.4950	10.92
10-	0.4640	9.90	0.4470	9.86
15-	0.3630	7.75	0.3450	7.61
20-	0.2970	6.34	0.2930	6.47
25-	0.2980	6.36	0.2770	6.11
30-	0.3020	6.45	0.2960	6.53
35-	0.3080	6.57	0.3210	7.08
40-	0.2890	6.17	0.2890	6.38
45-	0.2750	5.87	0.2690	5.94
50-	0.2360	5.04	0.2250	4.96
55-	0.1960	4.18	0.1840	4.06
60-	0.1630	3.48	0.1560	3.44
65-	0.1420	3.03	0.1400	3.09
70-	0.1270	2.71	0.1190	2.63
75-	0.0880	1.88	0.0830	1.83
80-	0.0440	0.94	0.0430	0.95
85- and over	0.0230	0.49	0.0250	0.55
TOTAL	4.6850	100.00	4.5320	100.00

NOTES

TO TABLES 7 A, B and C

(I) I.L. number 156 not used.

" " 172 includes malignant tumours of the uterus, unspecified (I.L. number 174).

" " 193 excludes benign and unspecified tumours of the central nervous system.

(II) Carcinoma in situ included.

TABLE 7 B
CANADA, MANITOBA :
MALE INCIDENCE RATES, 1960 - 62.

INTER-NATIONAL LIST No.	No. OF CASES IN WHOLE PERIOD ALL AGES	AGE UN-KNOWN	ALL AGES	AVERAGE ANNUAL INCIDENCE PER 100,000 — AGE IN YEARS 85- AND OVER	80-	75-	70-	65-	60-	55-	50-	45-	40-	35-	30-	25-	20-	15-	10-	5-	0-	INTER-NATIONAL LIST No.
140	182	3	12.9	87.0	83.3	87.1	81.4	54.0	45.0	18.7	25.4	19.4	13.8	2.2	3.3	1.1	0.0	0.0	0.0	0.0	0.0	140
141	9	0	0.6	0.0	0.0	0.0	5.2	9.4	2.0	0.0	2.8	0.0	0.0	0.0	0.0	0.0	0.0	0.0	0.0	0.0	0.0	141
142	30	0	2.1	14.5	22.7	7.6	5.2	7.0	6.1	3.4	2.8	1.2	4.6	2.2	1.1	0.0	2.2	1.8	0.0	0.0	0.0	142
143-4	27	0	1.9	29.0	37.9	11.4	5.2	9.4	8.2	5.1	2.8	0.0	0.0	0.0	1.1	0.0	0.0	0.0	0.7	0.0	0.0	143-4
146	6	0	0.4	0.0	0.0	0.0	0.0	2.3	2.0	5.1	0.0	0.0	1.2	0.0	0.0	0.0	0.0	0.0	0.0	0.0	0.0	146
145,147-8	13	1	0.9	72.5	15.2	11.4	2.6	2.3	4.1	0.0	1.4	1.2	1.2	0.0	0.0	0.0	0.0	0.0	0.0	0.0	0.0	145,147-8
150	43	0	3.1	72.5	37.9	37.9	23.6	11.7	6.1	8.5	1.4	0.0	0.0	2.2	4.4	3.4	0.0	0.9	0.0	0.0	0.0	150
151	399	4	28.4	333.3	356.1	257.6	217.8	98.6	100.2	51.0	28.2	23.0	4.6	2.2	0.0	0.0	0.0	0.9	0.0	0.0	0.0	151
152	16	0	1.1	14.5	7.6	11.4	10.5	2.3	6.1	0.0	2.8	1.2	0.0	0.0	0.0	0.0	0.0	0.0	0.0	0.0	0.0	152
153	339	1	24.1	362.3	219.7	223.5	165.4	77.5	114.5	40.8	19.8	17.0	10.4	6.5	3.3	1.1	2.2	0.0	0.0	0.0	0.0	153
154	185	0	13.2	202.9	181.8	98.5	73.5	63.4	32.7	32.3	19.8	7.3	6.9	4.3	0.0	0.0	0.0	0.0	0.0	0.0	0.0	154
155.0	35	0	2.5	14.5	22.7	15.2	15.7	9.4	10.2	11.9	1.4	1.2	1.2	0.0	1.1	0.0	0.0	0.0	0.0	0.0	0.6	155.0
155.1	30	0	2.1	29.0	30.3	7.6	13.1	11.7	2.0	5.1	8.5	2.4	0.0	0.0	0.0	0.0	0.0	0.0	0.0	0.0	0.0	155.1
157	169	2	12.0	115.9	90.9	128.8	73.5	58.7	34.8	37.4	19.8	2.4	2.3	1.1	1.1	0.0	0.0	0.0	0.0	0.6	0.0	157
160	12	0	0.9	0.0	0.0	7.6	7.9	9.4	2.0	1.7	0.0	0.0	0.0	1.1	0.0	0.0	0.0	0.0	0.0	0.0	0.0	160
161	54	0	3.8	0.0	30.3	34.1	28.9	14.1	18.4	3.4	8.5	7.3	1.2	0.0	0.0	0.0	0.0	0.0	0.0	0.0	0.0	161
162-3	612	1	43.5	231.9	287.9	238.6	325.5	281.7	204.5	115.6	48.0	27.9	17.3	7.6	3.3	0.0	0.0	0.0	0.0	0.0	0.0	162-3
170	7	0	0.5	0.0	7.6	0.0	2.6	7.0	2.0	1.7	0.0	0.0	0.0	0.0	0.0	0.0	0.0	0.0	0.0	0.0	0.6	170
177	563	0	40.1	956.5	704.5	477.3	367.5	173.7	81.8	15.3	15.5	3.6	0.0	0.0	0.0	0.0	0.0	0.0	0.0	0.0	0.6	177
178	39	1	2.8	0.0	7.6	0.0	5.2	0.0	4.1	3.4	2.8	6.1	3.5	7.6	4.4	7.8	1.1	1.8	0.0	0.0	0.6	178
179.0	11	0	0.8	0.0	7.6	7.6	5.2	2.3	0.0	3.4	1.4	0.0	1.2	0.0	0.0	1.1	0.0	0.0	0.0	0.0	0.0	179.0
180	105	3	7.5	72.5	60.6	64.4	28.9	23.5	16.4	23.8	15.5	13.3	3.5	1.1	0.0	0.0	0.0	0.0	0.0	0.0	1.8	180
181.0	209	1	14.9	173.9	166.7	132.6	84.0	75.1	65.4	22.1	22.6	6.1	2.3	5.4	2.2	0.0	0.0	0.0	0.0	0.0	0.0	181.0
190	22	0	1.6	14.5	7.6	7.6	5.2	4.7	10.2	0.0	2.8	4.8	1.2	0.0	1.1	1.1	0.0	0.0	0.0	0.0	0.0	190
191	683	17	48.6	594.2	356.1	337.1	309.7	199.5	108.4	120.7	60.7	47.3	43.8	20.6	9.9	13.4	1.1	0.9	0.0	0.0	0.0	191
192	22	0	1.6	14.5	15.2	3.8	7.9	7.0	2.0	1.7	1.4	2.4	2.3	1.1	0.0	0.0	0.0	0.0	0.0	0.0	2.4	192
193	113	0	8.0	29.0	0.0	11.4	10.5	18.8	30.7	10.2	19.8	20.6	6.9	3.2	6.6	4.5	1.1	3.7	3.6	3.2	6.0	193
194	12	0	0.9	14.5	7.6	0.0	0.0	7.0	8.2	0.0	1.4	0.0	0.0	2.2	0.0	0.0	0.0	0.0	0.0	0.0	0.0	194
195	11	1	0.8	0.0	0.0	3.8	10.5	0.0	0.0	0.0	0.0	2.4	3.5	1.1	0.0	2.2	4.5	0.9	1.4	0.6	1.2	195
196	26	0	1.8	0.0	7.6	7.6	2.6	4.7	4.1	1.7	4.2	0.0	2.3	3.2	1.1	1.1	2.2	1.8	0.0	0.6	0.0	196
197	25	0	1.8	0.0	0.6	7.6	2.6	2.3	4.1	6.8	7.1	2.4	2.3	3.2	3.3	2.2	1.1	2.8	1.4	0.6	0.6	197
200	78	1	5.5	43.5	53.0	26.5	31.5	18.8	14.3	6.8	4.2	2.4	6.9	3.2	6.6	4.5	9.0	3.7	0.0	0.6	0.6	200
201	56	0	4.0	29.0	7.6	18.9	10.5	4.7	6.1	5.1	4.2	7.3	0.0	3.2	0.0	0.0	0.0	0.0	0.0	0.6	0.0	201
203	49	0	3.5	43.5	22.7	26.5	18.4	16.4	18.4	10.2	5.6	1.2	0.0	2.2	5.5	0.0	2.2	0.9	2.2	4.5	5.4	203
204	150	0	10.7	72.5	75.8	60.6	57.7	39.9	24.5	23.8	18.4	6.1	3.5	6.5	5.5	0.0	0.0	0.0	0.7	0.0	0.6	204
202,205	16	0	1.1	14.5	0.0	0.0	2.6	4.7	8.2	1.7	1.4	1.2	2.3	0.0	1.1	0.0	0.0	0.0	0.0	0.0	0.6	202,205
OTHER	140	1	10.0	173.9	106.1	56.8	68.2	35.2	28.6	18.7	24.0	4.8	4.6	1.1	0.0	1.1	0.0	0.9	0.0	0.6	1.8	OTHER
140-205	4498	37	320.0	3753.6	3037.9	2424.2	2081.4	1368.5	1036.8	612.2	404.0	243.6	154.6	88.7	60.7	45.9	26.9	23.9	10.1	11.6	22.4	140-205
RATE PER CASE IN PERIOD	-	-	0.07	14.49	7.58	3.79	2.62	2.35	2.04	1.70	1.41	1.21	1.15	1.08	1.10	1.12	1.12	0.92	0.72	0.64	0.60	RATE PER CASE IN PERIOD

TABLE 7 C

CANADA, MANITOBA :

FEMALE INCIDENCE RATES, 1960 - 62.

INTER-NATIONAL LIST No.	AVERAGE ANNUAL INCIDENCE PER 100,000 — AGE IN YEARS																		ALL AGES	No. OF CASES IN WHOLE PERIOD		INTER-NATIONAL LIST No.
	0-	5-	10-	15-	20-	25-	30-	35-	40-	45-	50-	55-	60-	65-	70-	75-	80-	85- AND OVER		AGE UNKNOWN	ALL AGES	
140	0.0	0.0	0.0	0.0	0.0	0.0	0.0	0.0	0.0	1.2	0.0	1.8	4.3	0.0	8.4	4.0	7.8	13.3	0.7	0	10	140
141	0.0	0.0	0.0	0.0	0.0	0.0	0.0	0.0	0.0	1.2	1.5	1.8	4.3	0.0	0.0	4.0	15.5	0.0	0.6	0	8	141
142	0.0	0.0	1.5	0.0	0.0	4.8	4.5	3.1	2.3	3.7	7.4	5.4	4.3	7.1	2.8	4.0	7.8	26.7	2.6	0	36	142
143-4	0.0	0.0	0.0	0.0	0.0	0.0	0.0	0.0	0.0	3.7	0.0	1.8	4.3	7.1	8.4	12.0	0.0	13.3	1.0	0	13	143-4
146	0.0	0.0	0.0	0.0	0.0	0.0	0.0	0.0	0.0	1.2	0.0	1.8	0.0	2.4	0.0	0.0	0.0	0.0	0.2	0	3	146
145,147-8	0.0	0.7	0.0	0.0	0.0	0.0	0.0	1.0	1.2	1.2	0.0	0.0	4.3	0.0	5.6	0.0	15.5	0.0	0.8	0	11	145,147-8
150	0.0	0.0	0.0	0.0	0.0	0.0	1.1	0.0	1.2	1.2	3.0	1.8	4.3	2.4	25.2	8.0	31.0	13.3	1.8	3	24	150
151	0.0	0.0	0.0	0.0	0.0	1.2	1.1	6.2	2.3	8.7	3.0	36.2	47.0	76.2	92.4	132.5	209.3	186.7	14.9	3	203	151
152	0.0	0.0	0.0	0.0	0.0	1.2	0.0	0.0	1.2	0.0	3.0	1.8	2.1	4.8	2.8	4.0	0.0	26.7	0.9	0	12	152
153	0.0	0.0	0.7	0.0	1.1	0.0	5.6	8.3	12.7	31.0	56.3	54.3	55.6	109.5	190.5	156.6	201.6	280.0	25.7	5	350	153
154	0.0	0.0	0.0	0.0	1.1	1.2	0.0	4.2	5.8	9.9	25.2	23.6	32.1	47.6	53.2	60.2	69.8	106.7	10.2	3	138	154
155.0	0.0	0.0	0.0	0.0	0.0	0.0	0.0	0.0	0.0	1.2	1.5	3.6	2.1	4.8	8.4	20.1	31.0	26.7	1.6	0	22	155.0
155.1	0.0	0.0	0.0	0.0	0.0	0.0	1.1	0.0	3.5	1.2	5.9	7.2	6.4	31.0	33.6	36.1	54.3	93.3	4.4	0	60	155.1
157	0.0	0.7	0.0	0.0	0.0	0.0	1.1	1.0	0.0	1.2	8.9	27.2	23.5	26.2	64.4	60.2	131.8	173.3	8.5	0	116	157
160	0.0	0.0	0.0	0.0	0.0	0.0	1.1	0.0	0.0	0.0	1.5	0.0	0.0	2.4	0.0	4.0	7.8	13.3	0.5	0	7	160
161	0.0	0.0	0.0	0.0	0.0	0.0	1.1	1.0	0.0	0.0	0.0	0.0	2.1	0.0	0.0	4.0	7.8	0.0	0.3	0	4	161
162-3	0.0	0.0	0.0	0.0	0.0	0.0	4.5	1.0	1.2	2.5	5.9	19.9	27.8	35.7	50.4	60.2	54.3	66.7	7.1	1	97	162-3
170	0.0	0.0	0.0	0.0	2.3	10.8	15.8	53.0	100.3	164.8	161.5	163.0	170.9	197.6	187.7	313.3	248.1	253.3	63.0	3	857	170
171	0.0	0.0	0.0	0.0	8.0	28.9	76.6	114.2	90.0	90.5	72.6	48.9	53.4	50.0	44.8	48.2	38.8	40.0	38.2	1	519	171
172	0.0	0.0	0.0	0.0	0.0	0.0	6.8	9.3	15.0	29.7	45.9	63.4	51.3	66.7	50.4	24.1	46.5	53.3	15.0	0	204	172
173	0.0	0.0	0.0	0.0	0.0	0.0	0.0	1.0	0.0	0.0	0.0	0.0	0.0	0.0	0.0	0.0	0.0	0.0	0.1	0	1	173
175	0.0	0.0	0.0	1.0	3.4	1.2	2.3	16.6	11.5	37.2	51.9	56.2	47.0	64.3	42.0	60.2	100.8	13.3	16.4	1	223	175
176	0.0	0.7	0.0	0.0	0.0	0.0	0.0	1.0	0.0	8.7	5.9	7.2	6.4	14.3	8.4	28.1	38.9	0.0	2.5	0	34	176
180	1.9	0.7	2.2	1.0	2.3	3.6	1.1	2.1	1.2	1.2	7.4	3.6	21.4	14.3	11.2	12.0	23.3	26.7	3.8	0	52	180
181.0	0.0	0.0	0.0	0.0	0.0	0.0	0.0	0.0	0.0	1.2	3.0	1.8	4.3	7.1	28.0	24.1	54.3	53.3	2.9	1	40	181.0
190	0.0	0.0	0.0	1.9	1.1	2.4	1.1	0.0	3.5	2.5	3.0	3.6	6.4	2.4	5.6	12.0	7.8	26.7	2.1	2	28	190
191	0.6	0.7	0.7	0.0	2.3	3.6	10.1	17.7	35.8	32.2	50.4	77.9	89.7	138.1	190.5	289.2	294.6	506.7	36.3	9	493	191
192	1.9	0.0	0.7	0.0	0.0	1.2	1.0	1.0	0.0	1.2	0.0	3.6	2.1	0.0	2.8	0.0	38.8	0.0	0.7	0	10	192
193	4.4	3.4	2.2	1.0	3.4	2.4	3.4	3.1	9.2	19.8	19.3	14.5	21.4	23.8	5.6	16.1	7.8	0.0	7.3	0	99	193
194	0.0	0.0	2.2	1.0	0.0	3.6	3.4	4.2	4.6	6.2	7.4	10.9	4.3	7.1	11.2	4.0	0.0	0.0	3.4	2	46	194
195	0.6	0.0	0.0	1.9	0.6	0.0	0.0	0.0	2.3	0.0	3.0	1.8	0.0	0.0	0.0	0.0	0.0	0.0	0.6	0	8	195
196	0.6	0.7	2.2	1.0	2.3	3.6	0.0	0.0	0.0	2.5	0.0	0.0	0.0	2.4	2.8	0.0	0.0	0.0	0.9	0	12	196
197	0.6	0.7	2.2	1.9	1.1	0.0	0.0	2.1	1.2	5.0	4.4	12.7	8.9	11.9	5.6	4.0	38.8	13.3	1.2	0	16	197
200	0.0	0.0	0.0	0.0	3.4	0.0	0.0	0.0	4.6	5.0	8.9	3.6	10.7	2.4	8.4	16.1	0.0	0.0	3.5	0	48	200
201	0.6	0.0	0.0	2.9	3.4	2.4	0.0	4.2	3.5	0.0	1.5	3.6	8.5	2.4	5.6	4.0	0.0	13.3	2.4	0	32	201
203	0.0	0.0	0.0	0.0	0.0	0.0	0.0	0.0	0.0	0.0	4.4	3.6	8.5	19.0	19.6	24.1	0.0	0.0	2.3	0	31	203
204	3.2	2.7	1.5	1.9	1.1	3.6	5.6	2.1	4.6	8.7	4.4	7.2	15.0	21.4	30.8	64.3	54.3	40.0	7.0	0	95	204
202,205	0.0	0.0	0.0	0.0	0.0	0.0	0.0	0.0	1.2	1.2	5.9	1.8	8.5	0.0	5.6	12.0	0.0	0.0	1.2	0	16	202,205
OTHER	0.0	0.0	0.7	0.0	0.0	3.6	4.5	2.1	4.6	14.9	7.4	18.1	21.4	45.2	44.8	76.3	108.5	106.7	9.5	2	129	OTHER
140-205	14.6	10.8	14.2	14.5	30.7	75.8	149.3	258.6	326.4	501.9	591.1	695.7	775.6	1040.5	1257.7	1602.4	1907.0	2186.7	302.1	3	4107	140-205
RATE PER CASE IN PERIOD	0.63	0.67	0.75	0.97	1.14	1.20	1.13	1.04	1.15	1.24	1.48	1.81	2.14	2.38	2.80	4.02	7.75	13.33	0.07	-	-	RATE PER CASE IN PERIOD

CANADA, NEW BRUNSWICK

There are three clinics in the province of New Brunswick, the main one being in St. John. A statistical clerk from the main clinic visits the other two at regular intervals and gathers data on all new cases. These data are recorded in the Provincial Tumour Registry located at the clinic in St. John. The data can be regarded as complete.

Registry Title and Address : New Brunswick Provincial Tumour Registry, c/o Saint John General Hospital, Saint John, New Brunswick. Supported financially by the Provincial Government.

Registration. Registration is sought by registry staff from hospital in-patients and out-patients and from radiotherapy departments. Pathologists report cases in pathology departments, and the Provincial Registrar from death certificates. Doctors treating cases at home send in registrations.

Follow-up. All registrations are followed up for life.

Physical description. The Registry covers the Province of New Brunswick which is bordered by Quebec and Nova Scotia. It lies between latitudes 45⁰ and 48⁰ north and longitudes 69⁰ and 65⁰ west. The total registration area is 73,437 square kilometres.

Demographic Description. Total population of the area under survey 597,900. None of the population live in conurbations of more than 100,000.

Medical Services. Total number of hospital beds of all kinds 4,002. Total number of doctors in practice in registration area 513. Cancer causes approximately 16 % of all deaths.

TABLE 8 A
CANADA, NEW BRUNSWICK :
POPULATION (100,000s), 1961

AGE (in years)	MALES		FEMALES	
	No.	Per Cent	No.	Per Cent
0–	0.4040	13.36	0.3820	12.93
5–	0.3870	12.80	0.3720	12.59
10–	0.3700	12.24	0.3570	12.08
15–	0.2740	9.06	0.2610	8.83
20–	0.1880	6.22	0.1860	6.29
25–	0.1680	5.56	0.1680	5.69
30–	0.1670	5.52	0.1720	5.82
35–	0.1780	5.89	0.1820	6.16
40–	0.1700	5.62	0.1680	5.69
45–	0.1570	5.19	0.1490	5.04
50–	0.1360	4.50	0.1240	4.20
55–	0.1060	3.51	0.1030	3.49
60–	0.0890	2.94	0.0910	3.08
65–	0.0810	2.68	0.0810	2.74
70–	0.0640	2.12	0.0670	2.27
75–	0.0450	1.49	0.0470	1.59
80–	0.0250	0.83	0.0280	0.95
85– and over	0.0150	0.50	0.0170	0.58
TOTAL	3.0240	100.00	2.9550	100.00

NOTES

TO TABLES 8 A, B and C

(I)   I.L. number 193 excludes benign and unspecified tumours of the central nervous system.

(II)   Carcinoma in situ included.

TABLE 8 B
CANADA, NEW BRUNSWICK :
MALE INCIDENCE RATES, 1962 - 64.

INTER-NATIONAL LIST No.	AVERAGE ANNUAL INCIDENCE PER 100,000 — AGE IN YEARS																		ALL AGES	No. OF CASES IN WHOLE PERIOD		INTER-NATIONAL LIST No.
	0–	5–	10–	15–	20–	25–	30–	35–	40–	45–	50–	55–	60–	65–	70–	75–	80–	85– AND OVER		AGE UNKNOWN	ALL AGES	
140	0.0	0.0	0.0	0.0	0.0	0.0	4.0	9.4	13.7	29.7	36.8	34.6	59.9	90.5	171.9	118.5	293.3	244.4	19.2	0	174	140
141	0.0	0.0	0.0	0.0	0.0	0.0	0.0	0.0	0.0	0.0	2.5	3.1	7.5	4.1	5.2	0.0	13.3	0.0	0.8	0	7	141
142	0.0	0.0	0.0	0.0	1.8	2.0	2.0	1.9	0.0	4.2	0.0	3.1	3.7	4.1	5.2	7.4	0.0	0.0	1.2	0	11	142
143-4	0.0	0.0	0.0	0.0	0.0	0.0	0.0	1.9	0.0	8.5	4.9	6.3	0.0	12.3	26.0	37.0	53.3	133.3	3.5	0	32	143-4
146	0.0	0.0	0.0	0.0	0.0	0.0	0.0	0.0	0.0	0.0	2.5	0.0	3.7	0.0	0.0	0.0	0.0	0.0	0.3	0	3	146
145,147-8	0.0	0.0	0.0	1.2	0.0	0.0	0.0	0.0	0.0	0.0	0.0	0.0	0.0	0.0	0.0	7.4	0.0	0.0	0.1	0	1	145,147-8
150	0.0	0.0	0.0	0.0	0.0	0.0	0.0	0.0	2.0	2.1	2.5	6.3	15.0	12.3	10.4	7.4	40.0	0.0	2.0	0	18	150
151	0.0	0.0	0.0	0.0	1.8	0.0	8.0	5.6	13.7	17.0	46.6	56.6	89.9	107.0	125.0	237.0	306.7	155.6	21.6	0	196	151
152	0.0	0.0	0.0	0.0	0.0	0.0	2.0	0.0	0.0	0.0	0.0	0.0	11.2	8.2	10.4	14.8	13.3	0.0	1.2	0	11	152
153	0.0	0.0	0.0	0.0	0.0	2.0	8.0	0.0	11.8	19.1	19.6	40.9	74.9	107.0	145.8	125.9	160.0	88.9	16.3	0	148	153
154	0.0	0.0	0.0	0.0	0.0	2.0	4.0	0.0	5.9	12.7	17.2	47.2	33.7	70.0	83.3	103.7	146.7	88.9	11.6	0	105	154
155.0	0.8	0.0	0.0	0.0	0.7	0.0	0.0	0.0	0.0	0.0	9.8	0.0	0.0	4.1	0.0	0.0	0.0	0.0	0.7	0	6	155.0
155.1	0.0	0.0	0.0	0.0	0.0	2.0	0.0	0.0	0.0	0.0	4.9	3.1	3.7	12.3	10.4	37.0	0.0	22.2	1.8	0	16	155.1
156	0.0	0.0	0.0	0.0	0.0	0.0	0.0	0.0	0.0	4.2	0.0	0.0	0.0	12.3	10.4	7.4	53.3	0.0	1.0	0	9	156
157	0.0	0.0	0.0	0.0	0.0	0.0	0.0	0.0	0.0	6.4	19.6	18.9	26.2	37.0	83.3	59.3	66.7	88.9	7.3	0	66	157
160	0.0	0.0	0.0	0.0	0.8	0.0	0.0	0.0	0.0	2.1	0.0	3.1	3.7	0.0	5.2	7.4	26.7	0.0	0.8	0	7	160
161	0.0	0.0	0.0	0.0	0.0	0.0	0.0	0.0	0.0	2.1	9.8	15.7	22.5	20.6	10.4	14.8	26.7	0.0	3.0	0	27	161
162-3	0.0	0.0	0.0	0.0	1.8	0.0	4.0	5.6	13.7	25.5	34.3	69.2	108.6	152.3	135.4	66.7	53.3	44.4	18.5	0	168	162-3
170	0.0	0.0	0.0	0.0	0.0	0.0	0.0	0.0	0.0	0.0	0.0	0.0	0.0	4.1	0.0	0.0	0.0	0.0	0.1	0	1	170
177	0.0	0.0	0.0	0.0	1.8	2.0	6.0	0.0	0.0	4.2	17.2	12.6	78.7	152.3	265.6	377.8	573.3	333.3	25.6	0	232	177
178	0.0	0.0	0.0	1.2	0.0	2.0	0.0	3.7	0.0	2.1	0.0	6.3	3.7	8.2	6.0	7.4	0.0	0.0	1.4	0	13	178
179.0	0.0	0.0	0.9	0.0	0.0	0.0	0.0	0.0	0.0	4.2	2.5	6.3	3.7	0.0	15.6	0.0	13.3	22.2	1.4	0	13	179.0
180	2.5	0.9	0.9	2.4	0.0	2.0	4.0	0.0	5.9	6.4	14.7	22.0	22.5	32.9	15.6	37.0	26.7	22.2	6.0	0	54	180
181.0	0.0	0.0	0.0	0.0	0.0	2.0	0.0	3.7	5.9	6.4	17.2	18.9	86.1	61.7	72.9	207.4	200.0	155.6	13.6	0	123	181.0
190	0.0	0.0	1.8	0.0	1.8	0.0	2.0	1.9	3.9	0.0	0.0	0.0	3.7	16.5	15.6	14.8	13.3	0.0	1.8	0	16	190
191	0.0	0.0	0.0	0.0	1.8	2.0	8.0	24.3	47.1	80.7	139.7	213.8	303.4	428.0	546.9	659.3	973.3	1044.4	77.9	0	707	191
192	0.0	0.0	0.9	0.0	1.1	0.0	2.0	0.0	0.0	2.1	4.9	10.4	7.5	4.1	10.4	22.2	13.3	0.0	1.1	0	10	192
193	6.6	2.6	0.9	2.4	0.0	2.0	4.0	1.9	3.9	10.6	4.9	15.7	7.5	4.1	0.0	7.4	0.0	0.0	3.9	0	35	193
194	0.0	0.0	0.0	1.2	0.0	0.0	0.0	0.0	2.0	0.0	0.0	0.0	7.5	4.1	5.2	0.0	0.0	0.0	0.8	0	7	194
195	0.0	0.9	0.0	1.2	0.0	0.0	0.0	0.0	0.0	0.0	0.0	0.0	0.0	0.0	0.0	0.0	0.0	0.0	0.3	0	3	195
196	0.8	0.9	1.8	1.2	0.0	0.0	0.0	3.7	0.0	0.0	4.9	3.1	0.0	4.1	0.0	7.4	53.3	0.0	1.2	0	11	196
197	3.3	0.9	1.8	2.4	0.0	0.0	0.0	1.9	2.0	2.1	0.0	6.3	15.0	16.5	20.8	0.0	0.0	0.0	3.0	0	27	197
200	0.8	0.0	1.8	0.0	1.8	4.0	0.0	0.0	2.0	2.1	2.5	3.1	15.0	4.1	5.2	14.8	53.3	0.0	2.1	0	19	200
201	0.0	0.9	0.0	0.0	3.5	2.0	2.0	1.9	0.0	10.6	0.0	9.4	11.2	12.3	0.0	14.8	13.3	22.2	2.4	0	22	201
203	0.0	0.0	0.0	3.6	0.0	0.0	0.0	0.0	2.0	0.0	0.0	3.1	18.7	0.0	15.6	29.6	13.3	22.2	1.8	0	16	203
204	5.0	6.0	1.8	3.6	1.8	2.0	2.0	0.0	2.0	2.1	7.4	6.3	15.0	16.5	26.0	37.0	40.0	22.2	5.5	0	50	204
202,205	0.0	0.0	0.0	0.0	0.0	0.0	0.0	0.0	0.0	0.0	0.0	0.0	0.0	0.0	0.0	0.0	0.0	0.0	0.0	0	0	202,205
OTHER	0.0	0.9	0.0	0.0	0.0	0.0	0.0	3.7	7.8	12.7	9.8	3.1	15.0	24.7	31.3	7.4	13.3	22.2	4.1	0	37	OTHER
140-205	19.8	13.8	9.0	17.0	19.5	27.8	61.9	71.2	143.1	280.3	433.8	638.4	1071.2	1444.4	1885.4	2296.3	3146.7	2511.1	264.7	0	2401	140-205
RATE PER CASE IN PERIOD	0.83	0.86	0.90	1.22	1.77	1.98	2.00	1.87	1.96	2.12	2.45	3.14	3.75	4.12	5.21	7.41	13.33	22.22	0.11	-	-	RATE PER CASE IN PERIOD

TABLE 8 C

CANADA, NEW BRUNSWICK :
FEMALE INCIDENCE RATES, 1962 - 64.

AVERAGE ANNUAL INCIDENCE PER 100,000

INTER-NATIONAL LIST No.	0-	5-	10-	15-	20-	25-	30-	35-	40-	45-	50-	55-	60-	65-	70-	75-	80-	85- AND OVER	ALL AGES	No. OF CASES ALL AGES	AGE UNKNOWN	INTER-NATIONAL LIST No.
140	0.0	0.0	0.0	0.0	0.0	0.0	0.0	0.0	0.0	2.2	0.0	3.2	0.0	4.1	5.0	0.0	0.0	0.0	0.5	4	0	140
141	0.0	0.0	0.0	0.0	0.0	2.0	0.0	0.0	0.0	0.0	5.4	3.2	0.0	0.0	10.0	0.0	11.9	19.6	0.9	8	0	141
142	0.0	0.0	0.0	0.0	0.0	2.0	1.9	1.8	4.0	0.0	2.7	0.0	3.7	0.0	0.0	14.2	0.0	19.6	1.1	10	0	142
143-4	0.0	0.0	0.0	0.0	0.0	0.0	0.0	0.0	0.0	0.0	0.0	0.0	0.0	4.1	14.9	0.0	23.8	0.0	0.7	6	0	143-4
146	0.9	0.0	0.0	0.0	0.0	0.0	0.0	0.0	0.0	0.0	0.0	0.0	0.0	0.0	5.0	0.0	0.0	0.0	0.2	2	0	146
145,147-8	0.0	0.0	0.0	0.0	0.0	0.0	0.0	0.0	0.0	0.0	0.0	0.0	0.0	0.0	0.0	7.1	0.0	0.0	0.1	1	0	145,147-8
150	0.0	0.0	0.0	0.0	1.8	0.0	1.9	0.0	0.0	0.0	8.1	0.0	11.0	0.0	5.0	0.0	0.0	19.6	1.1	10	0	150
151	0.0	0.0	0.0	0.0	1.8	0.0	0.0	1.8	9.9	6.7	10.8	22.7	62.3	57.6	89.6	92.2	142.9	78.4	11.2	99	0	151
152	0.0	0.9	0.0	0.0	0.0	0.0	0.0	1.8	0.0	0.0	2.7	3.2	0.0	12.3	10.0	10.0	0.0	0.0	1.0	9	0	152
153	0.0	0.0	0.0	0.0	1.8	0.0	5.8	3.7	6.0	31.3	32.3	68.0	124.5	160.5	129.4	212.8	166.7	294.1	24.1	214	0	153
154	0.0	0.0	0.0	0.0	0.0	2.0	1.9	3.7	6.0	13.4	13.4	25.9	54.9	37.0	59.7	106.4	107.1	78.4	10.2	90	0	154
155.0	0.0	0.0	0.0	0.0	0.0	0.0	0.0	0.0	4.0	0.0	0.0	0.0	0.0	4.1	0.0	0.0	0.0	0.0	0.3	3	0	155.0
155.1	0.0	0.0	0.0	0.0	0.0	0.0	1.9	0.0	0.0	2.2	10.8	3.2	14.7	20.6	19.9	14.2	47.6	0.0	2.8	25	0	155.1
156	0.0	0.9	0.0	0.0	0.0	0.0	0.0	0.0	0.0	0.0	0.0	3.2	7.3	20.6	0.0	7.1	11.9	0.0	1.2	11	0	156
157	0.0	0.0	0.9	0.0	0.0	0.0	0.0	0.0	2.0	0.0	10.8	6.5	18.3	12.3	29.9	85.1	47.6	58.8	4.5	40	0	157
160	0.0	0.0	0.9	0.0	0.7	0.0	0.0	0.0	0.0	4.5	2.7	0.0	3.7	4.1	0.0	0.0	0.0	0.0	0.7	6	0	160
161	0.0	0.9	0.0	0.0	0.0	0.0	0.0	0.0	0.0	2.2	0.0	0.0	3.7	0.0	24.9	0.0	11.9	19.6	1.0	9	0	161
162-3	0.0	0.0	0.0	0.0	0.0	2.0	0.0	0.0	2.0	8.9	18.8	12.9	11.0	12.3	10.0	7.1	23.8	0.0	3.0	27	0	162-3
170	0.0	0.0	0.0	0.0	1.8	2.0	32.9	29.3	101.2	127.5	126.3	148.9	175.8	156.4	228.9	269.5	190.5	294.1	49.3	437	0	170
171	0.0	0.0	0.0	0.0	9.0	21.8	54.3	91.6	101.2	80.5	75.3	74.4	40.3	41.2	44.8	42.6	71.4	39.2	31.1	276	0	171
172	0.0	0.0	0.0	0.0	1.8	2.0	3.9	3.7	23.8	33.6	32.3	42.1	54.9	57.6	29.9	49.6	71.4	0.0	11.8	105	0	172
173	0.0	0.0	0.0	0.0	3.6	2.0	0.0	0.0	0.0	2.2	0.0	0.0	0.0	0.0	0.0	0.0	0.0	0.0	0.5	4	0	173
174	0.0	0.0	0.0	0.0	0.0	0.0	0.0	0.0	0.0	0.0	0.0	0.0	0.0	0.0	0.0	0.0	0.0	0.0	0.0	0	0	174
175	0.0	0.0	0.0	1.3	3.6	0.0	3.9	14.7	7.9	17.9	26.9	38.8	36.6	20.6	34.8	42.6	59.5	19.6	9.1	81	0	175
176	0.0	0.0	0.0	0.0	0.0	0.0	0.0	1.8	2.0	2.2	2.7	9.7	18.3	8.2	19.9	14.2	0.0	39.2	2.5	22	0	176
180	0.0	0.9	0.0	0.0	0.0	0.0	0.0	0.0	2.0	4.5	5.4	6.5	22.0	16.5	5.0	7.1	0.0	0.0	2.5	22	0	180
181.0	0.0	0.0	0.0	0.0	0.0	2.0	0.0	0.0	4.0	6.7	5.4	16.2	18.3	41.2	34.8	56.7	47.6	19.6	5.3	47	0	181.0
190	0.9	0.0	0.0	0.0	0.0	0.0	5.8	1.8	2.0	2.2	0.0	3.2	0.0	0.0	5.0	14.2	23.8	0.0	1.6	14	0	190
191	1.7	0.0	0.0	0.0	5.4	11.9	15.5	12.8	49.6	49.2	123.7	77.7	131.9	267.5	298.5	510.6	440.5	607.8	49.9	442	0	191
192	0.0	3.6	0.0	0.0	0.0	2.0	0.0	0.0	0.0	0.0	0.0	6.5	7.3	0.0	0.0	7.1	0.0	0.0	0.8	7	0	192
193	0.0	0.0	0.9	1.3	1.8	6.0	3.9	3.7	2.0	4.5	5.4	6.5	14.7	4.1	5.0	0.0	11.9	0.0	2.6	23	0	193
194	0.0	0.0	0.0	1.3	0.0	2.0	3.9	0.0	7.9	0.0	5.4	6.5	3.7	0.0	14.9	21.3	11.9	19.6	3.2	28	0	194
195	0.0	0.0	0.0	0.0	0.0	0.0	0.0	0.0	0.0	0.0	0.0	0.0	0.0	0.0	0.0	0.0	0.0	0.0	0.0	0	0	195
196	0.0	0.9	0.0	0.0	5.4	2.0	0.0	0.0	0.0	6.7	0.0	0.0	3.7	0.0	5.0	0.0	0.0	0.0	0.5	4	0	196
197	0.0	0.0	0.9	1.3	0.0	2.0	0.0	3.7	2.0	4.5	2.7	12.9	11.0	0.0	10.0	35.5	23.8	19.6	3.4	30	0	197
200	0.0	0.0	0.0	0.0	1.8	0.0	3.9	3.7	4.0	6.7	5.4	0.0	3.7	4.1	14.9	7.1	23.8	39.2	2.0	18	0	200
201	0.0	0.9	0.0	1.3	1.8	2.0	0.0	1.8	0.0	0.0	0.0	6.5	7.3	8.2	14.9	0.0	23.8	0.0	2.1	19	0	201
203	0.0	0.0	0.0	0.0	3.6	0.0	0.0	3.7	2.0	2.2	2.7	3.2	7.3	0.0	5.0	7.1	0.0	0.0	0.8	7	0	203
204	6.1	1.8	0.0	1.3	0.0	2.0	1.9	0.0	6.0	2.2	2.7	3.2	22.0	20.6	29.9	28.4	0.0	0.0	4.9	43	0	204
202,205	0.0	0.0	0.0	0.0	0.0	0.0	0.0	0.0	0.0	2.2	0.0	0.0	0.0	0.0	0.0	0.0	0.0	0.0	0.1	1	0	202,205
OTHER	0.9	0.0	0.0	0.0	0.0	0.0	1.9	1.8	2.0	2.2	16.1	0.0	14.7	12.3	19.9	35.5	11.9	58.8	3.5	31	0	OTHER
140-205	12.2	9.0	4.7	7.7	39.4	63.5	145.3	186.8	353.2	427.3	556.5	618.1	908.4	1008.2	1233.8	1695.0	1583.3	1745.1	252.1	2235	0	140-205
RATE PER CASE IN PERIOD	0.87	0.90	0.93	1.28	1.79	1.98	1.94	1.83	1.98	2.24	2.69	3.24	3.66	4.12	4.98	7.09	11.90	19.61	0.11	-	-	RATE PER CASE IN PERIOD

CANADA, NEWFOUNDLAND

A Provincial Cancer Registry in Newfoundland has been operating since 1956, but there are numerous unsolved problems which affect the completeness of the data. Due to its peculiar topography, there are numerous small population groups in Newfoundland which are completely isolated at some time during the year. It is estimated, however, that the Registry covers approximately 90 % of the malignant cases which occur annually. The data on these cases come from the doctors in the province on a special cancer registry form.

Registry Title and Address : Newfoundland Provincial Cancer Registry, c/o St. John's General Hospital, St. John's, Newfoundland.

Registration. Doctors register cases among hospital in-patients and out-patients, and from radiotherapy departments. Pathologists register cases from pathology departments, and the Provincial Registrar registers cases from death certificates. Doctors register cases they attend at home.

Follow-up. All registrations are followed up for life.

Physical description. The Registry covers the island of Newfoundland and Labrador. Newfoundland lies on the gulf of the St. Lawrence, between latitudes 47⁰ and 56⁰ North and longitudes 53⁰ and 59⁰ West. The total registration area is 404,519 square kilometres.

Demographic Description. Total population of area under survey 457,900. None of the population live in conurbations of more than 100,000.

Medical Services. Total number of hospital beds of all kinds 2,585. Total number of doctors in practice in registration area 310. Cancer causes approximately 17 % of all deaths.

TABLE 9 A
CANADA, NEWFOUNDLAND :
POPULATION (100,000s), 1961

NOTES

TO TABLES 9 A, B and C

(I)   I.L. number 193 excludes benign and unspecified tu-
      mours of the central nervous system.

(II) Carcinoma in situ included.

AGE (in years)	MALES		FEMALES	
	No.	Per Cent	No.	Per Cent
0-	0.3440	14.64	0.3330	14.94
5-	0.3260	13.87	0.3180	14.27
10-	0.3030	12.89	0.2920	13.10
15-	0.2200	9.36	0.2190	9.83
20-	0.1530	6.51	0.1490	6.68
25-	0.1400	5.96	0.1270	5.70
30-	0.1330	5.66	0.1230	5.52
35-	0.1300	5.53	0.1180	5.29
40-	0.1280	5.45	0.1130	5.07
45-	0.1140	4.85	0.1030	4.62
50-	0.0960	4.09	0.0800	3.59
55-	0.0700	2.98	0.0630	2.83
60-	0.0580	2.47	0.0560	2.51
65-	0.0490	2.09	0.0480	2.15
70-	0.0370	1.57	0.0370	1.66
75-	0.0280	1.19	0.0270	1.21
80-	0.0140	0.60	0.0140	0.63
85- and over	0.0070	0.30	0.0090	0.40
TOTAL	2.3500	100.00	2.2290	100.00

TABLE 9 B

CANADA, NEWFOUNDLAND :
MALE INCIDENCE RATES, 1960 - 62.

AVERAGE ANNUAL INCIDENCE PER 100,000 — AGE IN YEARS

INTERNATIONAL LIST No.	0-	5-	10-	15-	20-	25-	30-	35-	40-	45-	50-	55-	60-	65-	70-	75-	80-	85- AND OVER	ALL AGES	No. OF CASES — AGE UNKNOWN	No. OF CASES — ALL AGES
140	0.0	0.0	0.0	0.0	0.0	0.0	10.0	12.8	5.2	14.6	34.7	57.1	63.2	88.4	99.1	202.4	214.3	285.7	16.2	9	114
141	0.0	0.0	0.0	0.0	0.0	0.0	0.0	0.0	2.6	0.0	0.0	9.5	0.0	6.8	9.0	23.8	47.6	0.0	1.3	0	9
142	0.0	0.0	0.0	0.0	2.2	0.0	0.0	0.0	0.0	0.0	0.0	4.8	5.7	6.8	0.0	11.9	23.8	0.0	1.0	1	7
143-4	0.0	0.0	0.0	0.0	0.0	0.0	0.0	0.0	0.0	0.0	3.5	0.0	11.5	6.8	18.0	0.0	23.8	47.6	1.1	0	8
146	0.0	0.0	0.0	0.0	0.0	0.0	0.0	2.6	0.0	2.9	0.0	4.8	5.7	13.6	0.0	11.9	0.0	0.0	1.0	0	7
145,147-8	0.0	0.0	0.0	0.0	0.0	0.0	0.0	0.0	0.0	0.0	0.0	4.8	5.7	6.8	0.0	0.0	0.0	0.0	0.3	0	2
150	0.0	0.0	0.0	0.0	0.0	0.0	5.0	7.7	0.0	2.9	6.9	4.8	23.0	6.8	18.0	59.5	23.8	0.0	2.4	0	17
151	0.0	0.0	0.0	0.0	0.0	0.0	0.0	7.7	15.6	43.9	76.4	100.0	120.7	224.5	369.4	488.1	452.4	285.7	32.8	1	231
152	0.0	0.0	0.0	0.0	0.0	0.0	0.0	0.0	0.0	2.9	0.0	4.8	0.0	0.0	0.0	11.9	0.0	0.0	0.4	0	3
153	0.0	0.0	0.0	0.0	0.0	4.8	0.0	12.8	10.4	17.5	34.7	42.9	46.0	102.0	117.1	238.1	357.1	142.9	16.7	8	118
154	0.0	0.0	0.0	0.0	0.0	0.0	0.0	2.6	0.0	11.7	0.0	9.5	11.5	34.0	18.0	47.6	47.6	95.2	3.5	1	25
155.0	0.0	0.0	0.0	0.0	0.0	0.0	0.0	0.0	0.0	0.0	0.0	0.0	5.7	0.0	0.0	11.9	0.0	0.0	0.3	0	2
155.1	0.0	0.0	0.0	0.0	0.0	0.0	0.0	0.0	0.0	0.0	3.5	4.8	5.7	0.0	9.0	11.9	23.8	0.0	0.9	0	6
156	0.0	0.0	0.0	0.0	0.0	0.0	0.0	0.0	2.6	0.0	6.9	0.0	0.0	0.0	18.0	11.9	23.8	0.0	1.1	0	8
157	0.0	0.0	0.0	0.0	0.0	2.4	0.0	0.0	5.2	8.8	3.5	19.0	5.7	47.6	54.1	47.6	47.6	0.0	4.5	1	32
160	0.0	0.0	0.0	0.0	0.0	0.0	0.0	0.0	5.2	2.9	0.0	4.8	5.7	20.4	0.0	0.0	0.0	47.6	1.3	0	9
161	0.0	0.0	0.0	1.5	0.0	0.0	2.5	0.0	5.2	0.0	6.9	9.5	11.5	13.6	9.0	23.8	0.0	47.6	2.3	0	16
162-3	0.0	0.0	0.0	0.0	0.0	0.0	5.0	15.4	15.6	61.4	69.4	47.6	97.7	122.4	45.0	95.2	71.4	190.5	17.0	0	120
170	0.0	0.0	0.0	0.0	0.0	0.0	0.0	0.0	0.0	0.0	0.0	0.0	11.9	6.8	0.0	11.9	0.0	0.0	0.3	0	2
177	0.0	0.0	0.0	0.0	0.0	0.0	0.0	0.0	0.0	2.9	0.0	9.5	40.2	34.0	243.2	214.3	214.3	238.1	10.6	1	75
178	0.0	0.0	1.1	0.0	0.0	4.8	12.5	0.0	0.0	0.0	0.0	0.0	0.0	0.0	0.0	0.0	0.0	0.0	1.4	0	10
179.0	0.0	0.0	0.0	0.0	0.0	2.4	0.0	5.1	0.0	8.8	0.0	0.0	0.0	6.8	0.0	23.8	23.8	0.0	1.3	1	9
180	1.9	0.0	0.0	0.0	0.0	0.0	2.5	0.0	5.2	5.8	3.5	0.0	11.5	20.4	9.0	0.0	0.0	0.0	1.7	0	12
181.0	0.0	0.0	0.0	0.0	0.0	0.0	5.0	7.7	0.0	0.0	17.4	38.1	51.7	61.2	90.1	71.4	166.7	190.5	9.9	5	70
190	0.0	0.0	0.0	0.0	0.0	0.0	2.5	0.0	0.0	0.0	0.0	4.8	5.7	20.4	0.0	23.8	0.0	0.0	1.3	1	9
191	0.0	0.0	0.0	0.0	0.0	0.0	2.5	7.7	41.7	29.2	72.9	66.7	149.4	142.9	153.2	369.0	381.0	761.9	29.4	15	207
192	0.0	0.0	0.0	0.0	0.0	0.0	0.0	0.0	0.0	0.0	0.0	0.0	5.7	6.8	0.0	0.0	0.0	0.0	0.3	0	2
193	1.9	5.1	2.2	6.1	4.4	4.8	5.0	5.1	10.4	5.8	13.9	14.3	17.2	6.8	9.0	0.0	0.0	0.0	5.5	0	39
194	0.0	0.0	0.0	0.0	0.0	0.0	0.0	0.0	2.6	2.9	0.0	0.0	0.0	6.8	0.0	0.0	0.0	0.0	0.7	2	5
195	0.0	1.0	0.0	0.0	0.0	4.8	0.0	0.0	0.0	0.0	0.0	0.0	0.0	0.0	0.0	0.0	0.0	0.0	0.7	0	5
196	0.0	0.0	0.0	1.5	0.0	0.0	0.0	0.0	0.0	0.0	3.5	4.8	5.7	0.0	0.0	0.0	23.8	0.0	1.1	0	8
197	0.0	0.0	0.0	0.0	2.2	0.0	0.0	0.0	0.0	0.0	0.0	19.0	5.7	6.8	0.0	0.0	0.0	0.0	1.1	1	8
200	1.0	0.0	0.0	1.5	2.2	2.4	2.5	0.0	0.0	2.9	3.5	9.5	11.5	13.6	11.9	11.9	0.0	0.0	2.0	0	14
201	0.0	0.0	0.0	1.5	4.4	7.1	2.5	2.6	5.2	2.9	3.5	4.8	11.5	0.0	0.0	0.0	0.0	0.0	2.1	0	15
203	0.0	0.0	0.0	0.0	0.0	2.4	2.5	2.6	0.0	0.0	0.0	4.8	5.7	13.6	9.0	0.0	0.0	0.0	0.9	0	6
204	4.8	3.1	1.1	1.5	4.4	2.4	0.0	2.6	2.6	0.0	3.5	14.3	5.7	6.8	18.0	11.9	23.8	0.0	3.8	1	27
202,205	0.0	0.0	0.0	0.0	0.0	0.0	0.0	0.0	0.0	2.9	0.0	0.0	0.0	13.6	18.0	0.0	47.6	0.0	0.9	0	6
OTHER	1.0	0.0	0.0	0.0	0.0	0.0	0.0	0.0	0.0	2.9	3.5	4.8	17.2	27.2	27.0	95.2	95.2	47.6	3.8	0	27
140-205	10.7	9.2	4.4	13.6	19.6	35.7	60.2	87.2	135.4	233.9	371.5	523.8	775.9	1088.4	1360.4	2131.0	2333.3	2381.0	182.3	48	1285
RATE PER CASE IN PERIOD	0.97	1.02	1.10	1.52	2.18	2.38	2.51	2.56	2.60	2.92	3.47	4.76	5.75	6.80	9.01	11.90	23.81	47.62	0.14	-	-

TABLE 9 C
CANADA, NEWFOUNDLAND :
FEMALE INCIDENCE RATES, 1960 - 62.

AVERAGE ANNUAL INCIDENCE PER 100,000 — AGE IN YEARS

INTERNATIONAL LIST No.	0-	5-	10-	15-	20-	25-	30-	35-	40-	45-	50-	55-	60-	65-	70-	75-	80-	85- AND OVER	ALL AGES	Cases: AGE UNKNOWN	Cases: ALL AGES	INTERNATIONAL LIST No.
140	0.0	0.0	0.0	0.0	0.0	0.0	0.0	0.0	0.0	0.0	0.0	5.3	0.0	6.9	0.0	0.0	0.0	0.0	0.3	0	2	140
141	0.0	0.0	0.0	0.0	0.0	0.0	0.0	0.0	2.9	0.0	4.2	0.0	0.0	6.9	18.0	0.0	0.0	0.0	0.7	0	5	141
142	0.0	0.0	0.0	0.0	0.0	0.0	0.0	5.6	0.0	0.0	0.0	0.0	0.0	0.0	9.0	0.0	0.0	0.0	0.4	0	3	142
143-4	0.0	0.0	0.0	0.0	0.0	0.0	0.0	2.8	0.0	0.0	0.0	5.3	0.0	0.0	9.0	24.7	0.0	0.0	0.6	0	4	143-4
146	0.0	0.0	0.0	0.0	0.0	0.0	0.0	0.0	0.0	3.2	0.0	5.3	0.0	0.0	18.0	12.3	0.0	0.0	0.9	0	6	146
145,147-8	0.0	0.0	0.0	0.0	0.0	0.0	0.0	0.0	0.0	3.2	0.0	0.0	6.0	0.0	0.0	0.0	0.0	0.0	0.3	0	2	145,147-8
150	0.0	0.0	0.0	0.0	0.0	2.6	5.4	0.0	11.8	6.5	16.7	0.0	11.9	20.8	9.0	49.4	47.6	0.0	2.1	0	14	150
151	0.0	0.0	0.0	0.0	0.0	0.0	5.4	8.5	11.8	3.2	16.7	105.8	59.5	145.8	108.1	185.2	261.9	444.4	17.6	2	118	151
152	0.0	0.0	0.0	0.0	2.2	2.6	2.7	0.0	0.0	0.0	0.0	5.3	6.0	6.9	0.0	0.0	6.0	0.0	0.6	0	4	152
153	0.0	0.0	0.0	0.0	0.0	0.0	2.7	0.0	14.7	29.1	29.2	47.6	47.6	97.2	117.1	185.2	166.7	370.4	15.4	3	103	153
154	0.0	0.0	0.0	0.0	0.0	0.0	0.0	5.6	2.9	3.2	4.2	26.5	23.8	41.7	18.0	12.3	23.8	0.0	3.4	3	23	154
155.0	0.0	0.0	0.0	0.0	0.0	0.0	0.0	0.0	2.9	3.2	0.0	0.0	0.0	6.9	0.0	0.0	0.0	0.0	0.4	0	3	155.0
155.1	0.0	0.0	0.0	0.0	0.0	0.0	0.0	0.0	0.0	0.0	0.0	5.3	6.0	27.8	27.0	24.7	23.8	0.0	1.8	0	12	155.1
156	0.0	0.0	0.0	0.0	0.0	2.6	0.0	0.0	2.9	3.2	4.2	0.0	0.0	6.9	18.0	12.3	23.8	37.0	1.2	0	8	156
157	0.0	0.0	0.0	0.0	0.0	0.0	0.0	0.0	0.0	0.0	4.2	10.6	0.0	34.7	72.1	49.4	0.0	74.1	3.7	0	25	157
160	0.0	0.0	0.0	0.0	0.0	0.0	0.0	0.0	0.0	0.0	0.0	10.6	6.0	0.0	0.0	0.0	0.0	0.0	0.4	0	3	160
161	0.0	0.0	0.0	0.0	0.0	0.0	0.0	0.0	0.0	6.5	0.0	0.0	0.0	6.9	0.0	12.3	23.8	37.0	0.7	0	5	161
162-3	0.0	0.0	0.0	0.0	0.0	0.0	0.0	0.0	0.0	9.7	8.3	15.9	17.9	6.9	36.0	49.4	0.0	0.0	3.0	2	20	162-3
170	0.0	0.0	0.0	0.0	2.2	15.7	13.6	36.7	61.9	80.9	125.0	185.2	95.2	104.2	99.1	74.1	95.2	185.2	28.3	4	189	170
171	0.0	0.0	0.0	0.0	0.0	0.0	27.1	31.1	50.1	29.1	50.0	58.2	71.4	41.7	45.0	24.7	47.6	37.0	16.2	4	108	171
172	0.0	0.0	0.0	0.0	0.0	0.0	0.0	0.0	0.0	3.2	0.0	10.6	6.0	0.0	9.0	0.0	0.0	0.0	0.4	0	3	172
173	0.0	0.0	0.0	0.0	2.2	0.0	0.0	0.0	0.0	9.7	8.3	10.6	29.8	41.7	18.0	0.0	0.0	0.0	3.4	2	23	173
174	0.0	0.0	0.0	0.0	0.0	2.6	0.0	2.8	0.0	0.0	16.7	15.9	11.9	20.8	45.0	37.0	23.8	0.0	3.4	1	23	174
175	0.0	0.0	0.0	3.0	2.2	0.0	0.0	0.0	17.7	25.9	20.8	42.3	35.7	13.9	18.0	12.3	0.0	37.0	6.6	1	44	175
176	0.0	0.0	0.0	0.0	0.0	0.0	5.4	2.8	2.9	3.2	4.2	0.0	17.9	13.9	18.0	12.3	0.0	37.0	1.9	0	13	176
180	1.0	0.0	0.0	1.5	0.0	0.0	0.0	2.8	0.0	0.0	8.3	5.3	6.0	20.8	0.0	12.3	0.0	0.0	1.8	0	12	180
181.0	0.0	0.0	0.0	0.0	0.0	2.6	0.0	0.0	0.0	3.2	0.0	5.3	0.0	6.9	36.0	24.7	142.9	37.0	2.7	2	18	181.0
190	0.0	0.0	0.0	0.0	0.0	7.9	2.7	0.0	0.0	0.0	4.2	5.3	29.8	6.9	0.0	0.0	23.8	37.0	1.8	0	12	190
191	0.0	0.0	0.0	0.0	0.0	0.0	2.7	11.3	2.9	16.2	33.3	26.5	71.4	55.6	144.1	209.9	238.1	296.3	17.2	17	115	191
192	0.0	0.0	0.0	0.0	0.0	2.6	0.0	0.0	0.0	0.0	0.0	0.0	0.0	0.0	0.0	0.0	0.0	0.0	0.0	0	0	192
193	3.0	2.1	2.3	0.0	2.2	0.0	8.1	2.8	5.9	9.7	20.8	0.0	17.9	13.9	9.0	0.0	0.0	0.0	4.3	0	29	193
194	0.0	0.0	0.0	4.6	0.0	0.0	0.0	5.6	2.9	3.2	0.0	0.0	0.0	13.9	18.0	12.3	0.0	0.0	1.9	1	13	194
195	0.0	0.0	0.0	0.0	0.0	0.0	0.0	0.0	0.0	0.0	0.0	0.0	0.0	0.0	0.0	0.0	0.0	0.0	0.0	0	0	195
196	0.0	0.0	2.3	0.0	0.0	0.0	0.0	0.0	0.0	0.0	4.2	0.0	0.0	6.9	0.0	12.3	0.0	0.0	0.9	1	6	196
197	0.0	0.0	0.0	0.0	0.0	0.0	0.0	0.0	0.0	0.0	0.0	0.0	0.0	0.0	0.0	0.0	0.0	0.0	0.0	0	0	197
200	0.0	1.0	0.0	0.0	0.0	0.0	0.0	0.0	2.9	0.0	4.2	5.3	0.0	13.9	0.0	0.0	0.0	0.0	1.0	0	7	200
201	0.0	0.0	0.0	0.0	0.0	0.0	5.4	2.8	0.0	0.0	0.0	5.3	0.0	13.9	0.0	0.0	0.0	0.0	0.9	0	6	201
203	0.0	0.0	0.0	0.0	0.0	0.0	2.7	0.0	2.9	0.0	0.0	5.3	0.0	6.9	0.0	0.0	0.0	0.0	0.4	0	3	203
204	4.0	2.1	0.0	0.0	0.0	2.6	0.0	0.0	5.9	0.0	4.2	10.6	35.7	13.9	0.0	37.0	0.0	111.1	4.0	0	27	204
202,205	0.0	0.0	0.0	0.0	0.0	0.0	0.0	0.0	2.9	0.0	0.0	5.3	0.0	13.9	9.0	0.0	0.0	0.0	0.7	0	5	202,205
OTHER	0.0	0.0	0.0	0.0	0.0	2.6	0.0	0.0	5.9	6.5	8.3	10.6	11.9	13.9	9.0	98.8	23.8	74.1	3.7	0	25	OTHER
140-205	8.0	5.2	4.6	9.1	11.2	44.6	75.9	121.5	203.5	262.1	383.3	640.2	631.0	847.2	945.9	1185.2	1142.9	1814.8	155.7	36	1041	**140-205**
RATE PER CASE IN PERIOD	1.00	1.05	1.14	1.52	2.24	2.62	2.71	2.82	2.95	3.24	4.17	5.29	5.95	6.94	9.01	12.35	23.81	37.04	0.15	-	-	**RATE PER CASE IN PERIOD**

CANADA, SASKATCHEWAN

The province of Saskatchewan has had free cancer treatment services since 1944. There are two clinics, one in Saskatoon and one in Regina where all patients investigated for malignancy must be seen. As in Alberta, professional fees are paid for all cases on whom a malignant diagnosis is made. The data in this province can be regarded as complete.

Registry Title and Addrees : Saskatchewan Provincial Cancer Registry, c/o University Hospital, Saskatoon, and c/o Grey Nuns' Hospital, Regina. Supported by the Provincial Government.

Registration. Registrations are made by doctors from hospital in-patients and out-patients; from pathologists in pathology departments; by Provincial Registrars from death certificates; and by doctors attending cases at home.

Follow-up. All registrations are followed-up for life.

Physical description. The Registry covers the Province of Saskatchewan which lies between Alberta on the west and Manitoba on the east, between latitudes 49° and 60° North, and longitudes 110° and 102° West. Total registration area is 651,903 square kilometres.

Demographic Description. Total population of the area under survey 925,200. Twelve per cent of the population live in conurbations of more than 100,000.

Medical Services. Total number of hospital beds of all kinds 7,454. Total number of doctors in practice in registration area 933. Cancer causes approximately 17 % of all deaths.

Publications. Annual Report of Saskatchewan Cancer Commission.

TABLE 10 A
CANADA, SASKATCHEWAN :
POPULATION (100,000s), 1961

AGE (in years)	MALES No.	MALES Per Cent	FEMALES No.	FEMALES Per Cent
0 –	0.5830	12.16	0.5540	12.43
5 –	0.5480	11.43	0.5210	11.69
10 –	0.4810	10.03	0.4610	10.35
15 –	0.3740	7.80	0.3540	7.94
20 –	0.2900	6.05	0.2800	6.28
25 –	0.2850	5.94	0.2670	5.99
30 –	0.3020	6.30	0.2820	6.33
35 –	0.2980	6.21	0.2910	6.53
40 –	0.2880	6.01	0.2820	6.33
45 –	0.2700	5.63	0.2560	5.75
50 –	0.2380	4.96	0.2110	4.74
55 –	0.2020	4.21	0.1700	3.82
60 –	0.1640	3.42	0.1450	3.25
65 –	0.1520	3.17	0.1300	2.92
70 –	0.1420	2.96	0.1110	2.49
75 –	0.1030	2.15	0.0770	1.73
80 –	0.0510	1.06	0.0420	0.94
85 – and over	0.0250	0.52	0.0220	0.49
TOTAL	4.7960	100.00	4.4560	100.00

NOTES

TO TABLES 10 A, B and C

(I)   I. L. number 193 excludes benign and unspecified tumours of the central nervous system.

(II)   Carcinoma in situ included.

TABLE 10 B
CANADA, SASKATCHEWAN :
MALE INCIDENCE RATES, 1960 - 62.

AVERAGE ANNUAL INCIDENCE PER 100,000

International List No.	0-	5-	10-	15-	20-	25-	30-	35-	40-	45-	50-	55-	60-	65-	70-	75-	80-	85- and over	All Ages	No. of Cases — All Ages	No. of Cases — Age Unknown
140	0.0	0.0	0.0	0.0	1.1	7.0	4.4	13.4	20.8	38.3	64.4	72.6	69.1	133.8	131.5	97.1	163.4	106.7	26.1	376	0
141	0.0	0.0	0.0	0.0	0.0	0.0	0.0	0.0	2.3	1.2	0.0	0.0	4.1	2.2	4.7	0.0	0.0	26.7	0.7	10	0
142	0.0	0.0	0.0	0.0	2.3	2.3	5.5	2.2	4.6	4.9	2.8	1.7	6.1	4.4	0.0	6.5	6.5	26.7	2.2	32	0
143-4	0.0	0.0	0.0	0.0	0.0	0.0	0.0	0.0	1.2	1.2	1.4	9.9	2.0	4.4	9.4	9.7	6.5	40.0	1.5	22	0
146	0.0	0.0	0.0	0.0	0.0	0.0	0.0	0.0	0.0	1.2	1.4	1.7	4.1	0.0	0.0	0.0	0.0	0.0	0.4	6	0
145,147-9	0.0	0.0	0.0	0.0	0.0	1.2	0.0	0.0	1.2	2.5	2.8	0.0	6.1	8.8	4.7	9.7	6.5	40.0	1.1	16	0
150	0.0	0.0	0.0	0.0	0.0	1.2	2.2	3.4	5.8	12.3	5.6	0.0	20.3	13.2	16.4	42.1	26.1	0.0	3.5	50	0
151	0.0	0.0	0.0	0.0	0.0	1.2	2.2	3.4	5.8	12.3	22.4	62.7	75.2	118.4	164.3	178.0	248.4	186.7	23.8	343	0
152	0.0	0.0	0.0	0.0	0.0	0.0	0.0	0.0	1.2	1.2	1.2	0.0	2.0	0.0	0.0	9.7	6.5	0.0	0.4	6	0
153	0.0	0.0	0.0	0.0	0.0	1.2	2.2	2.2	8.1	12.3	16.8	38.0	46.7	74.6	98.6	158.6	117.6	213.3	16.6	239	0
154	0.0	0.0	0.0	0.0	0.0	0.0	0.0	0.0	3.5	16.0	28.0	34.7	46.7	76.8	115.0	145.6	98.0	80.0	16.0	230	0
155.0	0.0	0.0	0.7	0.0	0.0	0.0	0.0	0.0	0.0	3.7	1.4	0.0	8.1	4.4	0.0	9.7	6.5	13.3	1.1	16	0
155.1	0.0	0.0	0.0	0.0	0.0	0.0	0.0	0.0	0.0	0.0	1.4	6.6	0.0	15.4	11.7	22.7	13.1	40.0	2.0	29	0
156	0.0	0.0	0.0	0.0	0.0	0.0	0.0	2.2	1.2	0.0	1.4	0.0	4.1	2.2	14.1	9.7	6.5	0.0	1.0	15	0
157	0.0	0.0	0.0	0.0	0.0	0.0	0.0	0.0	0.0	6.2	5.6	21.5	40.7	30.7	65.7	45.3	104.6	53.3	8.3	120	0
160	0.0	0.0	0.0	0.0	0.0	0.0	0.0	0.0	0.0	1.2	0.0	1.7	2.0	4.4	4.7	0.0	0.0	0.0	0.5	7	0
161	0.0	0.0	0.0	0.0	1.1	1.2	0.0	0.0	0.0	2.5	0.0	1.7	0.0	8.8	7.0	3.2	0.0	0.0	0.8	11	0
162-3	0.0	0.0	0.0	1.8	1.1	1.2	1.1	5.6	12.7	23.5	39.2	77.6	115.9	136.0	150.2	119.7	104.6	120.0	24.9	358	0
170	0.0	0.0	0.0	0.0	0.0	0.0	0.0	0.0	0.0	0.0	0.0	0.0	0.0	4.4	4.7	3.2	0.0	0.0	0.3	5	0
177	0.0	0.0	0.0	0.0	1.1	0.0	0.0	8.9	5.8	1.2	5.6	41.3	105.7	206.1	394.4	569.6	699.3	786.7	47.7	686	0
178	0.0	0.0	0.0	0.0	0.0	5.8	3.3	0.0	1.2	1.2	1.4	3.3	2.0	2.2	2.3	0.0	0.0	0.0	2.1	30	0
179.0	0.0	0.0	0.0	0.0	0.0	0.0	0.0	0.0	1.2	1.2	0.0	0.0	2.0	6.6	0.0	12.9	13.1	13.3	0.9	13	0
180	1.1	0.0	0.0	0.0	0.0	0.0	2.2	2.2	10.4	8.6	15.4	21.5	14.2	26.3	32.9	48.5	26.1	66.7	7.2	103	0
181.0	0.0	0.0	0.0	0.0	0.0	3.5	3.3	4.5	4.6	12.3	16.8	36.3	38.6	89.9	112.7	116.5	130.7	266.7	16.5	237	0
190	0.0	0.0	0.0	0.0	1.1	0.0	11.0	1.1	1.2	6.2	2.8	5.0	8.1	6.6	11.7	9.7	13.1	26.7	2.6	37	0
191	0.0	0.0	0.0	0.0	0.0	3.5	11.0	12.3	32.4	63.0	93.8	163.4	237.8	368.4	495.3	705.5	934.6	920.0	83.1	1195	0
192	0.0	0.0	0.0	0.0	0.0	0.0	0.0	1.1	1.2	34.6	2.8	3.6	7.0	11.0	7.0	3.2	6.5	0.0	2.8	41	0
193	1.7	2.4	0.0	0.9	1.1	1.2	2.2	6.7	10.4	7.4	4.2	11.6	10.2	4.4	14.1	0.0	0.0	0.0	4.1	59	0
194	0.0	0.0	0.0	0.0	0.0	0.0	1.1	0.0	1.2	3.7	0.0	5.0	4.1	0.0	11.7	3.2	13.1	0.0	1.4	20	0
195	0.0	0.0	0.0	0.0	0.0	0.0	0.0	0.0	0.0	0.0	0.0	0.0	2.0	0.0	2.3	0.0	0.0	0.0	0.1	2	0
196	1.1	1.8	0.7	0.9	1.1	1.2	2.2	4.5	2.3	1.2	2.8	1.7	2.0	6.6	0.0	0.0	0.0	13.3	0.5	7	0
197	0.6	1.2	2.8	0.9	1.1	1.2	0.0	2.2	4.6	8.6	18.2	3.3	4.1	24.1	11.7	9.7	0.0	0.0	2.7	39	0
200	0.0	0.0	1.4	0.0	9.2	2.3	2.2	2.2	4.6	4.9	2.8	11.6	24.4	8.8	32.9	42.1	26.1	13.3	6.7	97	0
201	0.0	0.0	0.0	0.0	0.0	0.0	1.1	1.1	1.2	1.2	5.6	1.7	4.1	21.9	7.0	3.2	19.6	0.0	2.5	36	0
203	0.0	3.0	2.1	2.7	1.1	1.2	0.0	3.4	5.8	0.0	11.2	5.0	16.3	37.3	7.0	9.7	13.1	13.3	2.5	36	0
204	4.6	0.0	0.0	0.9	0.0	0.0	1.1	1.1	1.2	4.9	1.4	21.5	28.5	0.0	54.0	84.1	65.4	66.7	10.4	150	0
202,205	0.0	0.6	0.0	0.9	0.0	0.0	2.2	0.0	1.2	1.2	2.8	3.3	2.0	13.2	2.3	16.2	0.0	0.0	1.1	16	0
OTHER	1.7	0.0	0.0	0.0	0.0	0.0	1.1	0.0	1.2	1.2	2.8	5.0	8.1	13.2	9.4	6.5	13.1	13.3	2.2	32	0
140-205	12.0	9.7	8.3	8.9	20.7	29.2	49.7	80.5	150.5	292.6	382.4	673.3	967.5	1475.9	2011.7	2511.3	2888.9	3146.7	328.5	4727	0
RATE PER CASE IN PERIOD	0.57	0.61	0.69	0.89	1.15	1.17	1.10	1.12	1.16	1.23	1.40	1.65	2.03	2.19	2.35	3.24	6.54	13.33	0.07	-	-

AGE IN YEARS

TABLE 10 C
CANADA, SASKATCHEWAN :
FEMALE INCIDENCE RATES, 1960 - 62.

AVERAGE ANNUAL INCIDENCE PER 100,000

INTER-NATIONAL LIST No.	0-	5-	10-	15-	20-	25-	30-	35-	40-	45-	50-	55-	60-	65-	70-	75-	80-	85- AND OVER	ALL AGES	AGE UNKNOWN	ALL AGES	INTER-NATIONAL LIST No.
140	0.0	0.0	0.0	0.0	1.2	0.0	0.0	0.0	0.0	1.3	3.2	0.0	4.6	7.7	3.0	0.0	7.9	30.3	1.0	0	13	140
141	0.0	0.0	0.0	0.0	0.0	1.2	0.0	0.0	0.0	1.3	0.0	0.0	2.3	2.6	3.0	8.7	23.8	0.0	0.7	0	10	141
142	0.0	0.0	0.0	0.0	2.4	1.2	0.0	2.3	4.7	2.6	3.2	2.0	11.5	2.6	6.0	8.7	7.9	30.3	1.8	0	24	142
143-4	0.0	0.0	0.0	0.0	0.0	0.0	2.4	0.0	0.0	0.0	1.6	0.0	4.6	2.6	3.0	8.7	7.9	0.0	0.9	0	12	143-4
146	0.0	0.0	0.0	0.0	0.0	0.0	0.0	0.0	1.2	0.0	0.0	0.0	2.3	2.6	3.0	0.0	0.0	0.0	0.3	0	4	146
145,147-8	0.0	0.0	0.0	0.0	0.0	0.0	0.0	0.0	0.0	2.6	0.0	0.0	0.0	7.7	9.0	0.0	0.0	0.0	0.6	0	8	145,147-8
150	0.0	0.0	0.0	0.0	0.0	0.0	0.0	0.0	0.0	1.3	0.0	0.0	0.0	5.1	3.0	0.0	0.0	0.0	0.3	0	4	150
151	0.0	0.0	0.0	0.0	0.0	0.0	2.4	1.1	2.4	7.8	11.1	19.6	29.9	48.7	51.1	69.3	79.4	60.6	8.0	0	107	151
152	0.0	0.0	0.0	0.0	0.0	0.0	0.0	0.0	1.2	1.3	3.2	2.0	2.3	10.3	3.0	4.3	0.0	0.0	0.9	0	12	152
153	0.0	0.0	0.0	0.9	2.4	3.7	7.1	6.9	8.3	20.8	28.4	45.1	62.1	79.5	114.1	134.2	182.5	106.1	17.9	0	239	153
154	0.0	0.0	0.0	0.0	0.0	0.0	2.4	2.3	7.1	9.1	9.5	29.4	41.4	38.5	78.1	60.6	111.1	90.9	9.8	0	131	154
155.0	0.0	0.6	0.0	0.0	0.0	0.0	1.2	1.1	0.0	0.0	0.0	0.0	0.0	2.6	3.0	8.7	0.0	0.0	0.5	0	7	155.0
155.1	0.0	0.0	0.0	0.0	0.0	0.0	0.0	1.1	0.0	3.9	3.2	7.8	9.2	20.5	33.0	60.6	79.4	45.5	4.5	0	60	155.1
156	0.0	0.0	0.0	0.0	0.0	0.0	0.0	1.1	0.0	2.6	1.6	2.0	2.3	0.0	3.0	8.7	0.0	30.3	0.8	0	11	156
157	0.0	0.0	0.0	0.0	0.0	0.0	0.0	0.0	1.2	5.2	1.6	11.8	18.4	23.1	24.0	39.0	55.6	30.3	4.1	0	55	157
160	0.0	0.0	0.0	0.0	0.0	0.0	0.0	0.0	2.4	1.3	3.2	0.0	2.3	2.6	0.0	4.3	0.0	30.3	0.7	0	10	160
161	0.0	0.0	0.0	0.0	0.0	0.0	0.0	0.0	0.0	0.0	0.0	0.0	0.0	0.0	0.0	0.0	0.0	0.0	0.0	0	0	161
162-3	0.0	0.0	0.0	0.9	0.0	0.0	0.0	1.1	2.4	2.6	12.6	21.6	11.5	7.7	6.0	13.0	7.9	0.0	2.9	0	39	162-3
170	0.0	0.0	0.0	0.0	2.4	7.5	29.6	51.5	138.3	164.1	142.2	113.7	177.0	200.0	192.2	216.5	285.7	287.9	59.3	0	793	170
171	0.0	0.0	0.0	0.0	1.2	6.2	13.0	49.3	41.4	50.8	41.1	25.5	23.0	43.6	39.0	21.6	23.8	0.0	16.5	0	221	171
172	0.0	0.0	0.0	0.0	0.0	0.0	3.5	13.7	14.2	35.2	47.4	60.8	75.9	66.7	48.0	30.3	39.7	30.3	15.3	0	204	172
173	0.0	0.0	0.0	0.9	0.0	0.0	2.4	0.0	0.0	0.0	0.0	0.0	0.0	0.0	0.0	0.0	0.0	0.0	0.2	0	3	173
174	0.0	0.0	0.0	0.0	0.0	0.0	0.0	0.0	0.0	0.0	0.0	0.0	0.0	0.0	0.0	0.0	0.0	0.0	0.0	0	0	174
175	0.0	0.0	0.0	0.0	2.4	5.0	4.7	8.0	9.5	18.2	28.4	23.5	43.7	38.5	39.0	56.3	39.7	15.2	10.2	0	136	175
176	0.0	0.0	0.7	0.0	0.0	0.0	2.4	1.1	0.0	2.6	6.3	5.9	0.0	2.6	6.0	17.3	55.6	30.3	2.1	0	28	176
180	1.2	0.0	0.0	0.0	0.0	1.2	1.2	1.1	5.9	3.9	1.6	17.6	0.0	17.9	18.0	21.6	39.7	45.5	3.7	0	49	180
181.0	0.0	0.0	0.0	0.0	0.0	0.0	3.5	1.1	2.4	2.6	7.9	3.9	0.0	15.4	33.0	30.3	31.7	45.5	2.9	0	39	181.0
190	0.0	0.0	0.0	0.9	2.4	1.2	4.7	2.3	4.7	2.6	0.0	1.6	0.0	7.7	6.0	17.3	0.0	0.0	2.0	0	27	190
191	0.0	0.0	0.0	0.0	3.6	1.2	13.0	12.6	27.2	59.9	49.0	86.3	124.1	212.8	282.3	368.0	682.5	515.2	45.3	0	606	191
192	1.8	0.6	0.0	0.0	1.2	0.0	0.0	0.0	1.2	2.6	0.0	2.0	0.0	0.0	3.0	0.0	7.9	0.0	0.8	0	11	192
193	1.2	2.6	2.9	0.9	0.0	0.0	1.2	5.7	2.4	1.3	4.7	11.8	0.0	0.0	6.0	0.0	0.0	0.0	2.3	0	31	193
194	0.0	0.6	0.7	0.0	2.4	0.0	2.4	1.1	3.5	3.9	0.0	7.8	0.0	0.0	0.0	17.3	0.0	15.2	1.7	0	23	194
195	1.8	0.6	0.7	0.0	0.0	0.0	1.2	1.1	0.0	0.0	0.0	0.0	0.0	0.0	0.0	0.0	7.9	0.0	0.4	0	5	195
196	0.6	0.0	1.4	4.7	0.0	0.0	1.2	1.1	0.0	0.0	1.6	0.0	0.0	0.0	0.0	4.3	0.0	15.2	1.0	0	13	196
197	1.2	0.0	0.7	2.8	1.2	1.2	3.5	1.1	2.4	1.3	1.6	7.8	0.0	5.1	15.0	4.3	0.0	30.3	2.1	0	28	197
200	0.6	0.6	0.7	1.9	1.2	5.0	2.4	0.0	3.5	7.8	0.0	9.8	0.0	35.9	24.0	21.6	15.9	0.0	4.0	0	53	200
201	0.0	0.6	0.0	2.8	4.8	0.0	3.5	0.0	2.4	1.3	0.0	0.0	0.0	0.0	6.0	0.0	0.0	0.0	1.5	0	20	201
203	0.0	0.0	0.0	0.0	0.0	1.2	5.9	1.1	2.4	3.9	0.0	3.9	0.0	12.8	12.0	4.3	7.9	0.0	1.1	0	15	203
204	4.2	3.8	3.6	1.9	2.4	1.2	1.2	1.1	3.5	3.9	0.0	9.8	0.0	5.1	21.0	47.6	15.9	0.0	4.6	0	62	204
202,205	0.0	0.0	0.0	0.0	0.0	0.0	1.2	1.1	2.4	0.0	0.0	2.0	0.0	5.1	6.0	0.0	0.0	0.0	0.7	0	9	202,205
OTHER	0.0	0.0	0.0	0.0	0.0	1.2	0.0	1.1	3.5	2.6	0.0	3.9	0.0	7.7	21.0	26.0	15.9	15.2	2.1	0	28	OTHER
140-205	12.6	10.2	11.6	17.9	31.0	37.5	111.1	169.5	299.1	427.1	415.5	541.2	648.3	941.0	1123.1	1333.3	1825.4	1500.0	235.6	0	3150	140-205
RATE PER CASE IN PERIOD	0.60	0.64	0.72	0.94	1.19	1.25	1.18	1.15	1.18	1.30	1.58	1.96	2.30	2.56	3.00	4.33	7.94	15.15	0.07	-	-	RATE PER CASE IN PERIOD

CHILE

Registry Title and Address : Chile National Cancer Registry, Division del Cancer y Enfermedades Cronicas, Servicio Nacional de Salud, Agustinas 715, Santiago, Chile.

Physical Description. The Registry covers the whole of Chile, a country extending over much of western South America, whose eastern boundary, separating it from Argentina, is the Andes chain of mountains. It lies between latitudes 17^U 15' and 55^U 59' South, and longitudes 66° 30' and 75° 48' West. The total registration area is 741,600 square kilometres.

Demographic Description. Total population of area under survey is 7,743,900.

TABLE 11 A

CHILE :
POPULATION (100,000s), CENSUS 1960

AGE (in years)	MALES No.	MALES Per Cent	FEMALES No.	FEMALES Per Cent
0-	6.1230	16.11	5.9430	15.07
5-	5.1860	13.65	5.1030	12.94
10-	4.3580	11.47	4.3480	11.02
15-	3.6460	9.60	3.8080	9.65
20-	3.1080	8.18	3.3090	8.39
25-	2.6910	7.08	2.8640	7.26
30-	2.3500	6.18	2.5190	6.39
35-	2.0780	5.47	2.2550	5.72
40-	1.8500	4.87	2.0000	5.07
45-	1.7190	4.52	1.8090	4.59
50-	1.4480	3.81	1.5240	3.86
55-	1.1170	2.94	1.2010	3.04
60-	0.8590	2.26	0.9440	2.39
65-	0.6810	1.79	0.7520	1.91
70-	0.4310	1.13	0.5170	1.31
75-	0.2210	0.58	0.3220	0.82
80-	0.0940	0.25	0.1550	0.39
85- and over	0.0370	0.10	0.0690	0.17
TOTAL	37.9970	100.00	39.4420	100.00

NOTES

TO TABLES 11 A, B and C

(I)   Rates for 155.0, 155.1 and 179.0 are available for one year (1961) and for 181.0 for two years (1959 and 1961). They are as follows :

Age in years	Annual incidence per 100,000 Males 155.0	155.1	179.0	181.0	Females 155.0	155.1	181.0
0-4	0.0	0.2	0.0	0.0	0.0	0.0	0.0
5-9	0.0	0.0	0.0	0.0	0.0	0.0	0.0
10-14	0.2	0.0	0.0	0.0	0.0	0.0	0.1
15-19	1.1	0.0	0.0	0.0	0.0	0.0	0.1
20-24	1.3	0.0	0.6	0.0	0.0	0.6	0.0
25-29	0.7	0.0	0.0	0.2	0.3	0.7	0.0
30-34	0.9	0.0	0.0	0.0	0.4	0.0	0.4
35-39	1.4	1.0	0.5	0.0	0.4	1.3	0.0
40-44	1.1	1.1	1.1	0.8	5.0	4.0	0.3
45-49	1.2	3.5	1.7	1.2	3.3	9.4	0.8
50-54	4.1	3.5	1.4	1.4	8.5	13.1	2.3
55-59	9.8	6.3	1.8	3.1	11.7	17.5	2.1
60-64	10.5	8.1	9.3	5.2	12.7	28.6	6.4
65-69	16.2	11.7	7.3	14.0	13.3	47.9	2.0
70-74	23.2	7.0	13.9	20.9	11.6	46.4	6.8
75-79	4.5	22.6	45.2	22.6	18.6	15.5	4.7
80-84	21.3	10.6	21.3	26.6	0.0	19.4	9.7
85 and over	0.0	0.0	27.0	13.5	0.0	28.9	0.0
All ages	1.8	1.2	1.2	1.1	2.0	4.3	0.6

(II)   I.L. number 193 excludes benign and unspecified tumours of the central nervous system.

(III)   Carcinoma in situ included.

TABLE 11 B
CHILE :
MALE INCIDENCE RATES, 1959 - 61.

INTER-NATIONAL LIST No.	0–	5–	10–	15–	20–	25–	30–	35–	40–	45–	50–	55–	60–	65–	70–	75–	80–	85– AND OVER	ALL AGES	AGE UNKNOWN	ALL AGES	INTER-NATIONAL LIST No.
140	0.1	0.1	0.0	0.0	0.0	0.0	0.1	0.6	0.5	2.1	1.8	1.5	3.1	4.9	11.6	10.6	17.7	9.0	0.7	0	80	140
141	0.0	0.0	0.0	0.0	0.0	0.1	0.0	0.2	0.7	1.2	2.5	1.2	3.1	2.0	3.1	7.5	3.5	0.0	0.4	0	49	141
142	0.0	0.0	0.0	0.1	0.0	0.6	0.6	0.6	0.5	1.0	0.7	1.8	1.2	1.5	3.9	1.5	3.5	9.0	0.4	0	42	142
143-4	0.0	0.1	0.0	0.0	0.0	0.2	0.0	0.2	0.0	0.0	1.4	0.6	2.3	1.0	1.5	6.0	7.1	0.0	0.3	0	38	143-4
146	0.0	0.0	0.0	0.0	0.0	0.0	0.0	0.0	0.0	1.0	0.2	0.3	0.8	1.0	0.8	0.0	0.0	0.0	0.1	0	7	146
145,147-8	0.0	0.0	0.0	0.0	0.2	0.0	0.3	0.0	0.2	1.0	1.2	1.5	2.3	3.9	2.3	1.5	0.0	0.0	0.3	1	38	145,147-8
150	0.0	0.0	0.0	0.1	0.1	0.4	1.3	2.4	7.2	8.5	24.9	40.3	48.1	65.1	61.9	86.0	56.7	72.1	6.8	1	775	150
151	0.1	0.1	0.1	0.2	0.9	2.8	8.2	12.5	35.7	58.8	96.0	168.9	210.7	236.9	281.5	319.8	273.0	252.3	29.5	3	3368	151
152	0.0	0.0	0.0	0.0	0.0	0.1	0.1	0.0	0.2	0.4	0.7	0.6	0.0	0.4	1.5	0.0	0.0	0.0	0.1	0	15	152
153	0.0	0.1	0.0	0.3	0.3	0.4	0.0	1.1	2.0	3.5	6.9	12.5	13.6	20.6	19.3	24.1	35.5	45.0	2.2	1	252	153
154	0.0	0.0	0.0	0.3	0.8	0.4	0.4	1.3	2.3	2.3	7.6	10.7	17.5	15.7	15.5	10.6	21.3	63.1	2.1	1	236	154
155	0.1	0.1	0.1	0.5	0.8	0.6	1.1	1.8	1.8	5.2	5.3	12.5	20.2	25.9	24.0	22.6	21.3	9.0	2.6	0	299	155
156	0.1	0.1	0.5	0.8	0.9	0.4	1.3	0.6	3.8	3.3	7.1	12.5	23.6	19.1	15.5	19.6	14.2	18.0	2.3	0	266	156
157	0.0	0.0	0.1	0.0	0.2	0.1	0.1	0.2	1.8	3.5	5.8	11.6	16.7	19.6	26.3	25.6	24.8	36.0	2.1	1	244	157
160	0.0	0.0	0.0	0.3	0.2	0.0	0.3	0.0	0.2	0.6	0.9	1.2	0.8	1.0	2.3	1.5	3.5	0.0	0.2	0	26	160
161	0.0	0.0	0.0	0.0	0.1	0.0	0.1	0.0	2.0	5.6	3.7	9.3	11.3	11.7	9.3	0.0	0.0	0.0	1.4	0	154	161
162-3	0.1	0.1	0.1	0.2	0.3	0.5	1.7	4.5	11.4	18.0	30.4	46.0	66.0	68.0	79.7	60.3	49.6	90.1	8.5	0	971	162-3
170	0.0	0.0	0.0	0.0	0.0	0.2	0.1	0.3	0.7	0.6	0.7	1.2	0.4	1.0	0.8	3.0	7.1	9.0	0.2	0	28	170
177	0.4	0.0	0.2	0.1	0.2	0.1	0.4	0.5	1.3	2.5	9.4	14.6	35.3	72.9	122.2	167.4	209.2	225.2	6.3	0	713	177
178	0.0	0.1	0.0	0.4	1.7	3.1	5.5	4.3	3.1	2.7	2.1	1.5	2.3	6.4	7.7	9.0	7.1	18.0	1.8	0	205	178
179	0.4	0.0	0.0	0.0	0.5	0.0	0.0	0.8	1.6	1.7	1.6	3.6	7.4	9.3	9.3	21.1	17.7	9.0	1.0	0	117	179
180	0.4	0.0	0.0	0.0	0.1	0.1	0.3	0.8	1.8	1.9	3.5	6.9	4.3	7.3	7.0	10.6	7.1	0.0	1.1	0	120	180
181	0.0	0.1	0.1	0.1	0.0	0.1	0.1	0.6	1.3	1.4	1.4	4.8	3.1	9.8	14.7	12.1	17.7	18.0	0.9	0	104	181
190	0.1	0.0	0.2	0.5	0.4	0.2	0.4	0.8	0.7	0.2	1.6	3.3	1.9	4.4	5.4	9.0	14.2	18.0	0.6	0	73	190
191	1.0	0.1	0.2	0.5	0.3	0.4	0.7	1.3	0.9	3.9	3.9	6.9	7.0	13.2	20.9	15.1	31.9	54.1	1.6	0	188	191
192	1.0	0.1	0.0	0.1	0.1	0.1	0.0	0.0	0.4	0.4	0.5	0.3	1.2	0.5	0.8	1.5	9.0	9.0	0.3	0	35	192
193	0.4	0.3	0.2	0.8	0.6	1.0	0.6	1.0	1.1	0.8	1.4	1.2	3.9	0.0	0.0	3.0	3.5	9.0	0.7	0	82	193
194	0.0	0.0	0.2	0.2	0.2	0.6	0.4	0.3	0.9	1.6	1.4	3.3	3.9	4.4	4.6	1.5	3.5	9.0	0.6	0	74	194
195	0.1	0.1	0.0	0.1	0.1	0.0	0.4	0.0	0.2	0.2	0.2	0.3	0.0	0.0	0.0	0.0	0.0	0.0	0.1	0	11	195
196	0.1	0.4	0.5	1.9	0.5	0.5	1.0	1.6	3.1	3.3	9.4	6.9	9.7	7.8	10.8	15.1	10.6	9.0	2.0	0	229	196
197	0.1	0.1	0.0	0.2	0.1	0.2	0.0	0.6	0.2	0.2	0.7	0.2	1.6	2.4	3.1	3.0	7.1	0.0	0.3	0	39	197
200	0.4	0.7	0.3	0.8	0.5	0.2	0.6	1.3	0.2	1.2	1.8	4.2	2.7	0.5	3.9	7.5	3.5	0.0	0.9	0	99	200
201	0.1	0.8	0.8	1.4	1.5	2.2	3.0	2.6	4.1	3.5	3.0	2.7	3.9	3.9	1.5	6.0	3.5	9.0	1.7	0	197	201
203	0.0	0.0	0.0	0.1	0.3	0.0	0.1	0.3	0.7	2.3	1.2	3.6	5.4	2.9	3.9	6.0	0.0	0.0	0.6	0	69	203
204	2.1	2.9	3.3	3.1	2.4	3.7	3.0	3.8	3.4	4.3	5.5	6.9	5.0	6.4	7.0	7.5	7.1	9.0	3.4	0	388	204
202,205	0.2	0.1	0.2	0.3	0.0	0.1	0.0	0.3	0.0	0.6	0.5	0.6	0.8	0.5	0.0	0.0	0.0	0.0	0.2	0	23	202,205
OTHER	0.8	0.5	1.0	2.2	1.2	3.1	3.1	6.1	8.5	9.7	17.0	28.9	42.7	54.8	48.7	67.9	70.9	153.2	7.0	4	795	OTHER
140-205	6.4	6.5	7.7	14.8	15.4	22.8	35.7	53.6	105.0	158.8	263.8	435.4	573.5	707.3	832.2	963.8	953.9	1153.2	91.7	11	10449	140-205
RATE PER CASE IN PERIOD	0.05	0.06	0.08	0.09	0.11	0.12	0.14	0.16	0.18	0.19	0.23	0.30	0.39	0.49	0.77	1.51	3.55	9.01	0.01	-	-	RATE PER CASE IN PERIOD

AVERAGE ANNUAL INCIDENCE PER 100,000 — AGE IN YEARS — No. OF CASES IN WHOLE PERIOD

TABLE 11 C

CHILE :

FEMALE INCIDENCE RATES, 1959 - 61.

INTER-NATIONAL LIST No.	AVERAGE ANNUAL INCIDENCE PER 100,000 — AGE IN YEARS																			No. OF CASES IN WHOLE PERIOD		INTER-NATIONAL LIST No.
	0-	5-	10-	15-	20-	25-	30-	35-	40-	45-	50-	55-	60-	65-	70-	75-	80-	85- AND OVER	ALL AGES	AGE UNKNOWN	ALL AGES	
140	0.0	0.0	0.0	0.1	0.1	0.0	0.0	0.1	0.2	0.4	0.7	0.3	0.4	0.9	1.9	3.1	2.2	0.0	0.2	0	20	140
141	0.1	0.0	0.0	0.0	0.0	0.0	0.0	0.3	0.7	0.0	0.7	1.1	1.4	2.7	0.6	1.0	2.2	4.8	0.2	0	28	141
142	0.1	0.1	0.1	0.1	0.2	0.1	0.0	0.4	0.3	0.4	1.1	0.8	1.1	0.4	2.6	1.0	0.0	4.8	0.3	0	32	142
143-4	0.0	0.1	0.0	0.0	0.0	0.1	0.0	0.4	0.7	0.4	0.4	0.8	0.4	1.3	1.3	1.0	0.0	0.0	0.2	0	23	143-4
146	0.0	0.0	0.0	0.1	0.0	0.0	0.0	0.0	0.0	0.0	0.0	0.0	0.0	0.0	0.0	2.1	0.0	0.0	0.0	0	2	146
145,147-8	0.0	0.0	0.0	0.1	0.0	0.1	0.0	0.1	0.0	0.2	0.2	0.3	0.7	0.9	0.6	3.1	0.0	0.0	0.1	1	14	145,147-8
150	0.0	0.0	0.1	0.0	0.2	0.6	0.8	1.3	4.0	6.3	12.9	19.7	25.8	23.0	23.2	21.7	28.0	33.8	3.5	6	413	150
151	0.0	0.0	0.0	0.3	1.0	1.3	3.4	7.8	14.3	22.8	38.7	63.6	97.8	88.2	114.1	101.4	109.7	67.6	13.0	0	1542	151
152	0.0	0.0	0.0	0.0	0.0	0.1	0.3	0.0	0.0	0.2	0.4	0.0	0.7	0.9	0.6	0.0	0.0	0.0	0.1	1	11	152
153	0.0	0.1	0.0	0.1	0.1	0.2	0.9	2.2	2.3	5.0	8.3	11.9	18.0	13.7	22.6	22.8	28.0	33.8	2.6	3	310	153
154	0.0	0.1	0.0	0.2	0.2	0.5	1.3	1.5	3.5	7.6	9.0	13.6	13.1	11.1	12.3	14.5	23.7	19.3	2.5	0	292	154
155	0.0	0.1	0.0	0.1	0.2	0.5	0.8	1.2	6.3	10.9	19.5	26.9	36.0	48.3	44.5	45.5	17.2	33.8	5.4	0	644	155
156	0.2	0.1	0.0	0.4	0.1	0.3	1.5	1.9	4.8	3.9	9.0	11.1	14.1	23.9	19.3	17.6	17.2	14.5	2.7	0	319	156
157	0.0	0.1	0.0	0.2	0.0	0.3	0.5	0.6	2.7	2.6	6.6	9.4	12.0	11.1	15.5	15.5	8.6	4.8	1.8	0	209	157
160	0.0	0.0	0.0	0.0	0.0	0.1	0.4	0.0	0.0	0.0	0.7	1.4	0.7	0.9	2.6	5.2	4.3	0.0	0.3	0	30	160
161	0.0	0.0	0.0	0.2	0.1	0.3	0.0	0.4	0.2	1.3	1.5	1.1	1.1	0.4	2.6	1.0	4.3	0.0	0.3	0	34	161
162-3	0.0	0.1	0.1	0.1	0.3	0.3	0.7	1.8	2.8	6.1	9.8	14.2	17.3	19.9	25.1	17.6	8.6	29.0	2.8	2	332	162-3
170	0.1	0.1	0.2	0.9	0.5	2.1	10.5	21.9	40.0	43.5	49.7	61.9	75.6	70.0	62.5	54.9	64.5	72.5	14.9	6	1759	170
171	0.1	0.1	0.1	0.6	3.9	17.9	53.5	77.8	106.0	123.6	117.0	119.3	116.2	103.7	78.7	56.9	75.3	77.3	35.5	6	4202	171
172	0.0	0.0	0.0	0.1	0.0	0.2	0.7	2.2	4.0	6.1	10.7	12.8	18.4	10.2	11.6	9.3	2.2	4.8	2.4	1	279	172
173	0.0	0.0	0.0	0.4	0.8	1.2	1.3	1.6	1.2	1.3	0.4	0.8	1.1	0.9	0.0	0.0	0.0	0.0	0.6	0	69	173
174	0.1	0.1	0.2	0.0	0.5	1.6	4.6	6.7	9.7	12.5	15.7	15.3	20.8	15.5	14.2	16.6	15.1	19.3	4.2	0	498	174
175	0.0	0.0	0.0	0.4	0.6	1.0	0.5	1.3	3.2	6.4	5.5	7.5	6.0	7.5	2.6	3.1	15.1	0.0	1.5	0	183	175
176	0.0	0.1	0.2	0.2	0.3	0.2	1.9	2.7	3.5	5.0	6.3	8.6	10.9	14.6	11.6	11.4	6.5	4.8	2.1	0	249	176
180	0.4	0.3	0.1	0.1	0.1	0.3	0.3	0.4	1.7	0.9	1.7	3.6	2.8	4.0	5.2	2.1	6.5	4.8	0.8	0	91	180
181	0.0	0.0	0.1	0.1	0.0	0.0	0.3	0.0	0.8	1.1	2.6	1.9	4.2	4.9	4.5	4.1	4.3	4.8	0.6	0	71	181
190	0.1	0.1	0.1	0.1	0.2	0.6	0.3	0.9	0.3	0.9	1.3	3.3	3.5	4.9	5.8	2.1	6.5	9.7	0.7	0	81	190
191	0.2	0.1	0.3	0.4	0.3	0.6	1.3	2.1	2.7	3.9	3.5	8.3	8.8	9.3	11.6	11.4	23.7	29.0	1.9	0	219	191
192	0.8	0.5	0.2	0.1	0.0	0.1	0.9	0.1	0.0	0.6	0.9	0.6	0.4	0.4	0.0	2.1	4.3	9.7	0.3	0	34	192
193	0.2	0.1	0.4	0.5	0.1	0.9	0.9	0.6	1.8	0.6	0.9	0.8	1.4	0.4	0.6	0.0	0.0	0.0	0.6	0	69	193
194	0.0	0.0	0.1	0.2	0.4	0.6	1.9	1.3	2.2	4.8	3.3	5.3	8.5	7.1	9.7	9.3	4.3	14.5	1.5	0	177	194
195	0.0	0.0	0.0	0.2	0.0	0.0	0.1	0.0	0.3	0.0	0.0	0.6	0.0	0.0	0.0	1.0	0.0	0.0	0.1	0	8	195
196	0.2	0.3	0.8	0.8	0.4	0.7	0.9	1.6	1.8	2.6	5.7	4.2	5.6	8.9	6.4	3.1	6.5	4.8	1.5	0	173	196
197	0.0	0.1	0.2	0.3	0.4	0.3	0.1	0.7	0.2	0.4	0.7	1.9	1.8	0.0	0.0	0.0	4.3	0.0	0.2	0	25	197
200	0.2	0.1	0.4	0.7	0.7	0.3	0.1	0.0	0.8	0.4	1.3	1.9	2.1	3.1	0.6	4.1	0.0	0.0	0.6	0	70	200
201	0.1	0.3	0.2	0.9	1.5	1.5	1.5	1.2	1.5	1.1	2.4	1.1	2.5	0.9	2.6	4.1	0.0	0.0	1.0	0	113	201
203	0.0	0.0	0.0	0.0	0.0	0.0	0.1	0.0	0.8	0.2	0.7	1.4	3.5	2.2	0.6	0.0	0.0	0.0	0.3	1	31	203
204	2.1	1.3	1.9	2.2	2.1	2.6	1.7	2.4	3.0	4.2	2.8	6.7	6.0	4.4	6.4	4.1	2.2	4.8	2.5	0	301	204
202,205	0.2	0.1	0.1	0.0	0.1	0.2	0.1	0.4	0.3	0.4	0.2	0.3	0.7	0.0	0.0	0.0	0.0	0.0	0.2	0	20	202,205
OTHER	0.4	0.3	0.5	1.2	2.2	2.8	5.0	7.5	9.5	15.7	21.2	31.9	41.7	38.1	50.3	47.6	51.6	154.6	7.7	0	906	OTHER
140-205	5.4	4.3	5.9	11.3	17.4	40.6	98.3	153.7	238.2	303.3	373.1	475.2	583.0	559.0	575.1	521.7	539.8	661.8	117.3	21	13883	140-205
RATE PER CASE IN PERIOD	0.06	0.07	0.08	0.09	0.10	0.12	0.13	0.15	0.17	0.18	0.22	0.28	0.35	0.44	0.64	1.04	2.15	4.83	0.01	-	-	RATE PER CASE IN PERIOD

A study was undertaken with the aim of registering all the cases of cancer which were first diagnosed as such in Cali, Colombia, South America in a defined period. This was a joint programme of the Departments of Pathology and Preventive Medicine of the Medical School.

Figures are given only for residents of the urban area which is limited by the Cauca river on the east, the mountains on the west and by well demarcated north and south borders set by the municipality in official maps.

The city is located in the Valley of the Cauca River, 1000 metres above sea level. It is separated from the Pacific Ocean by the Western range of mountains of the Andes system and a tropical rainy forest. A road of 140 kilometres in distance connects Cali with the ocean. The latitude of the city is 3º27' N. The Valley which surrounds the city contains mainly sugar-cane plantations and cattle farms. The average temperature is 24º C.

The records of all medical institutions of the city were reviewed by medical students during the months of June, July and August of 1963 and 1964. Simultaneously, medical students made personal contacts with all the physicians known to have a private practice in Cali. They reviewed together the records and abstracted the necessary information on the cancer cases. The files of all pathologic anatomy, clinical pathology and X-ray laboratories were also examined for the same purpose. In the first survey all cases diagnosed between January 1st, 1962 and May 31st, 1963 were registered. In the second survey cases diagnosed between June 1st, 1963 and May 31st, 1964 were recorded. Duplicates were later eliminated. Also during the same study period all death certificates were being examined weekly for a special mortality survey. The cases of cancer thus found were later investigated in hospitals' and physicians' files. The records of a total of 483 physicians and 16 medical institutions were reviewed.

Special attention was given to the date of diagnosis. All cases diagnosed before January 1st, 1962, were eliminated. All cases of non-residents of Cali were eliminated. Of those remaining, 85 % were known residents of Cali and in 15 % information on the resident status was not available.

Next the cancer patients were grouped according to the primary site of origin of the tumour. The proportion of resident and non-resident cancer patients for each group was calculated from the special mortality study carried out in the same time period. In this study the resident status was investigated by home visits. These proportions were then applied to the corresponding groups of primary sites of the morbidity survey, choosing at random the cases to be eliminated.

Patients living permanently in Cali or having arrived in Cali to live, were considered residents. Patients coming to Cali for other reasons, including prolonged medical treatments, were considered non-residents.

A national census was carried out on July 15th, 1964. Our University was allowed to use the information from the beginning. University staff studied the completeness and quality of the census by means of a representative sample and found a proportion of under-registration of 0.5 %. Previous census was carried out on May 9th, 1951. Population at risk was estimated using the rate of growth and applying the age and sex proportions of the 1964 census.

All possible sources of diagnoses were explored. Only one physician in town refused collaboration. Approximately half of the cases were reported from more than one source. In large medical institutions cases were recorded from 2 or more of the following sources : records office, pathology department, X-ray department and cancer registry.

A high proportion of cases was confirmed histologically. All cases of doubtful histologic classification were personally reviewed by the senior author.

Pelayo Correa,
Guillermo Lanos.

Registry Title and Address : Cali, Colombia Cancer Survey, Departments of Pathology and Preventive Medicine, Facultad de Medicina, Universidad del Valle, Cali, Colombia, South America. Commenced January 1st, 1962. Supported financially by the Anna Fuller Fund.

Registration. Records were reviewed by medical students during June, July and August 1963 and 1964 for cases diagnosed between 1st January, 1962 and 31st May, 1963 and 1st June, 1963 and 31st May, 1964, from hospital in-patients and out-patients and from the radiotherapy departments of 16 Medical Institutions.
Records of clinical and anatomical pathology departments were similarly reviewed. Death certificates were examined weekly during the above period for a mortality survey and later investigated in hospitals' and physicians' files. All private practitioners (except one) reviewed case records with medical students during the same period. 483 physicians co-operated. It is possible that registration of cancer in children and cases of skin cancer are less than 90 % complete.

Follow-up. Approximately 30 % of cases are followed-up in the follow-up registry of one hospital until death.

Physical Description. Urban area of Cali, Colombia, South America, limited by the Cauca River to the east, the mountains on the west and by well demarcated north and south borders set by the municipality on official maps. The valley of the Cauca River is 1,000 metres above sea level and is separated from the Pacific Ocean by western range of mountains and tropical rain forest. The valley is mainly sugar cane plantations and cattle farms. The average temperature is 24 degrees centigrade. The area lies on latitudes 3o 27' North and longitudes 76o 31' West. The total registration area is 82.6 square kilometres.

Demographic Description. Total population of area under survey 578,440. The great majority of people are mestizos (mixture of Spanish and Indians) who migrated to Cali from mountainous areas of Colombia during the last 20 years. There is a minority of negroes. There are smaller proportions of Lebanese, Italian, German and Central European Jews, the exact proportions of which are not known. The main occupational composition of the population is : industry 50 %, commerce 20 %, agriculture 2 % and personal service 20 % approximately. The entire population lives in a conurbation of more than 100,000.

Medical Services. Total number of hospital beds of all kinds is 1,504 (1963). Total number of doctors in practice in registration area is approximately 500, excluding interns, residents in training in hospitals and non-praticing medical school staff. Cancer causes approximately 18.1 % of deaths in adults (those over 15 years of age). There are no figures available for children.

Publications. Correa and Llanos (1966); Correa, Llanos and Aguilera (1964); Velasquez (1965).

TABLE 12 A
COLOMBIA, CALI :
POPULATION (100,000s), 1963

NOTES

TO TABLES 12 A, B and C

(I)   Period of registration 1.1.62 to 31.5.64.

(II)   I.L. number 156 included in other sites.
       "   "   193 includes benign and unspecified tu-
              mours of the central nervous system.

(III) Carcinoma in situ excluded.

AGE (in years)	MALES		FEMALES	
	No.	Per Cent	No.	Per Cent
0 –	0.4788	17.38	0.4674	15.43
5 –	0.3994	14.50	0.4003	13.21
10 –	0.3120	11.32	0.3301	10.90
15 –	0.2584	9.38	0.3359	11.09
20 –	0.2414	8.76	0.3027	9.99
25 –	0.2139	7.76	0.2548	8.41
30 –	0.1989	7.22	0.2171	7.17
35 –	0.1661	6.03	0.1805	5.96
40 –	0.1301	4.72	0.1315	4.34
45 –	0.0998	3.62	0.1083	3.58
50 –	0.0859	3.12	0.0916	3.02
55 –	0.0575	2.09	0.0595	1.96
60 –	0.0483	1.75	0.0573	1.89
65 –	0.0256	0.93	0.0316	1.04
70 –	0.0172	0.62	0.0261	0.86
75 –	0.0118	0.43	0.0157	0.52
80 –	0.0054	0.20	0.0093	0.31
85 – and over	0.0047	0.17	0.0095	0.31
TOTAL	2.7552	100.00	3.0292	100.00

TABLE 12 B
COLOMBIA, CALI :
MALE INCIDENCE RATES, 1962 - 64.

AVERAGE ANNUAL INCIDENCE PER 100,000 — AGE IN YEARS

INTER-NATIONAL LIST No.	0–	5–	10–	15–	20–	25–	30–	35–	40–	45–	50–	55–	60–	65–	70–	75–	80–	85– AND OVER	ALL AGES	AGE UNKNOWN	ALL AGES (No. of cases)	INTER-NATIONAL LIST No.
140	0.0	0.0	0.0	0.0	0.0	0.0	0.0	0.0	3.2	0.0	0.0	7.2	8.6	16.2	48.1	0.0	76.6	0.0	1.1	0	7	140
141	0.0	0.0	0.0	0.0	0.0	0.0	0.0	0.0	0.0	12.4	4.8	0.0	17.1	16.2	0.0	70.1	76.6	176.1	1.8	0	12	141
142	0.0	0.0	0.0	0.0	0.0	0.0	2.1	0.0	0.0	0.0	4.8	7.2	17.1	0.0	0.0	35.1	76.6	0.0	1.1	0	7	142
143-4	0.0	0.0	0.0	0.0	0.0	0.0	0.0	0.0	0.0	0.0	9.6	7.2	8.6	0.0	24.1	0.0	0.0	0.0	0.8	0	5	143-4
146	0.0	0.0	0.0	0.0	0.0	0.0	0.0	0.0	0.0	0.0	0.0	0.0	0.0	0.0	0.0	0.0	0.0	0.0	0.0	0	0	146
145,147-8	0.0	0.0	0.0	0.0	0.0	0.0	0.0	0.0	0.0	8.3	19.3	0.0	34.3	0.0	0.0	0.0	0.0	88.0	1.7	0	11	145,147-8
150	0.0	0.0	0.0	0.0	0.0	0.0	2.1	0.0	38.2	0.0	4.8	14.4	42.8	32.3	48.1	0.0	76.6	88.0	2.3	9	15	150
151	0.0	0.0	0.0	1.6	1.7	0.0	4.2	17.4	0.0	58.0	110.8	57.6	265.6	355.6	529.3	385.7	229.9	0.0	24.9	0	166	151
152	0.0	0.0	0.0	0.0	0.0	0.0	0.0	0.0	0.0	8.3	0.0	7.2	0.0	0.0	24.1	0.0	76.6	0.0	0.8	0	5	152
153	0.0	0.0	0.0	1.6	1.7	1.9	2.1	2.5	0.0	4.1	14.5	7.2	8.6	48.5	48.1	35.1	0.0	0.0	2.7	1	18	153
154	0.0	0.0	0.0	1.6	0.0	0.0	0.0	0.0	0.0	4.1	0.0	0.0	17.1	16.2	0.0	0.0	76.6	0.0	1.1	0	7	154
155.0	0.0	0.0	0.0	0.0	0.0	3.9	0.0	0.0	0.0	8.3	4.8	7.2	25.7	32.3	0.0	70.1	0.0	0.0	2.0	0	13	155.0
155.1	0.0	0.0	0.0	0.0	0.0	0.0	0.0	0.0	0.0	8.3	4.8	21.6	8.6	32.3	24.1	0.0	0.0	0.0	1.5	0	10	155.1
157	0.0	0.0	0.0	0.0	0.0	0.0	0.0	0.0	0.0	0.0	0.0	7.2	8.6	64.7	0.0	35.1	0.0	0.0	1.1	0	7	157
160	0.0	0.0	0.0	0.0	0.0	0.0	0.0	0.0	0.0	0.0	0.0	0.0	8.6	0.0	0.0	0.0	0.0	0.0	0.2	0	1	160
161	0.0	0.0	0.0	0.0	0.0	0.0	0.0	5.0	3.2	4.1	24.1	21.6	42.8	16.2	96.2	0.0	76.6	176.1	3.9	1	26	161
162-3	0.0	0.0	0.0	0.0	0.0	0.0	0.0	0.0	6.4	24.9	9.6	43.2	94.2	113.1	120.3	70.1	76.6	88.0	6.8	2	45	162-3
170	0.0	0.0	0.0	0.0	0.0	0.0	0.0	0.0	0.0	0.0	0.0	0.0	8.6	0.0	0.0	0.0	0.0	0.0	0.2	0	1	170
177	0.0	0.0	0.0	0.0	0.0	0.0	6.2	0.0	0.0	4.1	14.5	43.2	85.7	226.3	312.7	350.7	689.6	88.0	10.5	3	70	177
178	0.0	0.0	0.0	0.0	0.0	1.9	0.0	5.0	0.0	8.3	0.0	0.0	8.6	16.2	0.0	0.0	0.0	0.0	1.5	0	10	178
179.0	0.9	0.0	0.0	0.0	0.0	0.0	0.0	2.5	0.0	4.1	0.0	21.6	8.6	16.2	72.2	35.1	153.3	88.0	2.3	1	15	179.0
180	0.0	0.0	0.0	0.0	0.0	0.0	6.2	0.0	0.0	8.3	14.5	0.0	25.7	16.2	24.1	0.0	0.0	0.0	1.7	0	11	180
181.0	0.0	0.0	0.0	0.0	0.0	0.0	6.2	0.0	6.4	0.0	14.5	14.4	77.1	97.0	216.5	140.3	76.6	0.0	5.9	0	39	181.0
190	0.0	0.0	1.3	0.0	0.0	1.9	4.2	5.0	3.2	0.0	4.8	0.0	17.1	16.2	72.2	0.0	76.6	88.0	2.4	0	16	190
191	0.0	0.0	0.0	0.0	0.0	1.9	2.1	7.5	28.6	41.5	43.4	107.9	282.7	129.3	312.7	175.3	306.5	88.0	18.0	8	120	191
192	0.9	0.0	1.3	0.0	0.0	1.9	0.0	2.5	0.0	0.0	4.8	7.2	0.0	0.0	24.1	0.0	0.0	0.0	0.9	0	6	192
193	4.3	4.1	0.0	0.0	1.7	1.9	0.0	2.5	6.4	0.0	14.5	0.0	8.6	0.0	0.0	0.0	0.0	0.0	2.9	0	19	193
194	0.0	0.0	0.0	0.0	1.7	1.9	2.1	2.5	3.2	8.3	4.8	28.8	34.3	16.2	0.0	0.0	0.0	0.0	2.6	0	17	194
195	0.0	0.0	0.0	0.0	0.0	0.0	0.0	0.0	0.0	0.0	0.0	0.0	0.0	0.0	0.0	0.0	0.0	0.0	0.0	0	0	195
196	0.0	2.1	5.3	4.8	0.0	0.0	4.2	0.0	3.2	12.4	9.6	0.0	8.6	16.2	24.1	0.0	0.0	0.0	2.4	0	16	196
197	0.0	1.0	0.0	3.2	13.7	1.9	0.0	5.0	3.2	16.6	4.8	14.4	17.1	16.2	24.1	0.0	153.3	0.0	3.3	1	22	197
200	2.6	3.1	1.3	0.0	1.7	0.0	2.1	0.0	6.4	8.3	9.6	7.2	0.0	16.2	24.1	35.1	76.6	0.0	3.5	0	23	200
201	0.9	0.0	2.7	1.6	0.0	0.0	0.0	0.0	0.0	0.0	0.0	0.0	8.6	0.0	0.0	0.0	0.0	0.0	2.6	0	17	201
203	0.0	0.0	0.0	0.0	0.0	0.0	2.1	0.0	0.0	4.1	9.6	7.2	0.0	0.0	0.0	35.1	0.0	0.0	0.3	0	2	203
204	3.5	2.1	1.3	8.0	1.7	1.9	4.2	0.0	6.4	4.1	9.6	7.2	0.0	0.0	0.0	35.1	76.6	0.0	3.6	0	24	204
202,205	0.0	0.0	0.0	1.6	1.7	0.0	4.2	0.0	0.0	0.0	0.0	0.0	0.0	16.2	0.0	0.0	0.0	0.0	1.2	1	8	202,205
OTHER	0.0	0.0	0.0	0.0	0.0	1.9	4.2	0.0	15.9	24.9	33.7	64.8	51.4	129.3	336.8	35.1	0.0	88.0	9.9	6	66	OTHER
140-205	13.0	13.5	13.3	24.0	25.7	25.1	52.0	57.3	136.8	286.1	404.6	532.5	1250.8	1487.0	2405.7	1507.9	2452.1	1056.5	128.7	33	857	140-205
RATE PER CASE IN PERIOD	0.86	1.04	1.33	1.60	1.71	1.93	2.08	2.49	3.18	4.15	4.82	7.20	8.57	16.16	24.06	35.07	76.63	88.04	0.15	-	-	RATE PER CASE IN PERIOD

TABLE 12 C

COLOMBIA, CALI :

FEMALE INCIDENCE RATES, 1962 - 64.

AVERAGE ANNUAL INCIDENCE PER 100,000 — AGE IN YEARS

INTER-NATIONAL LIST No.	0-	5-	10-	15-	20-	25-	30-	35-	40-	45-	50-	55-	60-	65-	70-	75-	80-	85- AND OVER	ALL AGES	No. OF CASES — AGE UNKNOWN	No. OF CASES — ALL AGES	INTER-NATIONAL LIST No.
140	0.0	0.0	0.0	1.2	0.0	0.0	0.0	0.0	3.1	0.0	0.0	0.0	7.2	39.3	0.0	0.0	0.0	0.0	0.8	0	6	140
141	0.0	0.0	0.0	0.0	0.0	0.0	0.0	0.0	0.0	0.0	13.6	7.0	7.2	0.0	0.0	52.7	0.0	0.0	1.0	0	7	141
142	0.0	1.0	0.0	1.2	0.0	3.2	5.7	6.9	0.0	3.8	4.5	0.0	7.2	0.0	0.0	0.0	0.0	0.0	1.8	0	13	142
143-4	0.0	0.0	0.0	0.0	0.0	0.0	0.0	0.0	0.0	0.0	4.5	0.0	7.2	13.1	31.7	26.4	44.5	43.6	1.1	0	8	143-4
146	0.0	0.0	0.0	0.0	0.0	0.0	0.0	0.0	0.0	0.0	0.0	0.0	0.0	0.0	0.0	0.0	0.0	0.0	0.0	0	0	146
145,147-8	0.0	0.0	0.0	1.2	0.0	0.0	0.0	0.0	0.0	7.6	4.5	7.0	7.2	0.0	15.9	26.4	0.0	87.1	1.0	0	7	145,147-8
150	0.0	0.0	0.0	0.0	0.0	0.0	0.0	0.0	0.0	0.0	0.0	0.0	7.2	0.0	0.0	0.0	0.0	0.0	0.5	0	4	150
151	0.0	0.0	0.0	0.0	0.0	3.2	5.7	2.3	31.5	30.6	67.8	62.6	86.7	130.9	158.5	52.7	44.5	43.6	12.3	6	90	151
152	0.0	0.0	0.0	0.0	0.0	0.0	0.0	0.0	0.0	0.0	0.0	0.0	0.0	13.1	15.9	0.0	0.0	0.0	0.3	1	2	152
153	0.0	0.0	0.0	0.0	0.0	1.6	0.0	0.0	6.3	3.8	0.0	7.0	21.7	0.0	15.9	26.4	44.5	43.6	1.6	0	12	153
154	0.0	0.0	0.0	0.0	0.0	0.0	3.8	2.3	3.1	0.0	9.0	0.0	14.4	0.0	0.0	0.0	0.0	0.0	1.2	0	9	154
155.0	0.9	0.0	0.0	1.2	0.0	0.0	1.9	2.3	3.1	15.3	9.0	0.0	7.2	39.3	111.0	0.0	0.0	0.0	2.6	2	19	155.0
155.1	0.0	0.0	0.0	0.0	0.0	0.0	1.9	4.6	9.4	15.3	45.2	20.9	14.4	39.3	111.0	26.4	0.0	0.0	4.8	0	35	155.1
157	0.0	0.0	0.0	0.0	0.0	0.0	0.0	2.3	3.1	0.0	4.5	13.9	0.0	13.1	31.7	26.4	44.5	0.0	2.2	0	16	157
160	0.0	0.0	0.0	0.0	0.0	0.0	0.0	0.0	0.0	0.0	0.0	0.0	7.2	0.0	0.0	0.0	44.5	0.0	0.4	1	3	160
161	0.0	0.0	0.0	0.0	0.0	0.0	0.0	0.0	0.0	0.0	4.5	7.0	7.2	0.0	0.0	0.0	44.5	0.0	0.5	0	4	161
162-3	0.0	0.0	0.0	0.0	0.0	3.2	1.9	25.2	0.0	7.6	18.1	97.4	21.7	13.1	31.7	0.0	44.5	43.6	1.9	3	14	162-3
170	0.0	0.0	0.0	0.0	0.0	3.2	11.4	25.2	53.5	80.2	108.4	97.4	93.9	91.7	63.4	263.6	44.5	43.6	18.3	0	134	170
171	0.0	0.0	0.0	0.0	1.4	17.9	78.1	133.0	229.7	263.6	225.9	340.1	353.8	248.8	317.1	105.4	89.0	87.1	62.0	6	454	171
172	0.0	0.0	0.0	0.0	1.4	1.6	3.8	6.9	12.6	11.5	27.1	13.9	28.9	52.4	31.7	52.7	0.0	0.0	4.6	0	34	172
173	0.0	0.0	0.0	0.0	0.0	1.6	1.9	4.6	0.0	0.0	0.0	7.0	0.0	0.0	0.0	0.0	0.0	0.0	0.7	0	5	173
174	0.0	0.0	0.0	0.0	0.0	0.0	0.0	0.0	0.0	0.0	0.0	0.0	0.0	0.0	0.0	0.0	0.0	0.0	0.0	0	0	174
175	0.0	0.0	1.3	3.7	2.7	6.5	11.4	0.0	25.2	34.4	54.2	41.7	28.9	13.1	15.9	26.4	0.0	43.6	8.3	2	61	175
176	0.0	0.0	0.0	0.0	0.0	0.0	1.9	4.6	15.7	0.0	4.5	34.8	21.7	26.2	63.4	0.0	0.0	0.0	3.3	1	24	176
180	2.7	0.0	0.0	0.0	0.0	0.0	1.9	4.6	3.1	3.8	0.0	0.0	0.0	0.0	0.0	26.4	0.0	0.0	1.0	0	7	180
181.0	0.0	0.0	0.0	0.0	0.0	0.0	1.9	0.0	3.1	0.0	9.0	27.8	14.4	26.2	15.9	26.4	44.5	0.0	2.3	2	17	181.0
190	0.0	0.0	0.0	0.0	2.7	1.6	9.5	4.6	6.3	11.5	4.5	0.0	7.2	39.3	0.0	0.0	0.0	0.0	1.8	1	13	190
191	0.0	0.0	0.0	0.0	0.0	0.0	0.0	6.9	22.0	45.8	63.2	118.2	166.1	170.2	95.1	105.4	311.5	217.8	16.8	4	123	191
192	2.7	0.0	0.0	0.0	0.0	0.0	0.0	0.0	0.0	3.8	0.0	0.0	0.0	0.0	0.0	0.0	0.0	0.0	0.5	0	4	192
193	1.8	1.0	1.3	0.0	2.7	3.2	1.9	0.0	3.1	3.8	9.0	0.0	0.0	0.0	0.0	0.0	0.0	0.0	1.4	0	10	193
194	0.0	0.0	0.0	0.0	1.4	3.2	1.9	18.3	3.1	19.1	18.1	27.8	14.4	13.1	31.7	0.0	0.0	0.0	4.4	0	32	194
195	0.0	1.0	0.0	0.0	0.0	0.0	0.0	0.0	0.0	0.0	0.0	0.0	0.0	0.0	0.0	0.0	0.0	0.0	0.3	0	2	195
196	0.9	0.0	3.8	1.2	1.4	0.0	0.0	0.0	3.1	0.0	0.0	0.0	7.2	0.0	0.0	0.0	0.0	0.0	1.0	0	7	196
197	0.0	2.1	0.0	1.2	1.4	3.2	0.0	0.0	0.0	0.0	0.0	7.0	7.2	0.0	15.9	0.0	0.0	43.6	1.4	0	10	197
200	0.9	0.0	1.3	1.2	1.4	0.0	0.0	0.0	12.6	0.0	0.0	13.9	7.2	39.3	47.6	0.0	0.0	0.0	2.2	0	16	200
201	0.0	0.0	0.0	1.2	0.0	3.2	1.9	0.0	0.0	0.0	9.0	7.0	7.2	0.0	0.0	0.0	0.0	0.0	1.2	0	9	201
203	0.0	0.0	0.0	1.2	0.0	0.0	0.0	0.0	0.0	0.0	4.5	0.0	0.0	13.1	0.0	0.0	0.0	0.0	0.3	0	2	203
204	0.9	1.0	2.5	1.2	0.0	1.6	0.0	2.3	3.1	0.0	4.5	7.0	14.4	13.1	0.0	26.4	0.0	0.0	1.4	0	10	204
202,205	0.0	1.0	0.0	0.0	0.0	0.0	0.0	0.0	0.0	0.0	0.0	0.0	0.0	0.0	0.0	0.0	0.0	0.0	0.5	0	4	202,205
OTHER	0.9	0.0	0.0	0.0	0.0	4.9	3.8	6.9	9.4	15.3	31.6	76.5	72.2	104.8	190.2	0.0	0.0	43.6	9.6	5	70	OTHER
140-205	11.5	6.2	10.0	14.8	15.0	60.1	148.7	238.4	462.6	576.9	758.9	945.8	1076.0	1152.3	1411.0	896.1	711.9	696.9	177.2	34	1297	140-205
RATE PER CASE IN PERIOD	0.89	1.03	1.25	1.23	1.37	1.62	1.91	2.29	3.15	3.82	4.52	6.95	7.22	13.09	15.85	26.36	44.49	43.56	0.14	-	-	RATE PER CASE IN PERIOD

JAMAICA, KINGSTON AND ST. ANDREW

In 1958, a Cancer Registry was started in Jamaica with the aim of outlining the pattern of cancer in the island, securing full registration of all cases, and making comparative epidemiological studies with other countries. The Registry is supported by the British Empire Cancer Campaign, and the Jamaica Cancer Society and at the beginning of the work, Professor John Knowelden kindly made himself available to study and advise on conditions in Jamaica. The Cancer Registry is situated in the Pathology Department of the University of the West Indies.

At the outset it was decided to secure full registration only in the Predominantly urban community of Kingston and St. Andrew (total population 419, 416 according to the 1960 census). This was done, as medical facilities are well developed in this area, the people are health conscious, and very few die without being seen by a medical pratitioner. In the rural areas, by contrast, medical facilities are poorly developed, health education is at a lower level, and many people die without even having been medically examined.

Two large general hospitals serve the Kingston and St. Andrew area - the Kingston Public Hospital (bed capacity about 500) and the Hospital of the West Indies (present bed capacity 460). Other specialised Government Hospitals are also situated in Kingston, i.e. the Sanatorium (in fact a Chest Hospital); the Mental Hospital, the Maternity Hospital and more recently the Children's Hospital. There are also three private nursing homes dealing with all types of cases having a total bed capacity of approximately 150.

Registration is obtained by the following means :

(1) The Registry staff personally visit all the wards of the two large general hospitals at least once per week, and interview all cancer patients or suspects, taking notes of the relevant investigations and particularly checking on the patients' permanent address. As specialist facilities for cancer treatment exist only in Kingston, many cancer cases are referred to the city for treatment; these country cases are recorded in the Registry, but only those permanently resident in Kingston and St. Andrew are used for incidence and epidemiological studies.

(2) Records are kept of all positive cancer biopsies in the histopathological Departments of both hospitals, and these reports with full details are available to the registry staff. The Registry also keeps on file slides from all cancer patients that have been biopsied. Two private pathologist do a small amount of histopathology for the nursing homes, and their slides are also available to the Registry.

(3) Other government institutions where cancer cases may occur (for example, Cancer of the lung in the Chest Hospital) are visited at less frequent intervals, and the private nursing homes are also periodically checked.

(4) The X-ray departments of the hospitals keep records of their suspicious cases, and these are available for checking by the registry staff.

(5) The Registrar General sends to the Registry a monthly list of all cancer deaths notified in Kingston and St. Andrew. These names are then checked by the Registry and if not already registered further investigations are made as to the adequacy of the diagnosis before the case is finally accepted.

(6) Notification cards are sent to private practitioners for them to notify their suspicious or definite cases to the Registry. In practice few practitioners have been co-operating in this, and personal effort and visits from the Registry staff are necessary to ferret out these cases that do not attend the general hospitals. On the whole, however, most cancer cases are referred at one time or other to the specialist hospitals where they are more easily available for

registration. Our records so far show that approximately 10 % of our cases were derived exclusively from private practitioners.

A certain amount of follow-up work is done, but this is limited owing to the large percentage of patients that never return to hospital after treatment, and the lack of the necessary machinery to pursue them to their domiciles.

G. Bras.

Registry Title and Address : The Cancer Registry, Pathology Department, University of West Indies, Kingston 7, Jamaica.
Commenced 1958. Principal sources of financial support are the British Empire Cancer Campaign and the Jamaica Cancer Society.

Registration. Registry staff register cases from hospital in-patients and out-patients, and also from pathology departments. Radiotherapy departments also register cases. Death certificate cases are registered by the Registrar General. Doctors and registry staff register cases attended at home. Registry staff also register cases in private nursing homes.

Follow-up. 9 % of registrations are followed-up (those re-admitted to hospital or coming to autopsy).

Physical Description. The city of Kingston and adjacent parish of St. Andrew is a seaboard city spreading over the coastal plain to the foothills of the Blue Mountains. Of St. Andrew roughly 50 % is below 1000 feet above sea-level, the remainder varying to over 5,000 feet. The area lies between latitudes 17o 43' and 18o 32' North and longitudes 76o 11' and 78o 21' West. The total registration area is 490 square kilometres.

Demographic Description. Total population of the area under survey 419,370. The population is 65 % black, 1 % white, 2 % East Indian, 1 % Chinese and Asiatic and 30 % mixed blood. 90 % of the population live in conurbations of more than 100,000.

Medical Services. Total number of hospital beds 2,089. Total number of doctors in practice in registration area 352. Cancer causes approximately 12.95 % of all deaths.

Publications. Bras and Watler (1965); Watler, Bras and McDonald (1959).

TABLE 13 A
JAMAICA, KINGSTON and St ANDREW :
POPULATION (100,000s), CENSUS 1960

AGE (in years)	MALES No.	MALES Per Cent	FEMALES No.	FEMALES Per Cent
0-	0.3237	17.06	0.3208	13.97
5-	0.2320	12.23	0.2393	10.42
10-	0.1703	8.97	0.1901	8.28
15-	0.1711	9.02	0.2282	9.94
20-	0.1786	9.41	0.2371	10.33
25-	0.1615	8.51	0.2165	9.43
30-	0.1314	6.92	0.1715	7.47
35-	0.1180	6.22	0.1574	6.85
40-	0.1034	5.45	0.1222	5.32
45-	0.0934	4.92	0.1108	4.83
50-	0.0739	3.89	0.0908	3.95
55-	0.0509	2.68	0.0656	2.86
60-	0.0369	1.94	0.0501	2.18
65-	0.0205	1.08	0.0328	1.43
70-	0.0145	0.76	0.0254	1.11
75-	0.0090	0.47	0.0177	0.77
80- and over	0.0084	0.44	0.0199	0.87
-	-	-	-	-
TOTAL	1.8975	100.00	2.2962	100.00

NOTES

TO TABLES 13 A, B and C

(I)   I.L. number 193 excludes benign and unspecified tumours of the central nervous system.
     "   "   205 included with other tumours.

(II)   Carcinoma in situ included.

TABLE 13 B
JAMAICA, KINGSTON and St ANDREW :
MALE INCIDENCE RATES, 1958 - 63.

AVERAGE ANNUAL INCIDENCE PER 100,000 — AGE IN YEARS

INTER-NATIONAL LIST No.	0–	5–	10–	15–	20–	25–	30–	35–	40–	45–	50–	55–	60–	65–	70–	75–	80–	85– AND OVER	ALL AGES	No. OF CASES AGE UNKNOWN	No. OF CASES ALL AGES	INTER-NATIONAL LIST No.
140	0.0	0.0	0.0	0.0	0.0	0.0	0.0	0.0	1.6	0.0	0.0	0.0	4.5	8.1	0.0	0.0	0.0		0.3	0	3	140
141	0.0	0.0	0.0	0.0	0.0	0.0	0.0	0.0	0.0	3.6	6.8	13.1	9.0	32.5	11.5	74.1	0.0		1.8	0	20	141
142	0.0	0.0	0.0	0.0	0.0	0.0	1.3	0.0	0.0	1.8	2.3	3.3	0.0	8.1	0.0	0.0	19.8		0.6	1	7	142
143-4	0.0	0.0	0.0	0.0	0.9	0.0	0.0	0.0	1.6	3.6	2.3	9.8	4.5	16.3	0.0	18.5	0.0		1.1	1	13	143-4
146	0.0	0.0	0.0	0.0	0.9	0.0	0.0	0.0	0.0	0.0	0.0	3.3	13.6	16.3	23.0	0.0	0.0		0.8	0	9	146
145,147-8	0.0	0.0	0.0	0.0	0.0	0.0	1.3	1.4	0.0	1.8	6.8	13.1	9.0	0.0	11.5	18.5	19.8		1.2	0	14	145,147-8
150	0.0	0.0	0.0	0.0	0.0	0.0	1.3	11.3	6.4	14.3	33.8	36.0	94.9	81.3	114.9	166.7	39.7		8.4	4	96	150
151	0.0	0.0	0.0	0.0	0.0	1.0	3.8	11.3	11.3	26.8	51.9	68.8	103.9	203.3	149.4	148.1	178.6		14.1	4	160	151
152	0.0	0.0	0.0	0.0	0.0	0.0	0.0	0.0	0.0	1.8	6.8	0.0	0.0	0.0	0.0	0.0	0.0		0.1	0	1	152
153	0.0	0.0	0.0	0.0	0.0	0.0	1.3	4.2	0.0	7.1	11.3	22.9	13.6	89.4	92.0	55.6	59.5		4.2	0	48	153
154	0.0	0.0	0.0	0.0	0.9	0.0	2.5	0.0	1.6	3.6	15.8	13.1	13.6	32.5	23.0	0.0	59.5		2.5	0	28	154
155.0	0.0	0.7	0.0	0.0	0.0	2.1	2.5	1.4	6.4	3.6	6.8	9.8	22.6	8.1	11.5	0.0	0.0		2.3	0	26	155.0
155.1	0.0	0.0	0.0	0.0	0.9	0.0	0.0	1.4	0.0	0.0	4.5	6.5	9.0	16.3	23.0	0.0	39.7		1.1	0	13	155.1
156	0.0	0.0	0.0	0.0	0.0	1.0	1.3	0.0	1.6	0.0	2.3	3.3	4.5	0.0	0.0	0.0	0.0		0.6	0	7	156
157	0.0	0.0	0.0	0.0	0.0	0.0	0.0	0.0	3.2	3.6	4.5	13.1	13.6	0.0	23.0	55.6	0.0		1.7	1	19	157
160	0.0	0.0	0.0	0.0	0.0	0.0	0.0	0.0	1.6	1.8	0.0	0.0	4.5	8.1	0.0	18.5	0.0		0.4	0	5	160
161	0.0	0.0	0.0	0.0	0.0	0.0	0.0	0.0	3.2	0.0	6.8	6.5	18.1	16.3	92.0	18.5	39.7		2.1	0	24	161
162-3	0.0	0.0	0.0	0.0	0.0	0.0	0.0	0.0	0.0	8.9	40.6	52.4	99.4	81.3	92.0	55.6	0.0		7.3	1	83	162-3
170	0.0	0.0	0.0	0.0	0.0	0.0	0.0	0.0	0.0	0.0	2.3	3.3	0.0	0.0	0.0	18.5	39.7		0.4	0	5	170
177	0.0	0.0	0.0	0.0	0.0	0.0	0.0	0.0	0.0	1.8	11.3	22.9	58.7	154.5	114.9	148.1	178.6		6.3	0	72	177
178	0.0	0.0	0.0	0.0	0.0	0.0	0.0	0.0	0.0	3.6	0.0	0.0	9.0	0.0	11.5	0.0	0.0		0.4	0	5	178
179	0.0	0.0	0.0	0.0	0.0	1.0	6.3	4.2	11.3	10.7	31.6	26.2	22.6	48.8	11.5	74.1	19.8		5.4	1	62	179
180	2.1	0.0	0.0	0.0	0.0	2.1	0.0	0.0	3.2	1.8	4.5	3.3	9.0	24.4	0.0	0.0	0.0		1.6	1	18	180
181	0.0	0.0	0.0	1.0	0.0	0.0	0.0	0.0	1.6	3.6	2.3	16.4	36.1	65.0	57.5	18.5	79.4		3.2	0	36	181
190	0.0	0.0	0.0	0.0	0.9	0.0	0.0	0.0	0.0	0.0	0.0	0.0	9.0	0.0	11.5	18.5	39.7		0.6	0	7	190
191	3.6	0.0	0.0	1.0	0.9	2.1	3.8	5.6	11.3	21.4	42.9	22.9	94.9	81.3	126.4	37.0	59.5		9.0	0	103	191
192	3.1	0.0	1.0	1.0	0.0	0.0	0.0	1.4	0.0	0.0	0.0	0.0	0.0	0.0	0.0	0.0	0.0		0.7	0	8	192
193	0.0	2.2	1.0	1.0	0.9	2.1	1.3	1.4	1.6	3.6	2.3	3.3	0.0	8.1	0.0	0.0	0.0		1.9	0	22	193
194	0.0	0.0	1.0	0.0	0.0	1.0	1.3	0.0	0.0	1.8	6.8	3.3	4.5	0.0	0.0	0.0	0.0		0.7	0	8	194
195	0.0	0.0	1.0	0.0	0.0	0.0	1.3	0.0	0.0	0.0	0.0	0.0	0.0	0.0	0.0	0.0	0.0		0.2	0	2	195
196	0.0	0.7	1.0	2.9	3.7	0.0	1.3	1.4	1.6	0.0	0.0	0.0	0.0	0.0	0.0	0.0	0.0		1.1	0	12	196
197	1.0	0.0	0.0	1.0	0.9	1.0	3.8	1.4	1.6	3.6	4.5	6.5	4.5	0.0	11.5	0.0	0.0		1.3	0	15	197
200	0.5	0.0	1.0	0.0	1.9	2.1	5.1	8.5	1.6	5.4	6.8	6.5	9.0	8.1	23.0	0.0	19.8		2.4	0	27	200
201	0.0	0.7	1.0	1.0	0.9	2.1	0.0	0.0	4.8	7.1	4.5	3.3	0.0	0.0	34.5	18.5	0.0		2.4	0	27	201
202	0.0	0.0	0.0	1.0	0.0	0.0	0.0	0.0	0.0	0.0	2.3	0.0	0.0	0.0	0.0	0.0	0.0		0.3	0	3	202
203	0.0	0.0	0.0	0.0	0.0	0.0	2.5	0.0	1.6	0.0	0.0	13.1	13.6	8.1	0.0	18.5	0.0		0.9	0	10	203
204	2.6	2.9	2.9	0.0	4.7	0.0	2.5	1.4	4.8	3.6	6.8	16.4	4.5	32.5	0.0	18.5	0.0		3.4	0	39	204
OTHER	0.0	0.0	0.0	0.0	0.9	0.0	0.0	2.8	4.8	8.9	20.3	26.2	31.6	40.7	69.0	74.1	39.7		4.7	1	53	OTHER
140-205	12.9	7.9	7.8	8.8	19.6	17.5	41.9	49.4	88.7	158.8	345.1	448.6	740.7	1089.4	1137.9	1074.1	932.5		97.5	15	1110	140-205
RATE PER CASE IN PERIOD	0.51	0.72	0.98	0.97	0.93	1.03	1.27	1.41	1.61	1.78	2.26	3.27	4.52	8.13	11.49	18.52	19.84		0.09	-		RATE PER CASE IN PERIOD

Note : Figures in column 80 — relate to the years 80 and over.

TABLE 13 C

JAMAICA, KINGSTON and St ANDREW :
FEMALE INCIDENCE RATES, 1958 - 63.

INTER-NATIONAL LIST No.	AVERAGE ANNUAL INCIDENCE PER 100,000 — AGE IN YEARS																		ALL AGES	No. OF CASES IN WHOLE PERIOD		INTER-NATIONAL LIST No.
	0-	5-	10-	15-	20-	25-	30-	35-	40-	45-	50-	55-	60-	65-	70-	75-	80-	85- AND OVER		AGE UN-KNOWN	ALL AGES	
140	0.0	0.0	0.0	0.0	0.0	0.0	0.0	0.0	0.0	0.0	3.7	0.0	0.0	5.1	6.6	0.0	0.0		0.3	0	4	140
141	0.0	0.0	0.0	0.7	0.0	0.8	1.0	0.0	2.7	0.0	0.0	2.5	0.0	5.1	13.1	9.4	0.0		0.7	0	10	141
142	0.0	0.0	0.0	0.0	0.0	0.0	1.0	1.1	0.0	1.5	1.8	5.1	3.3	15.2	6.6	0.0	0.0		0.8	0	11	142
143-4	0.0	0.0	0.0	0.0	0.0	0.0	0.0	0.0	2.7	3.0	5.5	5.1	3.3	10.2	6.6	9.4	8.4		1.1	0	15	143-4
146	0.0	0.0	0.0	0.0	0.0	0.8	0.0	0.0	0.0	1.5	1.8	0.0	0.0	5.1	6.6	0.0	0.0		0.4	0	5	146
145,147-8	0.0	0.0	0.0	0.0	0.0	0.0	0.0	1.1	0.0	0.0	3.7	0.0	0.0	0.0	0.0	0.0	0.0		0.2	1	3	145,147-8
150	0.0	0.0	0.0	0.0	0.0	0.0	1.0	0.0	1.4	1.5	9.2	17.8	33.3	20.3	45.9	47.1	33.5		3.3	3	46	150
151	0.0	0.0	0.0	0.0	0.7	0.8	1.9	5.3	2.7	13.5	16.5	25.4	39.0	55.9	91.9	65.9	41.9		6.6	0	91	151
152	0.0	0.0	0.0	0.0	0.0	0.0	0.0	0.0	0.0	0.0	0.0	0.0	0.0	0.0	0.0	0.0	0.0		0.0	0	0	152
153	0.0	0.0	0.0	0.0	0.0	0.0	0.0	0.0	6.8	7.5	16.5	30.5	53.2	30.5	59.1	56.5	83.8		5.8	2	80	153
154	0.0	0.0	0.0	0.0	0.0	1.5	1.0	4.2	4.1	6.0	16.5	25.4	3.3	10.2	13.1	28.2	41.9		3.7	0	51	154
155.0	0.0	0.0	0.0	0.0	0.0	0.0	1.0	2.1	1.4	3.0	1.8	2.5	16.6	0.0	13.1	0.0	0.0		0.8	0	11	155.0
155.1	0.0	0.0	0.0	1.5	0.0	1.5	0.0	0.0	0.0	4.5	9.2	5.1	0.0	10.2	13.1	37.7	8.4		1.7	0	24	155.1
156	0.0	0.0	0.0	0.0	0.0	0.0	0.0	1.1	0.0	1.5	0.0	0.0	0.0	0.0	0.0	0.0	0.0		0.1	0	2	156
157	0.0	0.7	0.0	0.7	0.0	0.0	0.0	1.1	1.4	1.5	1.8	0.0	3.3	0.0	13.1	28.2	33.5		1.0	0	14	157
160	0.0	0.0	0.0	0.0	0.0	0.0	0.0	1.1	1.4	1.5	3.7	0.0	3.3	0.0	13.1	0.0	0.0		0.7	1	10	160
161	0.0	0.0	0.0	0.0	0.0	0.0	0.0	0.0	0.0	0.0	0.0	0.0	0.0	5.1	13.1	9.4	0.0		0.1	0	2	161
162-3	0.0	0.0	0.0	0.0	0.0	0.0	0.0	3.2	4.1	3.0	1.8	7.6	10.0	20.3	13.1	0.0	8.4		1.7	2	24	162-3
170	0.0	0.0	0.0	0.0	2.1	5.4	20.4	27.5	43.6	78.2	101.0	61.0	76.5	142.3	78.7	141.2	117.3		22.9	3	315	170
171	0.0	0.0	0.0	0.0	4.9	12.3	34.0	48.7	92.7	97.8	165.2	149.9	159.7	167.7	144.4	150.7	92.1		37.9	6	522	171
172	0.0	0.0	0.0	0.0	0.0	0.8	0.0	3.2	1.4	15.0	3.7	20.3	23.3	20.3	19.7	0.0	8.4		2.9	0	40	172
173	0.0	0.0	0.0	1.5	2.1	0.0	1.0	1.1	2.7	1.5	5.5	5.1	10.0	0.0	6.6	0.0	0.0		1.5	0	20	173
174	0.0	0.0	0.0	0.0	0.0	0.0	0.0	0.0	0.0	0.0	0.0	0.0	0.0	0.0	0.0	0.0	0.0		0.0	0	0	174
175	0.0	0.7	0.9	0.7	0.7	3.8	2.9	7.4	10.9	19.6	20.2	17.8	26.6	25.4	26.2	18.8	8.4		5.7	0	78	175
176	0.0	0.0	0.0	0.0	1.4	2.3	1.9	3.2	1.4	3.0	5.5	7.6	6.7	10.2	32.8	0.0	8.4		2.1	0	29	176
180	1.6	0.0	1.8	0.7	0.7	0.8	0.0	1.1	1.4	1.5	0.0	2.5	0.0	0.0	6.6	0.0	0.0		0.9	0	13	180
181	0.0	0.0	0.0	0.0	0.7	0.8	1.0	0.0	1.4	1.5	3.7	22.9	6.7	20.3	26.2	28.2	0.0		2.3	2	32	181
190	0.0	0.0	0.0	0.0	0.0	0.0	0.0	0.0	0.0	4.5	3.7	2.5	6.7	0.0	6.6	0.0	0.0		0.9	1	12	190
191	0.0	0.0	0.0	0.7	0.0	0.8	2.9	4.2	9.5	15.0	18.4	25.4	33.3	61.0	85.3	75.3	117.3		7.9	6	109	191
192	3.6	0.0	0.9	0.0	0.0	0.0	0.0	1.1	0.0	0.0	0.0	2.5	0.0	0.0	6.6	0.0	0.0		0.7	0	10	192
193	0.0	0.0	0.0	0.7	0.0	1.5	1.9	1.1	1.4	0.0	5.5	5.1	0.0	0.0	13.1	0.0	0.0		0.8	0	11	193
194	0.0	0.0	0.0	0.0	1.4	0.8	0.0	4.2	2.7	3.0	1.8	2.5	6.7	5.1	0.0	0.0	0.0		1.5	0	20	194
195	0.0	0.0	0.9	2.2	0.0	0.0	0.0	0.0	1.5	1.5	1.8	0.0	0.0	0.0	0.0	0.0	0.0		0.1	0	9	195
196	0.0	0.7	0.9	0.0	0.0	1.5	0.0	0.0	0.0	1.5	1.8	0.0	3.3	0.0	0.0	0.0	0.0		0.7	0	9	196
197	0.5	0.0	0.0	0.7	0.7	2.3	1.0	1.1	1.4	3.0	3.7	0.0	3.3	10.2	13.1	0.0	33.5		1.7	0	24	197
200	1.0	0.0	0.0	0.0	0.0	0.8	2.9	2.1	2.7	6.0	7.3	10.2	0.0	10.2	6.6	0.0	8.4		2.0	1	28	200
201	0.0	0.0	0.0	0.0	0.0	0.0	0.0	0.0	0.0	1.5	0.0	2.5	0.0	0.0	6.6	0.0	0.0		0.2	0	3	201
202	0.0	0.0	0.0	0.0	0.0	0.0	0.0	0.0	0.0	3.0	0.0	0.0	0.0	0.0	0.0	0.0	0.0		0.1	0	2	202
203	0.0	0.0	0.0	0.0	0.0	0.0	0.0	0.0	0.0	4.5	3.7	0.0	6.7	5.1	6.6	9.4	0.0		0.7	0	9	203
204	2.6	2.1	0.9	2.2	1.4	0.8	0.0	3.2	4.1	4.5	1.8	0.0	6.7	10.2	26.2	9.4	0.0		2.5	0	34	204
OTHER	0.0	0.0	0.0	0.0	0.0	1.5	3.9	1.1	8.2	18.1	23.9	22.9	20.0	30.5	39.4	9.4	92.1		5.7	2	79	OTHER
140-205	9.4	4.2	6.1	11.0	17.6	41.6	81.6	130.2	214.1	333.9	471.7	487.8	585.5	716.5	853.0	725.0	753.8		130.9	30	1804	140-205
RATE PER CASE IN PERIOD	0.52	0.70	0.88	0.73	0.70	0.77	0.97	1.06	1.36	1.50	1.84	2.54	3.33	5.08	6.56	9.42	8.38		0.07	-	-	RATE PER CASE IN PERIOD

Note : Figures in column 80— relate to the years 80 and over.

PUERTO RICO

The Central Cancer Registry of Puerto Rico began in 1950 as a section of the Division of Cancer Control. It covers all cancer cases diagnosed by physicians in all hospitals and clinics in Puerto Rico. In addition to the legal requirements for reporting cancer cases, the Registry maintains a systematic search for unreported cases, including an annual check of all pathologists' registries,. and admission and records departments of all hospitals in the island.

Each record of the Central Cancer Registry consists of four basic documents : the clinical abstract which is completed by a medical record clerk of the Registry or hospital, or by the physician for the private case; a carbon copy of the biopsy report from the pathologist; a follow-up form with the up-to-date information of the case; and a photocopy of the death certificate from the Demographic Registry of the Department of Health, for the dead cases. It is important to mention that les than 10 % of all records remained with only the death certificate, and 91 % have either clinical abstract or biopsy report or both, at the beginning of the following year.

The Editing and Filing Unit of the Registry is very careful to avoid duplication of cases by means of different checks in its index system. Once the basic information of a case is edited, it is coded, and punched in an I.B.M. tabulation card following the method of a single punch for each column. Each coded sheet is reviewed against the record by a second clerk before it is sent for punching. Once all cards are made, a 15 % sample from these cards are checked for corrections of the punching; moreover, a general review of the whole year group cards is done against the accession book of the Editing Unit. For the purpose of tabulation, all the cards are processed in a 101 I.B.M. tabulation machine.

Isidro Martinez

Registry Title and Address : Puerto Rico Cancer Registry, Division of Cancer Control, Department of Health, Santurce, Puerto Rico, West Indies. Commenced 1950. Supported by Local and Federal Government funds.

Registration. Registrations are made from hospital in-patients and out-patients, radiotherapy and pathology departments, death certificates, and doctors attending cases at home. There is a systematic search for unreported cases by means of an annual check of the pathologists' registries, and the admission books of all hospitals and clinics in Puerto Rico. A group of dermatologists in the Island, however, do not agree to report cases with cancer of the skin.

Follow-up. All cases except carcinoma of the skin (about 15 %) are followed up every year for life.

Physical Description. Puerto Rico is a rectangular-shaped island east of Hispaniola. It is surrounded by the Atlantic Ocean in the north and the Caribbean Sea in the south. It lies between latitudes 17⁰ 50' and 18⁰ 30' North and longitudes 65⁰ 30' and 67⁰ 15' West. The total registration area is 8,897 square kilometres.

Demographic Description. Total population of area under survey 2,483,800. The population is 80 % white and mixed blood, and 20 % negro. It is 90 % Catholic and 10 % Protestant. The main occupational composition of those over 14 years of age is : industry and commerce 33.6 %, agriculture 7.4 %, unemployed 4.9 %, and not in labour force 53.4 %. Thirty per cent of the population live in conurbations of more than 100,000.

Medical Services. Total number of hospital beds 12,695. Total number of doctors in practice in registration area 2,500. There are some cultural and economic factors that might cause 5 % or more of the population to delay seeking medical advice unduly. Cancer causes approximately 13 % of all deaths.

Publications. Annual Reports.

TABLE 14 A
PUERTO RICO :
POPULATION (100,000s), MEAN 1962 - 63

AGE (in years)	MALES No.	MALES Per Cent	FEMALES No.	FEMALES Per Cent
0-	1.7965	14.76	1.7440	13.77
5-	1.6640	13.67	1.6180	12.77
10-	1.6240	13.34	1.5800	12.47
15-	1.2490	10.26	1.2830	10.13
20-	0.9655	7.93	1.0095	7.97
25-	0.7435	6.11	0.9080	7.17
30-	0.6205	5.10	0.8245	6.51
35-	0.6015	4.94	0.7150	5.65
40-	0.5995	4.93	0.6220	4.91
45-	0.5335	4.38	0.5780	4.56
50-	0.4675	3.84	0.4545	3.59
55-	0.3580	2.94	0.3415	2.70
60-	0.2880	2.37	0.3025	2.39
65-	0.2545	2.09	0.2490	1.97
70-	0.1840	1.51	0.1805	1.43
75- and over	0.2225	1.83	0.2560	2.02
-	-	-	-	-
-	-	-	-	-
TOTAL	12.1720	100.00	12.6660	100.00

NOTES

TO TABLES 14 A, B and C

(I) I.L. number 155.1 obtained by subtracting rates for 155.0 from rates for 155.

" " 193 excludes benign and unspecified tumours of the central nervous system.

(II) Carcinoma in situ included.

TABLE 14 B

PUERTO RICO :

MALE INCIDENCE RATES, 1962 - 63.

INTER-NATIONAL LIST No.	\multicolumn{17}{c}{AVERAGE ANNUAL INCIDENCE PER 100,000 — AGE IN YEARS}	ALL AGES	No. of cases in whole period — AGE UNKNOWN	No. of cases in whole period — ALL AGES	INTER-NATIONAL LIST No.
	0-	5-	10-	15-	20-	25-	30-	35-	40-	45-	50-	55-	60-	65-	70-	75-					
140	0.0	0.0	0.0	0.0	0.0	1.3	1.6	0.0	1.7	4.7	0.0	5.6	13.9	11.8	10.9	13.5	1.6	0	39	140
141	0.0	0.0	0.0	0.0	0.0	0.7	0.8	5.0	6.7	13.1	17.1	16.8	20.8	39.3	51.6	44.9	5.3	0	129	141
142	0.0	0.0	0.0	0.0	0.0	0.0	0.0	0.8	0.0	0.0	0.0	0.0	1.7	5.9	0.0	4.5	0.3	0	7	142
143-4	0.0	0.0	0.0	0.0	0.0	0.7	0.8	0.8	3.3	12.2	20.3	25.1	34.7	37.3	29.9	44.9	5.2	0	126	143-4
145,147-8	0.0	0.0	0.0	0.0	0.0	0.0	2.4	1.7	8.3	12.2	21.4	29.3	26.0	35.4	32.6	31.5	5.3	0	129	145,147-8
146	0.0	0.0	0.0	0.0	0.0	0.0	0.0	0.0	0.0	0.0	2.1	2.8	0.0	3.9	2.7	0.0	0.3	0	7	146
150	0.0	0.0	0.0	0.0	0.5	0.0	0.0	3.3	5.8	18.7	57.8	61.5	97.2	86.4	78.8	139.3	13.2	1	322	150
151	0.3	0.0	0.0	0.0	0.5	2.0	3.2	3.3	10.0	24.4	52.4	72.6	137.2	172.9	236.4	265.2	21.6	1	525	151
152	0.0	0.0	0.0	0.0	0.0	0.0	0.0	0.0	0.0	0.0	2.1	1.4	1.7	2.0	5.4	2.2	0.3	1	8	152
153	0.0	0.0	0.0	0.4	0.0	0.0	0.8	0.0	2.5	6.6	9.6	7.0	15.6	25.5	29.9	44.9	3.3	1	80	153
154	0.0	0.0	0.0	0.0	0.5	0.7	0.0	3.3	5.0	5.6	5.3	8.4	17.4	17.7	19.0	20.2	2.6	0	64	154
155.0	0.6	0.0	0.0	0.0	0.5	0.7	0.0	0.8	0.0	0.9	1.1	7.0	13.9	11.8	24.5	31.5	2.1	2	51	155.0
155.1	0.0	0.0	0.0	0.0	0.0	0.0	0.0	0.0	0.0	0.9	2.1	2.8	6.9	11.8	13.6	15.7	1.1	0	27	155.1
156	0.0	0.3	0.0	0.4	0.0	2.0	0.0	0.0	0.0	2.8	5.3	14.0	13.9	13.8	13.6	15.7	2.1	0	50	156
157	0.0	0.0	0.0	0.0	0.0	0.0	0.0	0.0	1.7	3.7	5.3	16.8	13.9	29.5	43.5	38.2	3.3	0	80	157
160	0.6	0.0	0.0	0.0	0.0	0.0	0.0	0.0	1.7	0.0	1.1	0.0	5.2	3.9	4.5	4.5	0.5	0	12	160
161	0.0	0.0	0.0	0.4	0.0	0.7	0.8	1.7	3.3	4.7	15.0	19.6	29.5	37.3	24.5	53.9	4.6	1	111	161
162-3	0.0	0.0	0.0	0.0	0.0	0.7	0.8	1.7	3.3	4.7	26.7	34.9	78.1	82.5	73.4	98.9	9.1	1	222	162-3
170	0.0	0.0	0.0	0.0	0.0	0.7	0.0	0.8	0.0	1.9	1.1	2.8	3.5	2.0	2.7	2.2	0.5	0	13	170
177	0.3	0.0	0.0	0.0	0.0	0.0	0.0	0.8	0.0	4.7	9.6	11.2	57.3	108.1	163.0	321.3	12.9	0	315	177
178	0.0	0.0	0.0	0.0	0.0	0.0	2.4	0.8	0.0	0.0	0.0	0.0	0.0	0.0	0.0	2.2	0.3	0	7	178
179.0	0.3	0.0	0.0	0.0	0.5	1.3	4.8	4.2	3.3	13.1	13.9	12.6	19.1	33.4	35.3	58.4	5.1	1	124	179.0
180	0.8	0.3	0.0	0.0	0.0	0.0	0.0	0.8	2.5	0.0	1.1	4.2	8.7	2.0	5.4	6.7	0.9	0	23	180
181.0	0.3	0.0	0.0	0.0	0.0	0.0	0.8	1.7	1.7	10.3	6.4	20.9	31.3	45.2	65.2	98.9	6.0	0	147	181.0
190	0.0	0.0	0.0	0.0	0.0	0.0	1.6	0.8	0.0	1.9	2.1	0.0	6.9	2.0	2.7	6.7	0.7	0	16	190
191	0.0	0.0	0.0	0.0	0.5	5.4	5.6	19.1	24.2	32.8	52.4	78.2	140.6	186.6	203.8	224.7	23.5	13	573	191
192	0.8	0.0	0.0	0.4	0.5	0.0	1.6	0.8	1.7	3.7	2.1	2.8	0.0	3.9	0.0	6.7	0.9	0	22	192
193	1.1	1.8	1.5	0.4	0.0	0.0	0.8	5.0	3.3	0.9	7.5	2.8	5.2	5.9	0.0	2.2	1.8	0	44	193
194	0.0	0.0	0.0	0.0	0.0	0.0	0.8	0.0	1.7	0.9	2.1	5.6	1.7	0.0	0.0	4.5	0.5	0	13	194
195	0.0	0.3	0.0	0.0	0.0	0.0	0.0	0.0	0.8	0.0	0.0	0.0	1.7	2.0	0.0	0.0	0.1	0	3	195
196	0.0	0.0	1.2	2.0	2.1	1.3	0.0	0.8	0.8	0.9	0.0	1.4	5.2	3.9	2.7	2.2	1.0	0	25	196
197	0.0	0.3	0.0	1.2	2.6	0.0	1.6	0.8	1.7	1.9	2.1	5.6	5.2	2.0	5.4	0.0	1.2	0	28	197
200	0.3	1.2	0.9	0.8	2.6	3.4	0.0	3.3	2.5	2.8	2.1	5.6	15.6	7.9	13.6	15.7	2.5	0	61	200
201	0.8	0.9	1.5	4.0	3.1	3.4	0.0	5.0	2.5	2.8	5.3	4.2	6.9	15.7	13.6	4.5	2.9	0	71	201
203	0.0	0.0	0.0	0.0	0.0	0.0	0.0	0.0	1.7	0.0	6.4	1.4	3.5	13.8	5.4	11.2	1.0	0	25	203
204	5.0	2.7	3.1	2.4	2.1	2.0	4.0	4.2	4.2	6.6	5.3	4.2	12.2	15.7	19.0	22.5	4.6	1	113	204
202,205	0.3	0.0	0.0	0.4	0.0	0.0	0.0	0.0	0.0	0.0	0.0	0.0	0.0	2.0	5.4	0.0	0.2	0	5	202,205
OTHER	0.6	0.6	0.0	0.0	0.5	1.3	1.6	1.7	4.2	4.7	9.6	29.3	26.0	37.3	67.9	80.9	6.1	2	148	OTHER
140-205	12.0	8.4	8.6	13.2	17.1	27.6	37.1	72.3	110.1	205.2	374.3	518.2	878.5	1117.9	1301.6	1741.6	154.7	25	3765	140-205
RATE PER CASE IN PERIOD	0.28	0.30	0.31	0.40	0.52	0.67	0.81	0.83	0.83	0.94	1.07	1.40	1.74	1.96	2.72	2.25	0.04			RATE PER CASE IN PERIOD

TABLE 14 C

PUERTO RICO :

FEMALE INCIDENCE RATES, 1962 - 63.

AVERAGE ANNUAL INCIDENCE PER 100,000 — AGE IN YEARS

INTER-NATIONAL LIST No.	0-	5-	10-	15-	20-	25-	30-	35-	40-	45-	50-	55-	60-	65-	70-	75-	80-	85- AND OVER	ALL AGES	AGE UNKNOWN	ALL AGES (cases)	INTER-NATIONAL LIST No.
140	0.0	0.0	0.6	0.0	0.0	0.0	0.0	0.0	0.8	0.9	1.1	0.0	3.3	2.0	2.8	9.8			0.6	0	14	140
141	0.0	0.0	0.0	0.0	0.0	0.0	0.0	0.7	4.0	0.9	7.7	1.5	3.3	16.1	13.9	19.5			1.6	0	40	141
142	0.0	0.0	0.0	0.0	0.0	0.0	0.0	0.7	0.0	0.9	0.0	1.5	1.7	4.0	2.8	0.0			0.3	0	7	142
143-4	0.3	0.0	0.0	0.0	0.0	0.0	0.0	0.7	1.6	3.5	4.4	1.5	11.6	16.1	22.2	25.4			2.0	1	50	143-4
146	0.0	0.0	0.3	0.0	0.5	0.0	0.6	0.0	0.0	0.0	0.0	0.0	0.0	4.0	13.9	9.8			0.2	0	6	146
145,147-8	0.0	0.0	0.0	0.0	0.0	0.0	0.0	0.7	1.6	1.7	2.2	4.4	21.5	16.1	13.9	9.8			1.6	0	41	145,147-8
150	0.3	0.0	0.0	0.0	0.0	0.0	0.0	2.1	5.6	3.5	14.3	16.1	36.4	38.2	74.8	68.4			5.6	2	143	150
151	0.0	0.0	0.0	0.0	0.5	1.1	1.8	3.5	8.0	6.9	18.7	22.0	52.9	94.4	110.8	173.8			10.7	1	271	151
152	0.0	0.0	0.3	0.0	0.0	0.0	0.0	0.7	0.8	1.7	3.3	0.0	1.7	0.0	5.5	3.9			0.5	0	13	152
153	0.0	0.0	0.3	0.0	0.0	1.1	1.2	0.7	3.2	4.3	11.0	5.9	11.6	30.1	33.2	58.6			3.7	1	94	153
154	0.0	0.0	0.0	0.0	0.0	0.0	1.8	0.7	4.0	2.6	6.6	10.2	9.9	16.1	24.9	29.3			2.5	0	63	154
155.0	0.3	0.0	0.0	0.0	0.0	0.0	0.0	0.0	1.6	0.9	3.3	2.9	3.3	10.0	5.5	7.8			0.9	0	22	155.0
155.1	0.0	0.0	0.0	0.0	0.0	0.0	0.0	0.0	1.6	2.6	4.4	10.2	13.2	22.1	13.9	29.3			2.2	0	55	155.1
156	0.0	0.0	0.0	0.0	0.0	0.6	0.5	1.4	0.0	2.6	2.2	7.3	5.0	12.0	11.1	17.6			1.4	0	36	156
157	0.0	0.0	0.3	0.0	0.0	0.0	0.0	0.0	2.4	0.0	2.2	5.9	11.6	22.1	19.4	33.2			2.1	0	52	157
160	0.0	0.0	0.0	0.0	0.0	0.0	0.5	0.7	0.0	0.0	0.0	0.0	1.7	4.0	8.3	5.9			0.4	0	11	160
161	0.0	0.0	0.0	0.0	0.5	0.0	0.0	0.0	1.6	1.7	2.2	5.9	5.0	4.0	11.1	9.8			1.0	0	25	161
162-3	0.0	0.0	0.0	0.0	0.0	0.0	1.3	2.1	2.4	5.2	8.8	16.1	16.5	36.1	24.9	35.2			3.5	0	89	162-3
170	0.0	0.0	0.0	0.0	0.5	2.8	8.5	15.4	27.3	35.5	38.5	36.6	54.5	70.3	74.8	70.3			12.2	1	309	170
171	0.0	0.0	0.0	0.0	4.5	17.1	39.4	80.4	102.1	132.4	84.7	124.5	163.6	114.5	94.2	144.5			36.6	2	928	171
172	0.0	0.0	0.0	0.0	0.5	0.0	1.2	1.4	1.6	3.5	12.1	11.7	6.6	20.1	16.6	11.7			2.2	0	56	172
173	0.0	0.0	0.0	0.0	0.0	0.0	0.0	0.0	0.8	0.9	0.0	0.0	0.0	0.0	0.0	0.0			0.1	0	2	173
174	0.0	0.0	0.0	0.0	0.0	0.0	0.0	1.4	2.4	0.0	5.5	7.3	1.7	4.0	5.5	11.7			1.1	1	27	174
175	0.0	0.3	0.0	1.2	2.0	1.7	1.8	2.8	1.6	13.8	13.2	11.7	24.8	20.1	8.3	13.7			3.6	1	92	175
176	0.0	0.0	0.0	0.0	0.0	0.0	0.6	1.4	6.4	3.5	1.1	11.7	8.3	18.1	19.4	43.0			2.7	1	68	176
180	2.3	0.3	0.0	0.0	0.0	0.6	0.0	0.7	1.6	0.0	0.0	4.4	3.3	6.0	0.0	3.9			0.9	0	23	180
181.0	0.0	0.0	0.0	0.8	0.0	0.0	0.0	0.7	1.6	4.3	9.9	5.9	16.5	24.1	13.9	43.0			2.8	0	71	181.0
190	0.0	0.0	0.0	0.0	0.0	0.6	0.0	0.7	1.6	3.5	2.2	0.0	3.3	2.0	5.5	2.0			0.6	0	14	190
191	0.3	0.3	0.3	1.2	2.0	5.5	4.9	16.8	26.5	30.3	50.6	90.8	119.0	178.7	196.7	367.2			26.1	14	662	191
192	0.9	0.3	0.0	0.0	0.0	0.0	0.6	0.0	0.0	2.6	1.1	0.0	1.7	4.0	5.5	2.0			0.6	0	15	192
193	1.1	1.9	0.6	1.2	1.0	0.6	1.2	2.1	1.6	3.5	3.3	8.8	3.3	6.0	2.8	0.0			1.7	0	44	193
194	0.3	0.0	0.0	1.2	0.5	1.1	5.5	4.9	3.2	0.9	5.5	7.3	3.3	6.0	5.5	11.7			2.0	0	50	194
195	0.0	0.3	0.6	0.0	0.0	0.6	0.6	0.0	0.0	1.7	0.0	1.5	0.0	0.0	0.0	0.0			0.2	0	4	195
196	0.9	0.0	0.9	1.2	1.0	0.0	0.6	0.7	0.8	0.0	0.0	0.0	3.3	0.0	2.8	2.0			0.4	0	11	196
197	0.0	0.0	0.0	0.8	1.0	0.0	0.0	1.4	1.6	1.7	1.1	0.0	11.6	16.1	11.1	2.0			0.8	0	20	197
200	0.0	0.3	0.6	0.0	0.5	0.6	1.2	1.4	0.8	3.5	5.5	8.8	9.9	2.0	8.3	9.8			1.3	1	32	200
201	0.0	0.0	0.6	0.8	0.0	0.6	0.6	1.4	0.0	2.6	1.1	2.9	3.3	2.0	8.3	9.8			1.5	0	39	201
203	0.0	0.0	0.0	3.1	0.0	1.1	2.4	1.4	2.4	4.3	5.5	5.9	6.6	4.0	5.5	3.9			0.5	0	12	203
204	2.0	2.2	0.6	0.0	2.0	0.0	0.0	0.0	0.8	0.0	0.0	0.0	0.0	4.0	22.2	9.8			2.9	1	73	204
202,205	0.3	0.0	0.0	0.0	0.0	0.0	0.0	0.0	0.8	0.0	0.0	0.0	3.3	2.0	2.8	0.0			0.2	0	4	202,205
OTHER	0.6	0.0	0.0	0.4	0.5	1.1	0.6	1.4	4.0	5.2	11.0	14.6	28.1	42.2	38.8	56.6			4.9	2	123	OTHER
140-205	9.5	5.9	5.7	10.9	17.8	35.8	78.2	149.7	229.1	293.3	344.3	465.6	679.3	891.6	941.8	1347.7			146.5	29	3711	140-205
RATE PER CASE IN PERIOD	0.29	0.31	0.32	0.39	0.50	0.55	0.61	0.70	0.80	0.87	1.10	1.46	1.65	2.01	2.77	1.95			0.04	-	-	RATE PER CASE IN PERIOD

History is made by the accomplishment of individual lay or professional people or a group of such people. Medical history is made in a similar way. The origin of the Connecticut Tumor Registry dates back to the year of 1930, when a progressive, interested and wide-awake public figure stimulated by a group of physicians decided to request the establishment of a cancer committee in New Haven, Connecticut. This committee was composed of lay and professional people who invested their time and efforts to determine the extent of the cancer problem as it existed at that time in New Haven. Due to their stimulation and interest, and with their active cooperation and help, the State Medical Society of Connecticut in 1933 appointed a committee on tumour study which was charged with evaluating the problem of cancer and to bring forth recommendations to improve this situation in Connecticut. By combining efforts, these organisations were able to have the legislature in 1935 approve a bill initiating a state-wide effort. The responsibility of pursuing this task was placed in the hands of the State Health Department.

Simultaneously, the American Society for the control of cancer organized a division in Connecticut in 1933. In this organization, surgeons, pathologists, and other physicians interested in studying the cancer problem combined their efforts.

The governor signed the bill which had been passed by the 1935 General Assembly and which reads as follows: ... "The State Department of Health is authorized to make investigations concerning cancer, the prevention and treatment thereof, and the mortality therefrom, and to take such action as it may deem will assist in bringing about a reduction in the mortality due thereto. "

The State Department of Health established a division of cancer research which was charged with the responsibility of fulfilling the mandate given to it by the legislature. Its first task was to gain a comprehensive picture of existing conditions. It tabulated cancer mortality data and analysed them according to age, sex, residence, nativity, and primary site of the tumour for the state as a whole. This analysis was completed in 1941 and went backs as far as the year 1920. It involved the examination of 32,510 death certificates with reclassification of the causes of death to conform to the international list of causes of death. Each of these deaths was recorded on a punch card and an alphabetical cross-index file was established to make it possible to locate any cancer death record with maximum ease and minimum expenditure of time. This file proved to be of great value in looking up follow-up information for hospitals.

Thereafter, and in order to carry out the study of morbidity due to cancer, it was necessary that accurate records of cancer cases be kept in all local hospitals. For this purpose, a standard tumor record was devised. A follow-up form was prepared to be used uniformly in all participating hospitals. In the beginning of 1941, a team composed of a physician, a statistician, and specially trained clerks visited each cooperating hospital and made abstracts of all cancer records diagnosed as of January 1935, up to that date. Copies of these records were taken to the Central Registry while the originals were kept at local hospital record rooms. With these records, it was possible to immediately start an analysis of five-year's experience for those patients on whom the information had been collected.

The original tumor record and follow-up form were developed with the help of the tumor committee of the Connecticut State Medical Society which also established guides for the adoption of Standard Nomenclature to be used by all hospitals in the state of Connecticut. This was accomplished with the help of pathologists, assisted by leading surgeons and radiologists. A specific code was devised and an instruction manual put into use at that time. This was used in the coding of all records early in 1950.

Legislature also made available to the State Health Department specific funds to support local registries and tumor clinics.

Through the years, the Connecticut Tumor Registry has grown in size and importance. By 1964, information on over 168,000 tumors had been collected. Approximately, 8,500 new cases are added yearly to the Registry. In addition, 1,000 second primaries are recorded and there are approximately 35,000 tumors under active follow-up. This number is growing due to the longer survival of patients with some types of cancer.

The Connecticut Registry provides an excellent opportunity to evaluate cancer therapy in terms of survival. It is a unique source of information in that it contains data on a large series of patients with cancer diagnosed during the indexed period and drawn from a defined population base. Thus, it is possible to study the survival experience of all patients known to have cancer seen in all hospitals in Connecticut or in all hospitals of a large community rather than just the experience of one institution or a selected series of patients exposed to a specific therapeutic cause. The Registry provides an opportunity to measure the trend in survival rates and to determine how much progress if any has been made in the menagement of patients. Furthermore, the number of cases available for analysis is large enough to permit evaluation of the interrelated influences on survival of such factors as age, sex, primary site, stage at diagnosis, urban and rural differences and method of treatment.

Presently, all hospitals in the state of Connecticut, non-profit, private and state, provide the Central Registry with the prepared abstract form of all new cases of cancer diagnosed and later with life-long follow-up of surviving cancer patients. In addition, the Public Health Statistics Section of the State Department of Health supplies the Cancer Registry with a copy of all death certificates on which mention of cancer has been made.'

This approach insures as complete a reporting as seems possible. During the last few years, the percentage of cancers reported by death certificates only has diminished to seven percent indicating that 93 percent of all patients are diagnosed and reported prior to death with all information necessary to determine the success of treatment.

Since some patients may seek medical attention out of state, arrangements are in effect with many research centers to notify the Connecticut Registry of patients with a Connecticut residency. For any which go unreported, death certificates are made available either through the Public Health Statistics Section of the State Health Department or through other vital statistics sections in the United States.

The data from the Connecticut Registry provide information on the incidence of cancer and its various sites by age and sex, rural and urban differences and many other characteristics which make up data on the number and geographic distribution of persons afflicted with cancer in a defined population group.

Registration procedure is as follows.

1. *Hospital*

The flow of the medical records of new admissions in all general hospitals of the state is almost uniform. The patient's chart reaches the medical record library and includes copies of any pathology reports, x-ray reports and information às to whether the patient has been an out-patient or an in-patient.

In most general hospitals, the separate tumor registry secretary then abstracts from these records the necessary information and creates a tumor record for the hospital files. A copy of this record is sent to the Connecticut Tumor Registry.

2. Connecticut Tumor Registry

The record from a hospital first reaches the quality-control unit. The members of this quality-control unit are well trained and experienced coders who check over the records received from the individual hospitals for accuracy and completeness of information and search for any discrepancies which may exist. If discrepancies are found, a person from the quality-control unit travels to the reporting hospital to discuss the individual case or cases with the tumor secretary or the medical records librarian.

As another quality control function, the hospitals are visited periodically and each registry is discussed with those responsible for its operation concerning the quality of the records, the information received and recorded, and the operation of the individual registry as it affects its affiliation with the Central Registry. This function of the quality-control unit is the external control exercised toward the good quality of reports recorded in the Central Registry. Internal checks on the quality of the coding is accomplished through recoding of a sample of records by a second coder and subsequent discussion of any discrepancies. When this method indicates low quality, a coder will be put through a retraining or refresher period. Further quality is assured through data processing methods described further on.

After complete checking by the members of the quality-control unit, the record is then given to the clerical supervisor who assigns one clerk to stamp the date of receipt and to alphabetize the records within hospital order.

New cases are then turned over to the visual index clerk who checks for a previous report concerning the patient. This could be a record from another hospital on the same tumor or a prior diagnosis of another tumor or there may be a death certificate in file.

Cases are then numbered and entered in the daily receipts book if there has been no previous report. If in earlier record has been found the new report receives the number already assigned to the earlier case.

Records are turned over to a coder who codes for four different punch cards :
1) the analytic card, 2) the index card, 3) the follow-up card, and 4) the allocation card. Cases are sent to data processing for punching and verification of the cards, edit checking and later computer quality control.

Case records are put in file in site and serial number order.

3. Follow-up

From the existing follow-up card, the follow-up form is prepared one year after the initial diagnosis and each year thereafter on its anniversary date. These forms are divided according to hospitals and sent at the beginning of each month. At the hospital, the tumor secretary fills out the forms and notes whether there has been a readmission to that hospital, or to any other hospital within the state known to the original hospital. It is also noted if there has been a recurrence or additional tumor treatment. The Registry will also obtain the follow-up information from the private physician treating and following his own patients.

When the tumor follow-up record is returned to the Connecticut Tumor Registry, a clerk stamps the date of receipt and separates the alive and dead cases.

On the routine alive patients, the data needed for follow-up is processed for a change in the coded card and punched in the data processing unit and re-intergrated into the Registry.

On death follow-up, the visual index strip is so marked and removed and the data processing card is changed.

Follow-up reports are then filed with the proper case for future recoding and updating of the analytic card.

4. Death Certificates

Photostatic copies of all death certificate with mention of cancer are routinely forwarded to the Connecticut Tumor Registry by the Public Health Statistics Section. When these are received monthly, they are stamped with the date of receipt and alphabetized. These are given to the visual index clerk who checks to see if there is a case record to match the death certificate. If there is a record the visual index strip is marked and the death certificate filed with the case.

Unmatched death certificates are indexed for future matching to newly received the death certificate is given a Registry number and put in analytic code.

If, however, the death occurred in a Connecticut hospital, a letter is sent requesting a tumor record for the patient. In this case a report is received or the hospital informs the Central Registry that cancer was not, in fact, present at death, thus removing the death certificate from Registry files.

If the death occurred elsewhere, an inquiry is sent to the physician certifying the death. Additional information thus received either removes it from the cancer category or enables the Registry to make up a tumor record.

When all sources of further inquiry have been exhausted, the death certificate remains in the Registry as a "non-analytic" case.

Henry Eisenberg

Registry Title and Address : Connecticut Tumor Registry, Connecticut State Department of Health, 79 Elm Street, Hartford, Connecticut, U.S.A. Commenced diagnosis in 1935 and started operation in 1941. Supported financially by the Federal Government and the State of Connecticut.

Registration. Cases are registered from all hospitals - private, public and non-profit making - in most large general hospitals by the tumor secretary. Out-patient cases are registered by the majority of reporting hospitals. The registry secretary reports cases from radiotherapy and pathology departments. Copies of death certificates with mention of cancer are supplied by the Public Health Statistics Section of the State Department of Health including Connecticut residents who die outside the state. At the special request of the State Registry doctors register cases attended at home. Research centres in other states supply information on Connecticut residents.

Follow-up. With the exception of superficial skin lesions all registrations are followed up till death. All "pre-malignant" and benign special interest tumours are followed up for 5 years.

Physical Description. The state of Connecticut is bounded by Massachusetts to the north, Rhode Island to the east, Long Island Sound to the south and New York to the west. It lies between latitudes 41º 15' and 42º 0' North and longitudes 71º 45' and 73º 30' West. The total registration area is 12,973 square kilometres.

Demographic Description. Total population of area under survey 2,603,690. The percentages of principal ethnic groups (foreign born or of foreign parentage) are : Italian 9.4 %, Canadian 4.8 %, Polish 4.6 %, Irish 3.0 %, German 2.5 %, all other 14.4 % and non-white 4.4. %. The main occupational composition is industry (mining, construction, manufacturing, forestry and fish) 49 %; commerce (rail, truck, communications, utilities, trade, finance, insurance, real estate, business and repair services) 29 %; agriculture 1 %; personal service (hotels, education, medical, health, recreation, entertainment) 17 %; Government 4 %. Seventy two per cent of the population live in conurbations of more than 100,000.

Medical Services. Total number of hospital beds of all kinds 9,566 (1963). Total number of doctors in practice in registration area 4,150 (1963). Cancer causes approximately 18 % of all deaths (1963).

Publications. Annual reports, "Cancer in Connecticut"
Campbell (1963); Greenberg (1959); Griswold, Wilder, Cutler and Pollack (1955).
    A list of the many reports based on data from the Registry is available from the Registry on request.

TABLE 15 A
U.S.A., CONNECTICUT :
POPULATION (100,000s), MEAN 1960 - 62

AGE (in years)	MALES		FEMALES	
	No.	Per Cent	No.	Per Cent
0 –	1.4319	11.21	1.3721	10.35
5 –	1.3213	10.34	1.2675	9.56
10 –	1.1763	9.21	1.1306	8.53
15 –	0.9019	7.06	0.8962	6.76
20 –	0.6937	5.43	0.7587	5.72
25 –	0.7587	5.94	0.7967	6.01
30 –	0.8615	6.74	0.8928	6.73
35 –	0.9313	7.29	0.9746	7.35
40 –	0.9248	7.24	0.9599	7.24
45 –	0.8540	6.68	0.8668	6.54
50 –	0.7170	5.61	0.7407	5.59
55 –	0.6083	4.76	0.6431	4.85
60 –	0.5030	3.94	0.5676	4.28
65 –	0.4334	3.39	0.5084	3.83
70 –	0.3208	2.51	0.3911	2.95
75 –	0.1901	1.49	0.2534	1.91
80 –	0.0959	0.75	0.1450	1.09
85 – and over	0.0544	0.43	0.0934	0.70
TOTAL	12.7783	100.00	13.2586	100.00

NOTES

TO TABLES 15 A, B and C

(I) I. L. number 193 excludes benign and unspecified tumours of the central nervous system.

(II) Carcinoma in situ excluded.

TABLE 15 B

U.S.A., CONNECTICUT :

MALE INCIDENCE RATES, 1960 - 62.

INTER-NATIONAL LIST No.	AVERAGE ANNUAL INCIDENCE PER 100,000 — AGE IN YEARS																		ALL AGES	No. OF CASES IN WHOLE PERIOD — AGE UNKNOWN	No. OF CASES IN WHOLE PERIOD — ALL AGES	INTER-NATIONAL LIST No.
	0-	5-	10-	15-	20-	25-	30-	35-	40-	45-	50-	55-	60-	65-	70-	75-	80-	85- AND OVER				
140	0.0	0.0	0.0	0.0	0.5	0.4	0.4	1.8	3.2	1.6	2.8	6.0	9.9	21.5	20.8	31.6	34.8	61.3	3.6	0	139	140
141	0.0	0.0	0.0	0.0	0.0	0.0	0.8	1.1	0.7	8.2	8.4	10.4	14.6	17.7	14.5	31.6	41.7	18.4	4.1	1	158	141
142	0.2	0.0	0.0	0.4	1.0	0.9	0.8	1.4	0.7	1.6	0.9	3.3	0.7	5.4	4.2	12.3	0.0	12.3	1.3	1	48	142
143-4	0.2	0.0	0.0	0.0	0.0	0.0	0.0	1.1	0.4	2.7	7.0	11.0	14.6	23.1	29.1	31.6	34.8	42.9	4.3	1	163	143-4
146	0.0	0.3	0.0	0.0	0.0	0.9	0.8	0.4	0.4	0.8	0.5	0.5	3.3	6.2	6.2	1.8	0.0	0.0	0.8	0	29	146
145,147-8	0.0	0.0	0.0	0.0	0.0	0.0	0.0	0.4	1.1	4.7	13.0	13.7	15.9	21.5	20.8	22.8	17.4	42.9	4.4	1	169	145,147-8
150	0.0	0.0	0.0	0.0	0.0	0.0	0.0	0.7	2.2	4.7	8.4	18.6	29.8	43.8	50.9	43.8	27.8	49.0	6.9	1	265	150
151	0.0	0.3	0.0	0.0	0.0	0.0	1.5	3.2	6.5	9.4	26.0	34.0	51.7	120.8	168.3	213.9	274.6	269.6	21.3	1	816	151
152	0.2	0.3	0.0	0.0	0.5	0.0	0.0	0.4	0.4	0.4	2.3	2.7	3.3	6.9	10.4	8.8	13.9	6.1	1.3	0	50	152
153	0.0	0.3	0.3	0.4	0.0	0.4	3.9	4.3	6.1	19.9	33.5	62.5	92.1	150.7	214.0	303.3	358.0	343.1	30.1	1	1154	153
154	0.0	0.0	0.0	0.0	0.0	0.4	0.0	1.1	4.7	10.9	23.2	46.0	59.6	95.4	108.1	170.1	177.3	177.7	17.6	2	676	154
155.0	0.0	0.5	0.0	0.0	0.0	0.9	0.4	0.7	0.4	1.2	2.8	5.5	8.0	17.7	26.0	7.0	27.8	30.6	2.7	0	104	155.0
155.1	0.0	0.0	0.0	0.0	0.0	0.0	0.0	1.1	1.1	0.8	2.3	3.8	6.6	15.4	28.1	28.1	20.9	36.8	2.7	0	105	155.1
156	0.0	0.0	0.0	0.0	0.0	0.0	0.0	0.0	0.0	0.4	2.8	2.7	4.0	11.5	10.4	14.0	17.4	36.8	1.6	0	62	156
157	0.0	0.0	0.0	0.0	0.0	0.9	0.0	2.1	4.3	3.9	11.2	25.8	35.8	64.6	61.3	89.4	128.6	134.8	10.6	0	408	157
160	0.0	0.0	0.0	0.0	0.6	0.0	0.4	0.0	0.4	1.2	0.0	1.1	3.3	3.1	2.1	1.8	10.4	12.3	0.6	0	24	160
161	0.0	0.0	0.0	0.0	0.0	0.0	0.4	0.7	5.8	8.6	15.8	29.6	35.1	39.2	35.3	45.6	62.6	18.4	8.2	0	315	161
162-3	0.0	0.0	0.0	0.0	0.5	0.0	3.1	7.9	18.4	40.6	74.8	163.3	224.7	270.7	318.0	271.8	232.9	134.8	49.4	9	1895	162-3
170	0.0	0.0	0.0	0.0	0.0	0.0	0.4	0.0	0.0	0.0	2.8	2.7	2.7	7.7	3.1	8.8	7.0	6.1	1.0	0	37	170
177	0.2	0.0	0.0	0.4	0.0	0.0	0.0	0.0	0.7	4.7	9.3	38.4	110.7	210.0	357.4	513.8	747.3	937.5	40.5	1	1552	177
178	0.5	0.3	0.0	1.5	1.9	6.6	4.6	8.9	3.6	1.2	1.4	0.5	2.7	1.5	2.1	5.3	7.0	0.0	2.4	0	93	178
179.0	0.0	0.0	0.0	0.7	0.0	0.4	0.0	0.0	0.4	0.8	0.9	2.2	5.3	3.1	5.2	3.5	10.4	6.1	0.9	0	33	179.0
180	1.6	0.3	0.0	2.2	0.5	0.0	1.2	1.4	4.3	6.6	10.7	18.1	27.2	37.7	34.3	49.1	59.1	18.4	7.1	2	274	180
181.0	0.0	0.0	0.0	0.4	1.0	0.0	4.3	2.9	5.8	12.1	20.0	40.6	67.6	98.4	160.0	147.3	253.7	190.0	19.8	1	759	181.0
190	0.0	0.8	0.6	0.7	1.4	3.5	3.9	6.4	5.4	4.7	6.5	4.0	4.0	3.1	8.3	8.8	7.0	24.5	3.3	0	127	190
191	0.0	0.8	0.6	1.1	1.0	3.1	13.5	19.7	37.1	52.3	81.8	99.7	168.3	165.4	224.4	266.5	326.7	416.7	47.2	108	1809	191
192	1.2	0.0	0.6	0.0	0.5	0.0	0.0	0.7	0.0	1.2	0.0	1.6	2.7	1.5	1.0	3.5	3.5	0.0	0.7	0	26	192
193	2.6	1.8	3.1	3.3	2.4	2.6	2.7	5.4	7.2	10.1	10.7	14.2	13.9	18.5	12.5	5.3	0.0	6.1	5.9	0	227	193
194	0.9	0.3	0.0	0.7	0.5	0.9	0.4	2.1	1.4	0.8	1.4	3.3	3.3	5.4	3.1	8.8	3.5	6.1	1.3	0	49	194
195	0.2	0.5	0.3	2.2	2.4	0.4	0.4	0.4	0.4	0.8	0.5	2.2	1.3	0.8	2.1	1.8	0.0	0.0	0.7	0	26	195
196	0.2	0.8	1.1	1.5	1.4	2.6	1.2	0.7	1.1	1.2	0.9	2.2	2.0	0.0	3.1	1.8	3.5	12.3	1.1	0	44	196
197	0.2	0.8	0.6	1.5	1.4	2.6	1.2	1.1	2.9	3.1	4.2	4.9	7.3	7.7	14.5	15.8	20.9	6.1	2.9	2	112	197
200	0.2	0.3	0.9	1.5	0.0	1.3	1.5	2.1	3.6	3.9	5.6	7.1	8.6	13.8	6.2	14.0	13.9	55.1	3.3	1	126	200
201	0.0	0.5	2.6	2.2	6.7	4.8	4.6	2.9	2.9	3.9	4.6	4.9	6.0	4.6	7.3	5.3	10.4	6.1	3.4	1	129	201
203	0.0	0.0	0.0	0.0	0.0	0.0	0.0	0.4	1.1	1.6	1.9	4.9	11.3	13.1	18.7	21.0	24.3	30.6	2.5	0	97	203
204	6.5	3.0	3.1	4.4	2.4	4.0	1.9	4.7	6.1	6.6	13.0	15.3	32.5	46.9	53.0	63.1	104.3	42.9	11.0	1	420	204
202,205	0.5	0.5	0.9	0.7	1.0	0.9	0.8	2.5	2.9	3.9	3.7	6.6	9.9	7.7	13.5	7.0	10.4	6.1	2.8	0	106	202,205
OTHER	1.6	0.5	0.0	0.4	1.0	0.9	1.9	3.6	6.8	10.5	19.5	29.6	41.1	63.1	114.3	131.5	93.8	159.3	14.4	0	553	OTHER
140-205	17.0	11.4	14.5	22.5	26.4	37.8	56.1	94.1	150.3	251.4	435.1	745.8	1141.2	1645.1	2172.7	2609.2	3187.3	3357.8	343.8	137	13179	140-205
RATE PER CASE IN PERIOD	0.23	0.25	0.28	0.37	0.48	0.44	0.39	0.36	0.36	0.39	0.46	0.55	0.66	0.77	1.04	1.75	3.48	6.13	0.03	-	-	RATE PER CASE IN PERIOD

TABLE 15 C
U.S.A., CONNECTICUT :
FEMALE INCIDENCE RATES, 1960 - 62.

AVERAGE ANNUAL INCIDENCE PER 100,000 — AGE IN YEARS

International List No.	0-	5-	10-	15-	20-	25-	30-	35-	40-	45-	50-	55-	60-	65-	70-	75-	80-	85- and over	All Ages	No. cases Age Unknown	No. cases All Ages
140	0.0	0.0	0.0	0.0	0.0	0.0	0.0	0.3	0.0	0.0	0.5	0.0	1.2	0.0	2.6	1.3	0.0	3.6	0.2	0	9
141	0.0	0.0	0.0	0.0	0.0	0.4	0.0	0.7	0.0	2.3	0.5	4.1	2.3	2.6	1.7	1.3	2.3	3.6	0.8	0	31
142	0.2	0.0	0.3	0.0	0.0	0.0	1.5	0.7	0.3	0.0	1.8	2.1	2.9	1.3	3.4	1.3	4.6	14.3	0.9	0	35
143-4	0.0	0.0	0.0	0.7	0.0	0.0	0.0	1.0	1.4	0.8	1.8	3.6	2.9	3.3	3.4	13.2	13.8	10.7	1.4	2	55
146	0.0	0.0	0.0	0.7	0.0	0.0	0.4	0.0	0.3	0.8	1.4	1.0	0.6	0.7	0.9	1.3	0.0	0.0	0.4	0	15
145,147-8	0.0	0.0	0.0	0.0	0.0	0.0	0.0	0.7	0.0	1.5	3.6	2.6	1.8	2.0	2.6	5.3	2.3	7.1	0.8	0	33
150	0.0	0.0	0.0	0.0	0.0	0.0	0.0	0.7	0.7	1.2	1.8	3.1	4.7	4.6	2.6	13.2	9.2	14.3	1.3	0	53
151	0.0	0.0	0.0	0.4	0.4	0.8	0.4	3.1	4.2	8.5	14.0	16.1	30.5	43.3	66.5	102.6	156.3	153.5	12.4	0	495
152	0.0	0.0	0.0	0.0	0.0	0.4	0.0	0.3	0.7	0.8	1.4	2.1	3.5	2.6	3.4	6.6	9.2	7.1	1.0	0	38
153	0.0	0.0	0.0	0.7	0.4	0.8	3.4	7.2	11.8	26.1	37.8	66.9	89.9	134.4	202.0	257.8	335.6	353.3	34.9	1	1387
154	0.0	0.0	0.0	0.4	0.9	0.4	1.3	3.4	3.5	9.2	22.5	29.0	43.5	55.1	59.7	94.7	114.9	96.4	13.5	0	535
155.0	0.0	0.0	0.0	0.0	0.0	0.0	0.0	0.0	0.0	1.2	0.9	1.1	1.2	5.2	6.8	11.8	16.1	14.3	1.4	0	54
155.1	0.0	0.0	0.0	0.0	0.0	0.4	0.3	0.0	0.3	0.8	4.5	3.1	12.3	16.4	28.1	32.9	57.5	71.4	4.2	0	169
156	0.2	0.0	0.0	0.0	0.0	0.0	0.0	0.0	0.0	1.2	3.2	1.6	3.5	3.9	6.0	11.8	9.2	21.4	1.3	0	52
157	0.0	0.0	0.3	0.0	0.0	0.4	0.3	0.3	1.4	5.8	8.1	9.3	22.3	32.1	57.1	59.2	73.6	89.2	7.9	1	314
160	0.5	0.0	0.0	0.0	0.0	0.0	0.3	0.3	1.0	1.2	0.9	0.5	0.6	1.3	3.4	3.9	0.0	7.1	0.6	0	23
161	0.0	0.0	0.0	0.0	0.0	0.0	0.3	0.7	2.1	1.5	0.9	2.1	2.9	2.0	0.9	1.3	0.0	0.0	0.7	0	28
162-3	0.0	0.0	0.0	0.4	0.4	0.4	1.1	3.8	7.6	12.3	13.1	18.7	27.6	30.2	40.9	31.6	41.4	82.1	8.6	0	341
170	0.0	0.0	0.0	0.4	1.3	6.3	24.6	56.8	93.8	133.4	155.3	180.4	175.6	212.4	234.4	285.5	333.3	414.0	74.0	7	2944
171	0.0	0.0	0.0	0.0	0.9	2.9	14.6	20.5	29.2	30.0	31.5	39.9	44.0	38.7	34.9	25.0	34.5	32.1	16.0	3	638
172	0.0	0.0	0.0	0.0	0.0	0.8	3.7	5.5	11.1	28.5	39.2	38.9	47.0	61.6	69.0	61.8	41.4	53.5	15.9	1	632
173	0.0	0.0	0.0	0.0	0.4	0.0	0.0	0.0	0.0	0.0	0.0	0.0	0.0	0.0	0.0	0.0	0.0	0.0	0.0	0	1
174	0.2	0.0	1.2	0.0	0.9	0.4	2.6	1.7	4.9	5.4	9.9	11.4	13.5	13.8	19.6	25.0	27.6	32.1	4.9	0	195
175	0.0	0.3	0.6	2.6	2.2	3.3	4.9	10.9	16.3	31.9	34.2	36.3	45.8	54.4	50.3	44.7	43.7	25.0	15.7	3	626
176	0.0	0.0	0.0	0.0	0.4	0.0	0.4	1.0	1.4	1.2	4.5	5.2	4.7	7.2	12.8	28.9	20.7	25.0	2.6	1	105
180	2.2	0.3	0.6	0.0	0.0	0.0	0.0	0.7	2.1	5.0	6.3	7.3	15.3	12.5	24.7	17.1	23.0	28.6	4.2	0	166
181.0	0.0	0.0	0.0	0.0	0.0	0.4	1.5	0.7	2.1	6.9	5.4	10.9	18.2	20.3	36.6	63.1	62.1	89.2	6.9	2	273
190	0.0	0.8	0.9	1.5	2.6	2.9	3.0	5.1	6.3	5.0	5.0	6.2	7.0	11.8	4.3	9.2	4.6	17.8	3.8	4	153
191	0.5	0.3	0.3	0.0	1.3	6.7	8.6	17.4	26.4	38.8	53.1	59.1	90.4	95.7	121.9	159.2	232.2	292.6	33.3	70	1324
192	0.5	0.3	1.2	0.0	0.4	0.0	0.0	0.0	0.3	0.4	1.4	1.0	0.6	0.7	4.3	1.3	6.9	3.6	0.6	0	24
193	0.0	0.0	0.6	0.7	0.9	2.1	3.4	3.1	3.5	7.3	8.1	7.8	12.3	9.8	11.1	5.3	4.6	0.0	4.3	0	172
194	1.2	0.3	0.6	1.5	3.1	4.2	4.5	4.4	6.3	4.6	5.4	2.1	2.9	7.2	7.7	7.9	13.8	28.6	3.5	0	139
195	0.0	0.5	1.2	2.2	0.4	0.4	0.4	1.0	1.0	0.0	1.4	1.0	2.3	0.0	4.3	2.6	0.0	0.0	0.7	0	27
196	0.2	0.0	1.2	1.1	0.0	0.4	0.7	0.3	1.0	0.4	0.9	0.5	4.7	3.9	4.3	2.6	4.6	0.0	1.0	0	39
197	0.5	0.0	0.0	0.4	2.2	2.1	0.7	1.0	2.4	3.8	2.3	4.7	4.7	7.9	7.7	7.9	6.9	7.1	2.5	2	98
200	0.2	0.0	0.9	3.3	0.0	0.4	2.2	0.7	4.9	2.7	2.3	4.1	8.2	7.2	16.2	15.8	18.4	7.1	2.7	0	108
201	0.2	0.0	0.0	0.0	3.1	1.7	0.0	1.7	1.4	2.3	2.3	1.0	4.1	4.6	2.6	1.3	4.6	14.3	1.9	0	76
203	0.0	2.1	1.8	1.1	0.0	0.0	0.4	0.7	0.3	1.2	2.3	3.1	13.5	13.8	15.3	10.5	9.2	10.7	2.4	0	94
204	4.1	0.8	0.9	1.8	1.8	0.4	0.4	3.1	2.1	2.3	5.9	7.3	11.2	22.3	27.3	38.1	27.6	35.7	5.6	0	224
202,205	3.4	0.3	0.9	1.5	3.5	0.4	0.4	1.4	2.8	4.6	4.5	5.7	10.6	10.5	14.5	14.5	23.0	32.1	4.0	0	160
OTHER	0.7	0.3	0.3	1.1	1.3	1.7	2.2	3.8	6.3	8.5	15.3	20.2	33.5	36.1	60.5	76.3	126.4	117.8	11.9	0	474
140-205	18.5	7.9	11.2	19.7	29.9	41.4	87.4	163.8	261.1	399.2	514.4	621.0	826.9	993.3	1275.9	1552.2	1914.9	2216.3	310.7	97	12359
RATE PER CASE IN PERIOD	0.24	0.26	0.29	0.37	0.44	0.42	0.37	0.34	0.35	0.38	0.45	0.52	0.59	0.66	0.85	1.32	2.30	3.57	0.03	-	-

USA, NEW YORK STATE LESS NEW YORK CITY

The reporting of cancer in New York State, exclusive of New York City, began on January 1, 1940. The Law provides that every physician shall report every case of cancer or other malignant disease under his care; that whenever cancer or other malignant disease is found in a tissue specimen examined in a laboratory, the person in charge or the person making the examination shall report the existence of cancer; and that the person in charge of every hospital, dispensary, asylum, or other similar public or private institution shall report every case of cancer or other malignant disease. Enactment of this legislation followed a recommendation made by the New York State Legislative Cancer Survey Commission in order that an adequate system of reporting cancer would in the course of time make available to the medical profession accurate information, instead of uncertain estimates, on (a) the true magnitude of the cancer problem, (b) the relative incidence of cancer in various sections of the State and among various social and economic groups, (c) the relation between cancer and such factors as occupation, (d) the extent of the alleged increase in cancer above that due to ageing of the population, (e) the accuracy of mortality statistics, (f) the true incidence of the various forms of cancer. In addition it was felt that there would thereby be furnished an invaluable index as to what sections of the population and what forms of cancer require the greatest attention and application of such control measures as education and the establishment of Tumor Clinics. This recommendation had previously received the endorsement of the Medical Society of the State of New York. Thus, from its inception, cancer morbidity reporting in New York State has had the active support of the medical profession.

Reports are now being received from three sources, namely (1) the physician, tumor clinic, or hospital; (2) the laboratory where the surgical specimen has been examined; and (3) from the death certificate. Because the primary purposes of the registry is to record the incidence of malignant neoplastic disease in a defined population, only the initial report is recorded for any single individual. Therefore, the second primary malignancy is being missed. The standard reporting form from the physician, tumor clinic, or hospital is kept as simple as possible to insure complete and accurate information. The individual is identified and basic characteristics of the individual and of the neoplasm are obtained. Laboratories are permitted to report by means of a carbon copy of the report which they would ordinarily make for the physician or for the hospital record. These reports are collected through the local full-time health officer who forwards them to the central registry. The year of receipt at the Bureau in Albany is considered the year of "onset" of the disease for the computation of age-specific rates.

Any death in New York State, exclusive of New York City, for which a diagnosis of malignant neoplastic disease is listed anywhere on the death certificate is checked to see whether the case has previously been reported. If it has not, then this death becomes a reported case as of the age at death. In 1964, 28.2 % of all reported cases were from this source.

An important question which occurs in reviewing the incidence data such as that obtained from a large central registry concerns the completeness of reporting. The question of how many cases of cancer are diagnosed among up-State residents, and yet never reported to the central registry must be ascertained. A study of the completeness of cancer reporting in New York State was done by the U.S. Public Health Service on a sample of 3,509 patients with a diagnosis of cancer receiving service in hospitals and tumor clinics during 1945. The results of this study indicated that when all 1945 and 1946 case and death reports had been totaled, between 84 % and 96 % of the cases of cancer of each of the major site groups diagnosed in 1945 and given hospital or tumour clinic service in that year had been reported. The average for all sites was 88.7 % reporting.

There is no reason to believe that this total figure for completeness of reporting has decreased over the years, since physicians have become more aware of the importance of cancer as a disease and of the need for reliable cancer statistics. The increasing volume of reports being received each year in the registry, together with the stable ratio of reports received per case indicates that the cancer registry, as maintained by the Bureau of Cancer Control, has a high per cent of total cases of malignant neoplasms being reported.

The diagnosis is considered confirmed histologically if the specimen has been examined at an approved laboratory, or if the death certificate indicates that an autopsy has been performed. Cases of unknown age constitute less than 1/2 % of the total.

As would be expected in the reporting of any chronic disease, an unusually large number of reports was received during 1940, the first year of reporting. Many of these were cases of long standing, and could not be considered "new", i.e., cases first diagnosed during that year. Since it took a few years for the registry to stabilize, the reports of the first few years are seldom used in analyzing trends.

The total volume of cancer reports has increased markedly in the 25 years of operation of the cancer registry until in 1964 alone, about 65,000 reports including death certificates were processed. A ratio of over two reports per case has been maintained annually. The majority of reports for new cases has come from physicians, tumor clinics, or hospitals. The number of reports received by death certificate only, has increased, and it is thought that two reasons are largely responsible. First, between 1947 and 1950, an administrative change was made so that death certificates were totally acceptable as cancer case reports if no previous report had been received. Prior to this time, health officers were instructed to obtain case reports on those cancer deaths not previously reported. Secondly, in recent years, there has been increased emphasis on special diagnostic techniques and more radical surgery which are more readily available in the large specialized hospitals. Consequently, more cancer patients who live in counties surrounding New York City are undoubtedly going to New York City hospitals for diagnosis and treatment. Since New York City is exempt from the cancer reporting Law, no report is received on these up-State residents until the time of death.

Our experience with cancer reporting in New York State indicates that reporting is practicable in areas where the medical profession is sympathetic with the aims of reporting. The completeness compares favourably with that of other reportable diseases. Cancer reporting has proved useful, first to indicate the total extent of the disease and the occurrence by site involved; secondly, to pursue epidemiologic investigations; and finally, to evaluate progress in cancer control programs including assistance to the local health officer by providing summary statistics.

Vincent H. Handy,
William S. Burnett.

Registry Title and Address : New York State Cancer Registry, Bureau of Cancer Control, State of New York Department of Health, 84 Holland Avenue, Albany, New York 12208, U.S.A. Commenced 1st January, 1940. Supported financially by New York State.

Registration. Cases are registered from hospital in-patients and out-patients by tumour clinic secretary or record room librarian, from pathology departments by pathologists, from death certificates from the State Health Department,

from doctors attending cases at home and from all other private or public institutions, under Public Health Law with effect from 1st June, 1954.

Follow-up. No cases are followed up.

Physical Description. The Registry covers New York State except New York
City. It is located in the north eastern part of the United States between Canada
and the Atlantic Ocean. A temperate climate, 10° to 27^oC in summer and -12°
to 5^oC in winter. Altitude of land ranges from sea level to over 5,000 feet; ge-
ological formation varies and includes limestone and sandy soil; rainfall varies
from 25 to 60 inches. It lies between latitudes 40° and 45° north and between
longitudes 72° and 80° west. The total registration area is 123,295 square
kilometres.

Demographic Description. Total population of area under survey 9,000,410.
The ethnic groups are white 86.5 %, negro 13.3 %, other 0.2 %. The main
occupational composition (employed males excluding armed forces) is industry
44.9 %; commerce 44.6 %; agriculture 4.1 %; personal service 6.4 %. Of
the total population 61.6 % live in conurbations of more than 100,000.

Medical Services. There are 38,738 general and cancer hospital beds (1965).
Total number of doctors in practice in registration area 14,329 (1963-64). Cancer caused approximately 17.06 % of all deaths in 1964.

Publications. Annual reports.
Ferber, Handy, Gerhardt and Solomon (1962).

TABLE 16 A
U.S.A., NEW YORK STATE
(excluding New York City) :
POPULATION (100, 000s), CENSUS 1960

AGE (in years)	MALES		FEMALES	
	No.	Per Cent	No.	Per Cent
0-	5.1184	11.62	4.9245	10.71
5-	4.7705	10.83	4.5826	9.97
10-	4.2362	9.62	4.0598	8.83
15-	2.9835	6.77	3.0836	6.71
20-	2.1077	4.79	2.4107	5.24
25-	2.4411	5.54	2.6631	5.79
30-	2.9930	6.80	3.2156	7.00
35-	3.2356	7.35	3.4265	7.45
40-	3.0598	6.95	3.1674	6.89
45-	2.8078	6.38	2.8553	6.21
50-	2.4852	5.64	2.5093	5.46
55-	2.1434	4.87	2.1889	4.76
60-	1.8156	4.12	1.9807	4.31
65-	1.5147	3.44	1.7627	3.83
70-	1.1245	2.55	1.3781	3.00
75-	0.6803	1.54	0.9084	1.98
80-	0.3396	0.77	0.5152	1.12
85- and over	0.1830	0.42	0.3318	0.72
TOTAL	44.0399	100.00	45.9642	100.00

NOTES

TO TABLES 16 A, B and C

(I) Cases occuring in subjects of unknown age are shown separately as in other registries; in calculating the age-specific incidence rates, however, these cases have been distributed among the subjects of known age.

(II) I.L. number 193 includes unspecified tumours of the central nervous system.

(III) Carcinoma in situ excluded from I.L. number 171; a very few similar lesions included at some other sites.

(IV) Second primary neoplasms occuring at either the same or another site not registered.

TABLE 16.B
U.S.A., NEW YORK STATE (excluding NEW YORK CITY) :
MALE INCIDENCE RATES, 1959 - 61.

AVERAGE ANNUAL INCIDENCE PER 100,000 — AGE IN YEARS

International List No.	0–	5–	10–	15–	20–	25–	30–	35–	40–	45–	50–	55–	60–	65–	70–	75–	80–	85– and over	All ages	Cases age unknown	Cases all ages	International List No.
140	0.0	0.1	0.0	0.0	0.0	0.1	0.7	1.0	2.0	2.0	5.2	8.9	9.2	13.9	22.8	24.5	41.2	41.9	3.4	3	454	140
141	0.1	0.0	0.0	0.0	0.0	0.0	0.3	0.5	0.9	1.5	4.6	6.1	10.6	12.5	13.6	13.7	18.6	21.9	2.4	1	323	141
142	0.1	0.1	0.0	0.4	0.0	0.4	1.3	0.7	1.1	1.4	1.2	3.0	3.1	2.0	5.0	4.4	8.8	9.1	1.1	0	144	142
143-4	0.0	0.0	0.0	0.0	0.0	0.0	0.0	0.6	1.1	3.2	5.9	7.6	10.6	8.8	20.2	25.5	26.5	43.7	3.1	2	405	143-4
146	0.0	0.0	0.0	0.2	0.2	0.0	0.1	0.1	0.4	1.4	0.7	1.2	2.6	1.5	2.4	0.5	0.0	5.5	0.5	1	67	146
145,147-8	0.0	0.0	0.0	0.1	0.0	0.0	0.0	0.1	0.4	2.7	7.1	9.5	9.7	12.1	16.6	15.2	16.7	12.8	2.7	2	362	145,147-8
150	0.0	0.0	0.0	0.0	0.0	0.0	0.1	0.2	1.1	3.4	6.7	11.2	18.4	28.6	32.3	37.7	50.1	49.2	5.0	1	658	150
151	0.0	0.1	0.0	0.0	0.2	0.1	0.8	2.7	6.1	10.2	16.1	28.3	54.2	82.1	124.8	160.7	185.5	173.0	16.5	1	2180	151
152	0.0	0.0	0.0	0.0	0.2	0.0	0.0	0.5	0.5	0.8	2.5	1.7	1.5	2.9	2.4	7.8	2.9	5.5	0.8	1	100	152
153	0.1	0.0	0.1	0.3	0.8	0.7	1.8	3.5	7.3	16.5	27.4	47.3	86.8	121.9	179.0	236.7	307.2	282.3	25.4	8	3361	153
154	0.1	0.1	0.0	0.0	0.0	0.1	1.6	2.4	4.0	8.5	21.9	35.5	58.0	81.0	103.5	155.3	158.0	151.2	16.2	6	2134	154
155.0	0.1	0.0	0.0	0.0	0.0	0.1	0.3	0.3	0.0	1.2	2.8	3.7	8.8	8.6	11.9	14.2	18.6	7.3	1.8	0	243	155.0
155.1	0.0	0.0	0.0	0.0	0.0	0.1	0.1	0.7	0.7	1.1	2.3	4.0	6.4	9.0	12.4	19.6	20.6	31.0	2.0	1	263	155.1
156	0.1	0.0	0.0	0.0	0.0	0.1	0.0	0.4	1.1	1.1	2.3	6.2	9.5	8.1	17.2	24.0	20.6	21.9	2.4	0	314	156
157	0.0	0.0	0.0	0.1	0.2	0.5	0.3	0.6	3.2	5.8	12.7	20.2	36.4	49.7	63.7	84.8	82.4	80.1	9.5	0	1258	157
160	0.1	0.0	0.0	0.0	0.0	0.0	0.4	0.4	0.9	0.8	0.8	2.8	3.1	2.4	5.0	6.4	5.9	3.6	0.9	0	114	160
161	0.0	0.0	0.0	0.0	0.0	0.3	0.2	0.6	1.7	5.0	10.9	14.9	23.9	34.3	30.5	31.8	19.6	25.5	5.5	1	733	161
162-3	0.1	0.0	0.1	0.0	0.3	0.7	2.2	5.6	14.1	33.7	74.2	131.7	199.0	253.3	273.6	235.7	187.5	134.8	43.9	1	5800	162-3
170	0.1	0.0	0.0	0.0	0.2	0.1	0.3	0.3	0.0	0.4	1.2	0.8	2.6	2.9	4.4	3.9	2.9	3.6	0.6	0	79	170
177	0.1	0.1	0.0	0.0	0.2	0.1	0.2	0.0	0.4	1.2	8.9	23.3	64.1	134.7	249.9	398.8	575.2	708.6	29.0	14	3830	177
178	0.1	0.1	0.2	0.8	3.0	4.1	6.3	4.2	4.9	3.0	2.5	1.1	1.1	1.1	1.5	1.0	2.0	1.8	2.1	1	277	178
179.0	0.1	0.0	0.0	0.0	0.6	0.0	0.0	0.1	0.3	0.7	1.6	1.7	2.2	4.0	6.5	6.4	3.9	7.3	0.8	0	106	179.0
180	1.1	0.7	0.2	0.3	0.6	0.0	0.3	0.8	2.4	6.9	10.3	15.1	22.6	29.0	28.8	33.3	26.5	18.2	5.7	1	759	180
181.0	0.1	0.0	0.0	0.4	0.2	0.7	1.2	3.9	3.9	9.6	15.4	29.1	52.1	85.8	117.1	157.8	156.1	194.9	16.1	2	2122	181.0
190	0.0	0.0	0.3	0.3	0.6	2.3	3.3	3.4	3.4	3.4	3.9	4.0	7.9	6.4	6.5	9.8	8.8	9.1	2.5	0	335	190
191	0.2	0.1	0.1	0.3	1.3	4.6	11.5	22.5	34.9	53.9	76.9	97.4	135.0	160.6	201.9	252.8	311.2	415.3	42.0	75	5554	191
192	0.2	0.1	0.0	0.2	0.0	0.1	0.1	0.2	0.4	0.5	0.8	1.1	1.8	1.5	2.7	2.4	2.0	1.8	0.5	0	65	192
193	3.6	3.7	2.1	1.7	1.3	2.9	4.1	4.4	6.5	7.6	12.1	16.0	16.7	15.0	10.1	9.3	2.0	0.0	6.0	0	790	193
194	0.0	0.1	0.1	0.6	1.3	1.1	0.2	0.4	1.5	1.9	1.9	3.6	2.4	3.7	3.3	2.4	3.9	3.6	1.1	0	148	194
195	0.7	0.3	0.8	0.1	0.3	0.3	0.2	0.3	0.3	0.5	0.4	1.7	0.9	0.9	1.8	2.4	1.0	0.0	0.5	0	70	195
196	0.1	0.3	0.1	0.2	0.6	0.5	0.4	0.5	0.9	1.1	1.1	1.9	2.4	4.6	6.8	4.4	7.9	12.8	1.2	0	163	196
197	0.3	0.1	0.7	0.7	0.9	1.1	0.6	0.7	1.2	2.1	1.9	4.2	4.2	4.2	5.6	5.9	13.7	16.4	1.6	1	206	197
200	0.2	1.0	1.2	2.0	1.1	2.6	2.8	3.7	6.1	6.2	8.6	11.5	18.0	24.6	27.6	29.4	29.4	20.0	6.0	1	787	200
201	0.0	0.6	1.3	2.7	5.1	4.0	3.8	4.3	2.8	4.6	5.2	5.8	3.5	7.3	8.9	6.4	7.9	5.5	3.3	1	432	201
203	0.0	0.0	0.1	0.0	0.0	0.0	0.6	0.4	1.3	2.0	3.5	4.8	7.9	13.4	13.0	14.2	8.8	7.3	2.2	0	285	203
204	6.6	4.6	2.9	3.2	1.6	2.5	2.5	3.3	3.6	5.9	9.7	14.0	23.7	42.3	52.8	57.3	72.6	71.0	9.8	1	1289	204
202,205	0.3	0.1	0.1	0.3	0.2	0.8	0.3	0.5	1.2	1.2	0.8	2.6	2.4	3.7	3.3	2.0	3.9	1.8	0.9	0	118	202,205
OTHER	0.1	0.2	0.1	0.9	1.7	1.1	2.0	2.5	5.1	9.0	16.2	24.7	37.6	46.9	61.7	68.1	83.4	85.6	10.4	3	1375	OTHER
140-205	14.0	12.3	9.9	17.1	21.5	32.5	51.2	76.5	127.8	222.2	388.0	608.2	962.0	1325.5	1751.0	2166.7	2494.1	2684.9	285.4	128	37703	140-205
RATE PER CASE IN PERIOD	0.07	0.07	0.08	0.11	0.16	0.14	0.11	0.10	0.11	0.12	0.13	0.16	0.18	0.22	0.30	0.49	0.98	1.82	0.01	-	-	RATE PER CASE IN PERIOD

TABLE 16 C

U.S.A., NEW YORK STATE (excluding NEW YORK CITY) :

FEMALE INCIDENCE RATES, 1959 - 61.

AVERAGE ANNUAL INCIDENCE PER 100,000 — AGE IN YEARS

INTERNATIONAL LIST No.	0-	5-	10-	15-	20-	25-	30-	35-	40-	45-	50-	55-	60-	65-	70-	75-	80-	85- AND OVER	ALL AGES	AGE UNKNOWN (cases)	ALL AGES (cases)	INTERNATIONAL LIST No.
140	0.0	0.0	0.0	0.0	0.0	0.0	0.2	0.3	0.1	0.1	0.7	0.2	0.5	0.8	2.4	1.5	1.9	4.0	0.3	0	41	140
141	0.1	0.0	0.0	0.1	0.0	0.0	0.1	0.1	0.6	1.1	1.7	2.1	3.0	2.5	4.4	5.1	2.6	5.0	0.9	0	118	141
142	0.0	0.0	0.1	0.1	0.0	1.5	0.3	0.9	0.8	1.8	0.9	2.3	2.2	3.6	3.1	3.7	3.2	5.0	1.0	1	136	142
143-4	0.0	0.0	0.0	0.1	0.1	0.0	0.2	0.3	0.7	1.6	1.9	1.7	1.5	3.0	3.1	4.8	6.5	8.0	0.9	1	122	143-4
146	0.0	0.1	0.0	0.0	0.0	0.0	0.0	0.1	0.2	0.6	0.5	0.5	0.2	0.6	1.2	0.4	1.3	0.0	0.2	1	27	146
145,147-8	0.0	0.0	0.0	0.0	0.0	0.0	0.1	0.0	0.4	0.9	1.2	1.5	1.7	1.7	1.7	2.6	2.6	4.0	0.5	1	74	145,147-8
150	0.0	0.0	0.0	0.1	0.0	0.0	0.0	0.2	0.6	0.6	2.7	3.2	4.0	4.3	6.8	10.6	9.7	19.1	1.4	1	193	150
151	0.0	0.0	0.0	0.0	0.0	0.3	0.8	1.7	3.5	6.0	7.4	11.0	18.7	39.7	56.4	79.3	127.5	105.5	9.5	1	1311	151
152	0.0	0.0	0.0	0.0	0.0	0.0	0.1	0.3	0.2	0.7	0.5	1.7	3.0	2.5	2.2	5.5	3.2	2.0	0.6	1	89	152
153	0.1	0.0	0.1	0.2	0.7	1.6	1.8	5.7	9.3	17.4	36.4	53.9	81.8	111.6	154.3	207.3	258.2	267.2	28.3	11	3908	153
154	0.0	0.0	0.0	0.0	0.0	0.8	1.1	1.8	4.9	9.6	16.9	23.0	36.2	46.5	60.0	75.6	92.3	94.4	11.6	4	1594	154
155.0	0.1	0.0	0.0	0.0	0.1	0.0	0.2	0.3	0.8	0.6	1.1	2.0	3.5	3.0	8.2	6.2	9.7	15.1	1.2	0	163	155.0
155.1	0.0	0.1	0.0	0.3	0.0	0.1	0.1	0.1	0.3	1.8	2.7	7.8	11.4	16.1	20.6	27.9	35.6	27.1	3.5	0	489	155.1
156	0.1	0.0	0.0	0.0	0.0	0.3	0.5	0.2	0.7	1.1	0.9	2.9	7.2	7.4	11.1	16.1	16.8	21.1	1.9	0	268	156
157	0.1	0.1	0.0	0.0	0.1	0.3	0.2	0.4	1.2	3.9	6.8	12.0	18.3	27.8	43.1	57.2	58.2	80.4	6.8	0	943	157
160	0.0	0.0	0.0	0.0	0.1	0.1	0.5	0.0	0.5	0.7	1.1	1.2	1.3	1.1	2.2	4.4	7.1	4.0	0.6	0	85	160
161	0.0	0.0	0.0	0.2	0.0	0.1	0.0	0.0	0.7	1.4	1.3	1.7	1.2	1.5	1.9	1.5	1.9	2.0	0.5	0	75	161
162-3	0.0	0.0	0.0	0.1	0.0	0.4	0.5	1.9	5.6	8.9	10.8	13.9	19.0	21.6	28.1	33.4	36.2	38.2	6.2	1	857	162-3
170	0.1	0.0	0.0	0.1	0.6	5.4	17.7	38.7	76.6	119.1	123.7	134.9	158.9	189.1	216.0	242.6	296.3	327.5	61.4	15	8466	170
171	0.0	0.0	0.0	0.2	1.7	6.9	13.5	21.0	31.7	33.6	38.0	39.1	39.0	40.3	42.8	44.0	40.8	43.2	17.4	17	2395	171
172	0.0	0.0	0.0	0.0	0.3	0.8	0.9	3.3	9.3	17.9	31.2	47.4	63.6	62.4	58.3	59.1	47.9	34.2	14.9	8	2056	172
173	0.0	0.0	0.0	0.1	0.3	0.5	0.2	0.2	0.3	0.1	0.3	0.3	0.0	0.2	0.0	0.0	0.0	0.0	0.1	0	20	173
174	0.0	0.0	0.0	0.0	0.0	0.1	0.6	1.0	1.1	2.8	2.9	2.9	7.2	8.5	8.0	7.0	16.8	15.1	2.0	0	273	174
175	0.1	0.1	0.2	0.6	1.4	2.1	2.8	6.8	12.0	23.5	27.5	32.0	40.4	41.2	43.5	44.0	31.7	32.1	12.4	3	1707	175
176	0.1	0.0	0.0	0.1	0.0	0.4	0.4	1.0	2.0	2.1	4.1	4.1	6.4	9.6	13.3	22.0	15.5	27.1	2.7	1	369	176
180	1.2	0.8	0.0	0.1	0.1	0.3	0.7	1.6	1.6	2.8	4.8	8.5	10.9	13.2	14.5	17.6	18.1	12.1	3.4	1	469	180
181.0	0.0	0.1	0.1	0.5	1.5	2.5	0.8	0.8	0.9	2.2	4.5	5.6	10.8	24.8	34.3	44.8	41.4	70.3	5.1	2	708	181.0
190	0.3	0.3	0.2	0.8	0.3	0.5	2.7	3.5	4.3	2.6	4.3	4.4	5.0	5.5	5.3	7.0	10.4	14.1	2.6	2	358	190
191	0.2	0.0	0.2	0.8	2.1	5.9	11.1	16.9	24.6	34.3	52.2	59.1	79.6	100.6	122.6	154.5	227.1	221.0	30.3	44	4173	191
192	0.3	0.0	0.0	0.0	0.0	0.0	0.0	0.1	0.3	0.1	0.3	0.2	0.8	2.1	0.5	0.4	1.9	0.0	0.2	1	34	192
193	3.0	3.1	2.0	2.2	1.7	1.6	2.2	3.7	3.9	7.7	8.2	9.9	13.3	9.8	5.8	2.9	4.5	0.0	4.5	1	619	193
194	0.0	0.1	0.2	1.6	1.8	4.0	5.0	3.8	4.0	5.1	3.7	4.6	4.2	4.7	7.5	7.0	7.8	2.0	2.9	3	403	194
195	0.2	0.2	0.7	0.3	0.1	0.5	0.4	0.2	0.4	0.9	0.4	0.8	0.5	0.2	0.5	0.4	1.9	1.0	0.3	0	46	195
196	0.5	0.1	0.3	0.8	0.3	0.9	1.1	1.2	0.2	0.6	0.8	2.0	1.0	1.3	3.9	3.3	1.3	4.0	0.7	0	102	196
197	0.2	0.3	0.6	0.2	0.7	0.9	1.5	1.8	1.4	1.8	1.9	1.7	3.5	4.5	4.6	6.2	7.1	6.0	1.5	0	201	197
200	0.2	0.2	0.8	1.9	1.2	3.9	2.8	1.7	3.2	4.7	6.4	8.8	9.8	17.0	18.1	20.5	17.5	15.1	4.1	1	565	200
201	0.0	0.2	0.6	1.9	2.4	2.3	2.4	1.7	2.6	1.8	2.0	2.4	3.0	5.1	3.4	5.1	4.5	2.0	2.0	1	276	201
203	0.0	0.0	0.0	1.7	0.0	0.3	0.1	0.1	0.8	1.4	2.8	3.8	8.2	7.9	6.8	11.0	7.1	2.0	1.7	1	229	203
204	5.6	4.1	1.8	1.7	1.2	2.3	2.4	2.2	2.6	4.3	6.1	8.1	14.5	17.8	30.0	41.1	45.9	38.2	6.8	1	935	204
202,205	0.5	0.0	0.2	0.0	0.0	0.3	0.3	0.5	0.9	1.3	1.2	0.6	2.7	2.5	3.1	3.3	0.6	2.0	0.8	0	106	202,205
OTHER	0.3	0.0	0.2	0.2	0.4	0.8	0.7	1.9	4.8	7.7	12.6	17.5	25.2	33.1	43.1	52.8	74.4	81.4	8.8	7	1209	OTHER
140-205	12.8	9.6	7.6	13.5	18.8	44.8	74.9	126.5	221.0	336.8	435.2	541.1	723.6	896.7	1097.6	1339.7	1595.5	1652.6	262.6	130	36212	140-205
RATE PER CASE IN PERIOD	0.07	0.07	0.08	0.11	0.14	0.13	0.10	0.10	0.11	0.12	0.13	0.15	0.17	0.19	0.24	0.37	0.65	1.00	0.01	–	–	RATE PER CASE IN PERIOD

ISRAEL

The Ministry of Health started registration of cases of cancer on 1st January, 1960, in the Division of Chronic Diseases and Rehabilitation with the Israel Cancer Association participating actively in this project and carrying a considerable part of the financial burden.

Cancer registration by the Ministry of Health was preceded by an assembly and work up of a card file of hospitalized cancer patients in the Central Bureau of Statistics, Health Section, using notification of death and of discharges from hospitals for all diagnoses, supplied to that institute as required by law. With the consent and co-operation of the Central Bureau of Statistics, this activity was wound up at the end of 1959 and the aforementioned action was incorporated in the work of the Cancer Registration section at the Ministry of Health.

The chances for success of our new undertaking were considered promising because :

1) Cancer registration in Israel can take full advantage of the well developed and organized medical services. Eighty per cent of the population are health insured, and high quality services are practically accessible to everyone. Seventeen institutes of pathology (among them two for Forensic Medicine) serve between them the whole country, and frequent meetings and consultations among pathologists aim at a uniformly high professional level. Physicians in this country are well informed and their understanding co-operation could be anticipated.

2) The registration covers the whole population, the characteristics of which are known for a variety of demographic details. On 22nd May, 1961, a Census of Population and Housing was held. The results of this census are used for correction of population estimates in the pre-census period and serve as the basis of later estimates. For political and geographical reasons immigration, emigration and tourism is well documented.

Compulsory notification of cases of cancer was not thought necessary. Instead, it was thought possible to get the desired information by :
  a) seeking the co-operation of physicians;
  b) an administrative order to hospitals to send in ready available data;
  c) the continued utilization of information reaching the Central Bureau of Statistics as required by law.

Consequently, the Cancer Registry in the Ministry of Health receives :
A. Directly from medical agencies :
  1) Copies of pathology reports concerning malignancies and premalignant conditions (biopsies, surgical specimens, autopsies, cytology) from all institutes of pathology.
  2) Copies of case summaries of cancer patients, from all departments of all hospitals (first and subsequent admissions).
  3) Monthly lists of new patients seen at oncological out-patient departments.
  4) Individual reports by regional chest clinics on patients seen with primary or secondary malignancies.
  5) Since 1st January, 1963, copies of death certificates carrying the diagnosis of malignancy (as main or as additional diagnosis) sent by the District Health Offices.
B. Via the Central Bureau of Statistics :
  6) Monthly lists of deaths, arranged by list number of main diagnosis.
  7) Hospital discharge notifications concerning cancer patients.
C. Upon special request :
  8) Forms fillet out by general practitioners.

Identification of subjects (and elimination of multiple registration) is one of our main problems. Indentification procedure includes :
  1) Matching with an alphabetically arranged file of patients' names

110

in phonetic transcript, which serves to solve some of the confusion caused by spelling European names in Hebrew letters, and of Hebrew and Arabic names in Latin characters.

    2) Using an auxiliary file of deaths arranged by date and place of death.

    3) Giving attention to other identifying features such as site, age, dates of hospitalizations, date of operation, number of patient file in hospital, and, most important, identity number (which, however, is not used routinely on medical documents).

This rather cumbersome procedure of intake, matching and checking is justified by the high percentage of coverage of diagnosed cases achieved already in the first years of operation of the Registry. Moreover, experience has shown that none of the many independent sources can be relied upon to yield all its cases.

Registration applies to the following neoplasms :

    1) all malignant neoplasms - Number 140-205 of the International Standard Classification of Diseases, 1955 Revision;

    2) benign tumours with premalignant significance (e.g. papilloma of the bladder);

    3) benign and undefined tumours of the nervous system;

    4) all tumours undefined whether malignant or not.

The Registry aims to get hold of the best possible diagnosis, the highest confirmation and the most accurate date of diagnosis (for establishing incidence and survival) for each case. This means requests for information from pathological institutions, from physicians in hospitals, from general practitioners in Sick Fund clinics and private practice, and, most important, of explaining the purposes of cancer registration to the doctors who write the case summaries. This educational effort results in a marked improvement of the quality of case summaries.

The establishment of the date of diagnosis was extremely important in the first years, when all cases were "new" to the Registry. It was here that the cancer file of previously hospitalized patients in the Central Bureau of Statistics was of great help in our endeavour to separate newly diagnosed from those re-appearing as hospitalized or dying. In spite of all these measures there certainly is an unknown number of cases that are erroneously counted as newly diagnosed. This is bound to happen in any new cancer register. On the other hand, cases may come to the attention of the register only some years later, especially those remaining ambulatory for a long time (chronic leukaemia, carcinoma of prostate, skin cancer) and these will have to be added to the incidence of previous years.

It is with these reservations in mind that the number of new cases for the four-year period 1960-1963 is published; these are the very first years of the register, and the last year may still be incomplete. The only justification lies in the fact that the numbers of cases reported for each site, by sex and age group, are fairly constant for the single years. An exception is skin cancer which shows a definite rise due to better coverage, and there is still doubt whether this group - which is the largest in numbers - has reached the same level of coverage as others.

A number of problems arise in the day-to-day work of a cancer registry, and agreement on how to deal with them would certainly be welcome. In the following paragraphs those which have a bearing on the tables are described along with the definitions used.

A. Year of incidence.

    1. The year of diagnosis of malignancy is the year of incidence.

    2. This principle was also applied for cases where in former years a tumour has been excised at the same place and been diagnosed as benign, re-

gardless of whether the second operation may or may not lead to a revision of the first slide and a correction of the first diagnosis.

3. On the other hand, for tumours first diagnosed as "undefined, whether malignant or not", and later confirmed as malignant, the year of the first diagnosis is taken as the year of incidence.

4. Those few deaths which remained with insufficient information (see part "D") are added to the incidence of the same year unless medical consideration decide against, for example : "state after radical mastectomy" in a woman over 70 is counted as diagnosed in pre-registration time, as this type of operation is most unlikely at that age.

B. Classification of diagnosis.

Classification is guided by the "International Classification of Diseases, 1955 Revision, W.H.O. Geneva 1957." However, according to our experience, the actual assignment of a specific list number has to be made very often according to the judgement of the reviewer in the register, and certain arbitrary rules had to be set for dealing with questioned diagnosis, as follows :

1. "Carcinomatosis, probably of ... (e.g. ovarian) origin" with no better confirmation possible, is classified under the list number of the "probable" site.

2. Cases for which the pathologist has found difficulty in giving a clear-cut diagnosis (e.g. "cancer involving stomach and pancreas arising either in stomach or in pancreas") are assigned the list number of the first mentioned organ.

3. With regard to the lack of familiarity of physicians with the implication as to classification of the wording of either diagnoses, "tumour of" is interpreted as "malignant tumour of" if this is the obvious meaning.

4. Cancer of lip (list number 140) and cancer of the skin and lip (list number 191.0) are combined under 140. Reported malignancies of this localization only very rarely allow differentiations between these two sites.

5. List number 142 "Malignant Neoplasms of Salivary Glands" should include, according to the definition, "mixed tumours (malignant) of salivary glands". This does not agree with the definition of the "Standard Nomenclature of Diseases and Operations" (used in most of our hospitals), where it includes "mixed salivary gland tumour"; that is, all those not specified as benign.

6. Malignant neoplasms of the "Cardiac region" are classified as stomach (list number 151) unless there is histological proof that the tumour originates in the oesophagus (list number 150). This is done because experience has shown that the majority of histologically proven malignant tumours of this region, even if termed by the clinician as "cancer of oesophagus", is described by the pathologist as "adenocarcinoma, originating in the gastric mucosa and invading the oesophagus".

Whenever serious doubt arises as to the correctness of the diagnosis a second opinion is asked from the physician or the pathologist, or both.

The possibility of later changes in diagnosis, especially for those of the last reported year, must be kept in mind. The tables presented are the result of all information which reached the Registry by October, 1964. Later information is likely to change the classification of quite a number of cases, known at that date only by secondary site (list numbers 156, 165, 198, 199), into those with a well-defined primary site. In addition, some of the cases which at the end of October, 1964, were registered as undefined, whether malignant or not (list numbers 230-239), may later turn out to be malignant.

C. Microscopic confirmation.

Cases are regarded as having microscopic confirmation when :

1. cytological or histological description is given in pathology reports or case summaries;

2. microscopic confirmation can be assumed although we have no actual

112

copy or description of the findings : a) cases with specific diagnosis, unless there is reasonable doubt whether a biopsy has been taken; b) all cases where radical surgery has been performed;

3. the macroscopic diagnosis of malignancy has been made at the autopsy, where no previous microscopic confirmation exists, but there is a remark in the report that material has been taken for histological examination. The work up of these cases may take a long time - even years - and a special effort may have to be made to get the final histological diagnosis.

D. Registration upon notification from Central Bureau of Statistics only.

Very few cases remainded under this heading, the only information available being from the monthly list of deaths supplied by the Bureau. This is due to various factors :

1. By special permission of the Bureau it is possible to get access to the original death certificates. This supplies in many cases sufficient information to decide that the case was diagnosed before start of cancer registration in the Ministry of Health.

2. For deaths occurring in hospitals and unknown to the Registry our request for information is effective.

3. For deaths from or with cancer occurring at home and unknown to the Registry, a few essential questions are asked from the general practitioners who signed the death certificates. In the first years the response was not satisfactory because of the great time lag between the date of death and our enquiry on the basis of the monthly list. Since the beginning of 1963, immediate notification by the District Health Office (from where the death certificate is sent to the Bureau) makes it possible to contact the physician at a time when the case is still fresh in his memory, with the result that the response is almost complete.

E. Annual incidence rates.

1. The annual incidence rates refer to newly detected cases among the resident population of Israel, during the years 1960-1963. Not included, therefore, are tourists, diplomatic personnel and, most important, immigrants diagnosed as having cancer in the country of origin.

For the purpose of computing incidence rates, the mean population was calculated as the mean of the estimated mid-year averages for each of the four years. This procedure was thought necessary with regard to the rapidly changing population structure in our immigrant country.

2. Age.
   a) The exact date of birth is unknown to a considerable part of our population and even age is not certain, especially in the higher age groups. This fact must be kept in mind for interpretation of population statistics in our country. The Central Bureau of Statistics publishes age groups divided only up to 75 years and over, but upon our special request a further breakdown was tabulated in order to enable the computation of rates up to age 85 years and over.
   b) The Cancer Registry prefers to use the age as stated - if at all - in one of the administrative documents (hospital discharge notification, death certificate) rather than that in the medical reports, when there are differences.
   c) For the purpose of calculating incidence rates, the number of cases with "age unknown" was distributed proportionally for each site.

As a final remark we want to state that the incidence rates for the population as a whole are the resultant of possibly very great differences in morbidity from cancer of specific sites among the various ethnic groups. The establishment of these differences as they exist today and the observation of the future development of the cancer morbidity pattern belong to the main tasks of the Israel Cancer Registry.

It is a pleasure to record our gratitude to Dr. Huppert, Head of the Health Section in the Central Bureau of Statistics, for his expert advice and assistance.

Ruth Steinitz.

Registry Title and Address : Israel Cancer Registry, Division of Chronic Diseases and Rehabilitation, Ministry of Health, Jerusalem, Israel. Commenced 1st January, 1960. Supported financially by the Israel Cancer Association and the Ministry of Health.

Registration. Cases are registered from hospital in-patients and out-patients, and from radiotherapy and pathology departments by clerical staff; from death certificates by the District Health Offices and Central Bureau of Statistics; and by special request, from doctors attending cases at home, and from the Central Bureau of Statistics. Special groups for which registration is thought to be less than 90 % complete are old people and Moslems; cancer of skin, and cancer of prostate; and patients attending out-patient clinics only.

Follow-up. It is intended to follow-up until death all cases, except skin cancer, although no evaluation is possible at this date.

Physical Description. The Registry covers the area enclosed by the political boundaries of the State of Israel, which are Lebanon to the north, Syria to the north and north east, Jordan and the Dead Sea to the east, Egypt and the Red Sea to the south east, Gaza strip and the Mediterranean Sea to the West. There are three main different subtropical climates : Mediterranean in the coastal area, continental in the mountainous region, and desert. Altitude varies from 397 metres below to 1,208 metres above sea level. The area lies between latitudes 30^0 and 33^0 north, and longitudes 34^0 and $35^038'$ east. The total registration area is 20,700 square kilometres.

Demographic Description. Total population of area under survey 2,243,790. The religious groups are Jews 87.3 %, Moslems 8.9 %, Christians 2.5 %. Ethnic divisions are Israeli 39.4 %, Asian 13.8 %, African 14.9 %, European and American 31.9 % (December 1964). The main occupational composition (male) is industry 27.0 %; commerce 7.9 %; agriculture 14.3 %; personal service 7.7 %. Of the total population 33.3 % live in conurbations of more than 100,000.

Medical Services. Total number of hospital beds of all kinds 7,622. Total number of doctors in practice in registration area 5,928. Groups which may delay seeking, or abstain from seeking medical advice are Moslems, non-Jewish women, old people. Cancer causes approximately 18 % of all deaths.

Publications. Steinitz (1963, 1965); Steinitz and Tzur (1965).

TABLE 17 A
ISRAEL :
POPULATION (100, 000s), MEAN 1960 - 63

AGE (in years)	MALES		FEMALES	
	No.	Per Cent	No.	Per Cent
0-	1.4123	12.41	1.3326	12.05
5-	1.4078	12.37	1.3232	11.97
10-	1.3224	11.62	1.2355	11.17
15-	1.0168	8.94	0.9376	8.48
20-	0.7843	6.89	0.7442	6.73
25-	0.7502	6.59	0.7496	6.78
30-	0.6845	6.01	0.7262	6.57
35-	0.6859	6.03	0.7362	6.66
40-	0.6174	5.43	0.6141	5.55
45-	0.6073	5.34	0.6433	5.82
50-	0.6440	5.66	0.6084	5.50
55-	0.5026	4.42	0.4393	3.97
60-	0.3808	3.35	0.3704	3.35
65-	0.2408	2.12	0.2298	2.08
70-	0.1651	1.45	0.1786	1.62
75-	0.0863	0.76	0.0994	0.90
80-	0.0460	0.40	0.0567	0.51
85- and over	0.0254	0.22	0.0329	0.30
TOTAL	11.3799	100.00	11.0580	100.00

NOTES

TO TABLES 17 A, B and C

(I)   I.L. number 193 includes benign and unspecified tumours of the central nervous system.

(II)   Carcinoma in situ excluded.

TABLE 17 B
ISRAEL :
MALE INCIDENCE RATES, 1960 - 63

Int. List No.	\[AVERAGE ANNUAL INCIDENCE PER 100,000 — AGE IN YEARS\] 0-	5-	10-	15-	20-	25-	30-	35-	40-	45-	50-	55-	60-	65-	70-	75-	80-	85- and over	All Ages	\[No. of Cases in Whole Period\] Age Unknown	All Ages	Int. List No.
140	0.2	0.0	0.0	0.7	1.6	1.7	3.7	4.7	3.2	7.0	7.0	16.4	9.8	12.5	21.2	29.0	16.3	0.0	3.8	6	173	140
141	0.0	0.0	0.0	0.0	0.0	0.0	0.4	0.0	0.8	0.4	1.2	1.0	2.0	2.1	1.5	5.8	0.0	0.0	0.4	1	18	141
142	0.0	0.4	0.8	0.7	1.3	0.0	0.4	0.0	0.4	1.6	3.1	1.5	3.9	3.9	4.5	0.0	0.0	0.0	0.9	0	40	142
143-4	0.0	0.0	0.0	0.2	0.3	0.3	0.4	1.5	1.2	2.9	2.7	1.5	3.3	4.2	12.1	2.9	0.0	0.0	1.0	0	46	143-4
146	0.0	0.0	0.4	0.5	0.6	0.0	1.5	0.4	0.8	3.7	3.9	3.0	5.9	2.1	9.1	2.9	0.0	9.8	1.3	1	59	146
145,147-8	0.0	0.0	0.0	0.2	0.0	0.0	0.4	0.0	1.2	0.4	1.9	2.5	0.7	0.0	3.0	5.8	5.4	9.8	0.5	3	25	145,147-8
150	0.0	0.0	0.0	0.0	0.3	0.7	1.1	0.4	1.2	2.1	3.9	8.0	14.4	14.5	30.3	49.2	87.0	108.3	3.0	1	137	150
151	0.0	0.0	0.2	0.0	0.3	0.0	0.4	4.4	10.1	14.0	31.1	66.7	126.1	168.2	234.7	330.2	407.6	265.7	22.5	9	1026	151
152	0.0	0.4	0.0	0.0	0.0	0.0	0.0	0.4	0.0	1.2	0.4	3.1	2.6	3.1	1.5	2.9	0.0	9.8	0.5	1	21	152
153	0.0	0.0	0.0	0.5	0.3	1.0	3.3	1.8	6.5	9.5	17.5	28.4	39.4	64.4	84.8	95.6	92.4	78.7	8.9	8	407	153
154	0.2	0.0	0.0	0.0	1.0	1.0	1.5	1.8	2.0	9.5	10.5	12.4	32.2	48.8	56.0	69.5	70.7	49.2	6.1	7	277	154
155.0	0.2	0.0	0.0	0.0	0.6	0.0	0.4	0.4	2.0	2.5	2.7	6.0	8.5	11.4	13.6	8.7	21.7	29.5	1.7	1	79	155.0
155.1	0.0	0.0	0.0	0.0	0.0	0.0	0.4	1.5	1.2	1.2	5.4	6.0	11.2	18.7	30.3	37.7	43.5	39.4	2.5	1	115	155.1
156	0.0	0.0	0.0	0.0	0.0	0.0	0.0	0.4	1.2	0.4	2.3	4.0	9.8	20.8	18.2	17.4	70.7	19.7	2.0	4	91	156
157	0.0	0.0	0.7	0.0	0.0	0.3	0.7	1.1	2.4	7.0	11.6	28.4	39.4	61.3	57.5	72.4	65.2	68.9	7.1	4	321	157
160	0.0	0.0	0.0	0.0	0.0	0.0	0.0	1.1	0.0	1.2	2.3	2.5	2.0	2.1	3.0	0.0	0.0	0.0	0.5	0	24	160
161	0.0	0.2	0.0	0.2	0.0	0.3	0.4	1.1	1.6	9.9	13.2	28.8	38.7	36.3	60.6	60.8	70.7	39.4	6.6	4	302	161
162-3	0.0	0.0	0.0	0.0	0.3	0.7	0.7	4.0	6.1	17.3	44.6	82.1	130.0	150.5	201.4	205.7	212.0	206.7	21.2	3	963	162-3
170	0.0	0.0	0.0	0.0	0.3	0.0	0.4	0.4	1.2	2.9	1.2	2.5	3.9	12.5	12.1	11.6	16.3	0.0	1.2	1	54	170
177	0.0	0.0	0.0	0.0	0.0	0.0	0.4	0.4	1.2	1.2	5.0	12.9	42.7	93.4	142.3	208.6	315.2	295.3	10.2	7	463	177
178	0.0	0.0	0.0	0.7	1.9	2.0	3.3	2.6	4.0	2.1	1.9	2.5	1.3	1.0	1.5	5.8	5.4	9.8	1.4	1	64	178
179.0	0.0	0.0	0.0	0.0	0.0	0.0	0.0	0.0	0.0	0.4	0.4	0.0	0.0	1.0	0.0	0.0	0.0	0.0	0.1	0	3	179.0
180	2.3	0.2	0.0	0.0	0.0	0.0	0.4	1.1	3.6	4.9	12.4	12.4	26.9	47.8	48.5	49.2	21.7	49.2	5.3	1	242	180
181.0	0.2	0.2	0.0	0.0	0.6	0.0	0.4	1.5	2.8	9.5	17.9	38.3	53.2	62.3	93.9	113.0	114.1	108.3	9.8	11	446	181.0
190	0.0	0.4	0.2	0.0	2.9	1.7	0.7	5.5	4.9	3.3	6.6	8.0	2.6	5.2	1.5	2.9	5.4	0.0	2.2	0	101	190
191	0.2	0.4	0.8	2.2	4.5	4.3	11.0	19.3	34.8	52.7	90.8	96.5	161.5	137.0	202.9	197.0	255.4	305.1	33.6	102	1528	191
192	1.1	0.4	0.2	0.0	0.3	0.3	0.0	0.4	1.2	2.9	2.3	4.0	3.3	4.2	4.5	2.9	0.0	0.0	1.1	3	52	192
193	6.4	4.1	4.9	6.1	4.8	4.7	9.9	8.0	10.5	18.1	19.0	19.9	32.2	26.0	21.2	8.7	0.0	9.8	9.8	7	446	193
194	0.0	0.2	0.6	0.5	1.3	1.0	1.1	1.5	1.6	0.8	2.3	4.5	8.5	10.4	10.6	14.5	21.7	0.0	1.8	1	81	194
195	0.4	0.2	1.1	2.5	1.0	0.3	0.0	0.7	0.8	1.2	1.9	1.5	1.3	1.0	0.0	0.0	0.0	0.0	0.5	0	21	195
196	0.2	0.7	1.1	1.2	1.0	0.3	0.4	1.1	0.4	2.1	1.2	1.5	1.3	3.1	4.5	8.7	5.4	0.0	1.2	1	53	196
197	0.7	1.1	2.6	1.2	1.0	2.0	1.1	1.8	2.0	1.6	6.2	4.5	9.8	5.2	10.6	26.1	5.4	9.8	2.5	3	113	197
200	3.9	3.9	2.6	4.9	7.7	5.7	4.7	6.6	6.9	7.0	14.8	12.4	20.4	38.4	36.3	55.0	43.5	39.4	8.3	7	377	200
201	0.0	0.7	0.8	2.2	3.5	4.0	3.3	4.7	1.6	2.1	5.0	6.0	5.9	8.3	6.1	5.8	10.9	0.0	2.7	0	121	201
203	0.0	0.0	0.2	0.0	0.0	0.0	0.4	1.8	1.2	0.8	4.3	7.0	9.8	15.6	13.6	8.7	21.7	0.0	1.8	0	83	203
204	5.0	5.5	3.8	3.9	2.6	2.3	5.1	3.3	4.5	7.0	10.9	21.9	24.3	36.3	60.6	49.2	48.9	78.7	8.4	2	381	204
202,205	1.4	0.0	0.4	0.0	0.0	0.0	0.0	0.0	0.0	0.0	0.4	1.0	0.0	1.0	4.5	0.0	0.0	0.0	0.4	0	17	202,205
OTHER	1.1	0.7	0.4	0.0	1.6	1.7	0.7	2.6	7.7	8.2	10.1	16.4	28.2	52.9	66.6	113.0	119.6	108.3	7.9	19	358	OTHER
140-205	23.0	19.0	18.7	27.8	40.2	36.0	58.1	87.8	132.0	220.6	380.0	574.0	917.1	1183.6	1585.4	1877.2	2168.5	1948.8	200.5	221	9128	140-205
RATE PER CASE IN PERIOD	0.18	0.18	0.19	0.25	0.32	0.33	0.37	0.36	0.40	0.41	0.39	0.50	0.66	1.04	1.51	2.90	5.43	9.84	0.02	-	-	RATE PER CASE IN PERIOD

TABLE 17 C
ISRAEL :
FEMALE INCIDENCE RATES, 1960 - 63.

AVERAGE ANNUAL INCIDENCE PER 100,000

INTERNATIONAL LIST No.	0–	5–	10–	15–	20–	25–	30–	35–	40–	45–	50–	55–	60–	65–	70–	75–	80–	85– AND OVER	ALL AGES	No. OF CASES — AGE UNKNOWN	No. OF CASES — ALL AGES	INTERNATIONAL LIST No.
140	0.0	0.0	0.0	0.0	0.0	0.3	1.0	0.7	0.8	0.4	2.5	1.7	5.4	4.4	8.4	15.1	4.4	15.2	1.0	1	46	140
141	0.0	0.2	0.0	0.0	0.0	0.0	0.0	0.3	0.0	0.8	0.8	0.0	2.0	0.0	4.2	12.6	13.2	0.0	0.5	0	20	141
142	0.2	0.2	0.2	0.0	1.3	0.0	1.7	1.4	2.8	1.2	2.1	1.1	2.0	5.4	1.4	0.0	4.4	7.6	1.0	0	44	142
143–4	0.0	0.0	0.6	0.3	0.3	0.3	0.0	0.3	0.4	0.4	2.5	4.6	3.4	2.2	2.8	2.5	17.6	7.6	0.8	1	36	143–4
146	0.0	0.0	0.6	0.5	1.0	0.0	0.0	0.0	1.6	1.9	0.8	3.4	1.3	4.4	0.0	0.0	0.0	7.6	0.7	1	30	146
145,147–8	0.0	0.0	0.0	0.0	0.0	0.0	0.0	0.0	0.0	0.8	0.8	1.1	0.0	4.4	0.0	0.0	0.0	15.2	0.3	0	14	145,147–8
150	0.0	0.0	0.0	0.0	0.0	0.7	0.3	0.0	1.6	0.4	3.3	4.0	10.1	12.0	28.0	17.6	30.9	30.4	2.0	4	89	150
151	0.0	0.0	0.0	0.0	0.0	0.3	3.8	5.1	5.3	15.2	16.4	35.9	49.3	102.3	151.2	208.8	260.1	167.2	14.1	3	625	151
152	0.0	0.0	0.0	0.5	0.0	0.3	0.0	0.0	0.4	0.4	1.2	1.7	3.4	4.4	4.2	0.0	4.4	0.0	0.5	10	22	152
153	0.0	0.0	0.6	0.0	0.0	1.0	3.1	6.1	5.7	20.2	21.0	21.6	45.9	45.7	98.0	98.1	194.0	98.8	10.8	10	476	153
154	0.0	0.0	0.0	0.5	0.0	0.3	2.1	3.1	4.5	6.6	18.5	30.7	31.0	39.2	39.2	47.8	35.3	68.4	6.7	6	295	154
155.0	0.4	0.0	0.0	0.0	0.0	0.0	0.3	0.7	0.0	2.7	3.7	2.8	2.7	2.2	2.8	7.5	8.8	0.0	0.9	1	40	155.0
155.1	0.0	0.0	0.0	0.8	0.9	0.3	0.0	1.4	1.6	7.4	14.0	15.4	36.4	53.3	72.8	88.0	75.0	60.8	6.9	3	307	155.1
156	0.0	0.0	0.0	0.0	0.3	0.3	0.0	0.3	0.8	1.6	5.8	2.8	7.4	10.9	21.0	47.8	52.9	60.8	2.4	1	104	156
157	0.0	0.0	0.0	0.3	0.0	0.0	0.7	1.7	0.8	5.4	11.1	8.5	24.3	38.1	49.0	55.3	75.0	38.0	4.9	2	216	157
160	0.0	0.0	0.0	0.0	0.0	0.0	0.3	0.3	1.2	0.4	0.8	1.7	0.0	0.0	0.0	2.5	8.8	0.0	0.3	0	14	160
161	0.0	0.0	0.0	0.3	0.0	0.0	0.3	0.3	1.2	1.6	0.8	5.1	2.0	3.3	2.8	0.0	8.8	0.0	0.7	0	32	161
162–3	0.2	0.0	0.2	0.0	0.3	0.7	0.7	1.4	4.1	8.9	10.3	17.1	25.6	57.7	57.4	85.5	52.9	83.6	6.5	1	288	162–3
170	0.0	0.0	0.2	0.8	1.0	6.7	24.4	53.7	97.7	126.3	156.6	149.7	166.7	143.6	141.4	143.4	136.7	106.4	46.8	23	2070	170
171	0.0	0.0	0.0	0.0	0.3	0.3	2.8	9.2	12.6	14.0	17.7	15.9	22.9	17.4	23.8	5.0	0.0	0.0	5.5	1	245	171
172	0.0	0.0	0.0	0.0	0.0	1.3	2.8	5.1	6.9	23.7	27.1	37.6	46.6	46.8	43.4	20.1	22.0	0.0	9.0	4	397	172
173	0.0	0.0	0.0	0.0	0.7	1.0	0.7	0.0	0.4	0.4	0.8	0.0	0.0	0.0	0.0	0.0	0.0	0.0	0.2	0	11	173
174	0.0	0.0	0.0	0.0	0.0	0.0	0.0	0.3	2.4	1.6	3.3	3.4	4.0	2.2	8.4	17.6	8.8	38.0	1.2	0	53	174
175	0.0	0.4	0.8	2.7	1.3	1.0	3.1	11.9	11.4	29.9	35.3	34.7	45.2	50.0	30.8	42.8	22.0	7.6	10.9	4	481	175
176	0.0	0.0	0.4	0.0	0.0	0.3	0.0	0.3	0.4	0.4	2.5	5.7	10.8	7.6	14.0	15.1	26.5	0.0	1.5	0	65	176
180	2.1	0.4	0.4	0.0	0.3	1.3	0.7	1.7	3.3	4.3	7.0	11.4	17.5	21.8	16.8	20.1	13.2	22.8	3.5	2	157	180
181.0	0.0	0.4	0.0	0.0	0.0	0.0	0.0	0.7	0.8	2.7	4.1	4.0	9.4	15.2	14.0	30.2	52.9	30.4	2.2	3	99	181.0
190	0.0	0.4	0.0	1.1	1.7	3.3	6.2	2.0	6.9	5.4	4.5	6.3	6.1	9.8	8.4	5.0	8.8	7.6	2.9	3	128	190
191	0.4	0.6	1.2	1.6	3.7	6.7	12.4	20.4	35.0	47.0	69.9	86.5	114.7	133.8	179.2	166.0	194.0	266.0	30.2	100	1338	191
192	1.1	3.0	0.0	0.0	0.0	0.0	1.0	0.7	0.8	1.2	2.1	3.4	4.0	4.4	1.4	7.5	4.4	0.0	1.0	1	46	192
193	5.3	2.6	0.8	5.1	3.7	7.3	5.5	6.8	13.8	15.5	22.2	25.6	22.3	29.4	15.4	15.1	0.0	15.2	9.1	6	403	193
194	0.4	0.4	0.8	4.0	3.0	2.7	4.8	5.1	3.7	6.6	5.8	7.4	16.2	13.1	18.2	7.5	13.2	15.2	4.1	3	180	194
195	0.2	0.9	1.6	1.6	0.3	0.7	1.4	0.3	1.2	1.2	0.4	0.0	2.7	0.0	1.4	0.0	0.0	0.0	0.4	0	18	195
196	0.9	1.7	0.6	1.1	0.0	2.7	1.4	0.3	0.8	1.2	0.8	0.0	0.7	1.1	1.4	0.0	4.4	0.0	0.9	0	38	196
197	1.9	2.1	1.0	1.3	2.4	2.0	4.1	2.0	1.2	2.3	3.7	1.7	7.4	6.5	4.2	5.0	13.2	22.8	2.4	2	105	197
200	0.4	0.9	1.6	1.1	4.0	2.0	3.1	3.4	4.1	7.4	8.6	12.0	24.3	20.7	29.4	32.7	44.1	7.6	5.5	5	244	200
201	0.0	0.9	0.0	1.1	2.0	2.3	3.8	4.8	2.4	2.3	2.5	2.3	3.4	4.4	5.6	2.5	0.0	0.0	2.1	2	95	201
203	3.0	3.8	0.0	0.3	0.0	3.3	2.8	0.0	1.6	0.0	4.9	9.1	8.8	12.0	19.6	12.6	8.8	7.6	1.8	2	81	203
204	0.4	0.4	3.8	3.2	2.4	0.3	0.0	3.7	4.5	5.1	16.0	13.1	16.9	25.0	23.8	22.6	83.8	53.2	6.6	2	291	204
202,205	0.2	0.2	0.2	0.5	0.0	0.3	0.0	0.0	0.4	0.0	0.8	3.4	1.3	2.2	2.8	0.0	0.0	0.0	0.5	0	23	202,205
OTHER	0.2	0.2	0.4	1.1	1.0	2.0	2.1	2.0	4.9	8.2	20.5	25.6	56.0	62.0	85.4	95.6	180.8	182.4	10.7	11	472	OTHER
140–205	16.9	16.1	16.8	27.5	31.9	49.7	96.4	157.2	250.4	382.8	533.4	618.0	860.6	1015.0	1230.4	1355.6	1675.5	1443.8	220.2	210	9738	140–205
RATE PER CASE IN PERIOD	0.19	0.19	0.20	0.27	0.34	0.33	0.34	0.34	0.41	0.39	0.41	0.57	0.67	1.09	1.40	2.52	4.41	7.60	0.02	–	–	RATE PER CASE IN PERIOD

AGE IN YEARS

JAPAN, MIYAGI PREFECTURE

The Department of Public Health, Tohoku University School of Medicine has carried out Cancer Registration in Miyagi Prefecture (1,743,195 enumerated as of the 1960 population census) which is located in the northeastern part of Honshu, the mainland of Japan. In Japan, except for Miyagi Prefecture and Hiroshima City, there is no other district where such a survey is being continuously conducted.

The registration office is organized in our department. We commenced this survey in 1951, and it continued until 1953, but was then discontinued for a while. It was commenced again in 1959 with the financial assistance of the National Cancer Institute, U.S.A., and is still being carried out at present.

Miyagi Prefecture is located on the Pacific coast and a large quantity of rice is produced in this district, but the industry is still under-developed. The capital of this prefecture is Sendai City with a population of 425,272 (as of 1960). It is the largest city of 6 prefectures in the northeastern part of mainland, and the centre of culture and administration, where Tohoku University School of Medicine is located. Many patients among the residents of the neighbouring prefectures as well as those of Miyagi Prefecture tend to come to Tohoku University Hospital, whereas the number of patients among the residents of Miyagi Prefecture who go out to the hospitals in the neighbouring prefectures is assumed to be very small. In our survey, only the residents in Miyagi Prefecture are considered to be the subjects. There are about 130 hospitals (in Japan, a "hospital" is defined as a medical institution with 20 or more beds), and 950 medical clinics in Miyagi Prefectures. Almost all of the medical clinics are under private management. We write letters of favour to the hospitals and medical clinics at the beginning of a year, and request the physicians to submit a report concerning the following items of information each time on each cancer patient they treat.

Name of Patient,
Sex and Occupation,
Date of birth,
Present Residence,
Permanent Address (HONSEKI)
Date of First Onset of Initial Complaint,
Preceding Diagnosis and Treatment,
Date of Diagnosis
Method of Diagnostic Confirmation,
Diagnosis, and (if patient deceased)
Date of Death.

For patients in Tohoku University Hospital and National Sendai Hospital, some more detailed information is also requested.

In spite of our earnest request, however, there are some cases about which no information is sent. At the beginning of the following year, we send a list of the reported cancer patients to each hospital and medical clinic, and ask the physicians to enter if there were any omissions in their reports. To some of the hospitals or medical clinics the staff of our department go and check the medical record and complete the survey cards. The staff of the Department of Pathology, Tohoku University School of Medicine have examined a great many histological specimens sent from the hospitals not only in Miyagi Prefecture but also from other prefectures. Utilizing these lists also, we make efforts to find cancer patients who reside in Miyagi Prefecture.

The number of deaths in Miyagi Prefecture for 1963 was 11,705, all of their death certificates being copied in our department, and of these 1,935 were cancer deaths. The cases mentioned as "cancer" in death certificates, but not reported as cancer patients from hospitals and clinics, are added to the number of incidence. In such a case, the year of onset is estimated by "the interval between onset and death" in the death certificates, and is presumed to be the year of new diagnosis. Accordingly, cancer incidence data for a certain year may change a little as time passes.

The figures given below show the total for the years 1959 and 1960 (4, 873 for both sexes) and the proportion notified only by death certificate.

	Number of patients	Death certificate only	Percentage
Male	2, 494	576	23. 1
Female	2, 379	491	20. 6

It is of geat regret that in our registration there still are many cases to be found as cancer only by death certificates, and such a fact should be reformed in the future. There may be some omitted cases which could not be found by any of the mentioned procedures, but the number is unknown.

Mitsuo Segi.

Registry Title and Address : Miyagi Prefecture Cancer Survey, Department of Public Health, Tohoku University School of Medicine, Miyagi Prefecture, Honshu, Japan. Commenced in 1951-1953. Re-commenced in 1959. Supported financially by the National Cancer Institute, U.S.A.

Registration. Cases are registered from hospital in-patients and out-patients by physicians, from radiotherapy and pathology departments by physicians, from death certificates by clerical staff, by doctors attending cases at home, and from histological specimens sent from other Prefectures.

Follow-up. No cases are followed up.

Physical Description. The area covered by the Registry is Miyagi Prefecture, Northern Ilonshu, Japan. Ilonshu, the main island of Japan, is situated in the North Pacific Ocean. It lies between latitudes 37⁰46' and 39⁰ north, and longitudes 140⁰41' and 140⁰17' east. The total registration area is 7, 286 square kilometres.

Demographic Description. Total population of area under survey 1, 743, 170. Only Japanese nationals are included in the registration population. The main occupational composition (of total employed persons) is industry 16. 1 %; commerce 22. 1 %; agriculture 46. 1 %; personal service 15. 7 %. Of the total population 24. 4 % live in conurbations of more than 100, 000.

Medical Services. Total number of hospital beds of all kinds 22, 996 (1962). Total number of doctors in practice in registration area 2, 046 (1962). Cancer causes approximately 16. 2 % of all deaths (1963).

Publications. Annual reports of health statistics (in Japanese), Health Department of Miyagi Prefecture.

Segi, Fukushima, Fuhisaku, Kurihara, Saito, Asano and Nagaike (1957).

TABLE 18 A
JAPAN, MIYAGI PREFECTURE :
POPULATION (100, 000s), 1960

AGE (in years)	MALES		FEMALES	
	No.	Per Cent	No.	Per Cent
0-	0.8268	9.74	0.7881	8.81
5-	1.0332	12.18	0.9946	11.12
10-	1.1225	13.23	1.0796	12.07
15-	0.7819	9.21	0.8039	8.99
20-	0.6772	7.98	0.7559	8.45
25-	0.7033	8.29	0.7588	8.48
30-	0.6881	8.11	0.7178	8.02
35-	0.5257	6.20	0.6099	6.82
40-	0.4173	4.92	0.4961	5.55
45-	0.3887	4.58	0.4551	5.09
50-	0.3566	4.20	0.3766	4.21
55-	0.3070	3.62	0.3156	3.53
60-	0.2449	2.89	0.2569	2.87
65-	0.1893	2.23	0.2083	2.33
70-	0.1281	1.51	0.1600	1.79
75-	0.0621	0.73	0.0988	1.10
80-	0.0249	0.29	0.0506	0.57
85- and over	0.0081	0.10	0.0194	0.22
TOTAL	8.4857	100.00	8.9460	100.00

NOTES

TO TABLES 18 A, B and C

(I)   I.L. number 193 excludes benign and unspecified tumours of the central nervous system.

(II)   Carcinoma in situ included.

TABLE 18 B
JAPAN, MIYAGI PREFECTURE :
MALE INCIDENCE RATES, 1959 - 60.

INTER-NATIONAL LIST No.	0-	5-	10-	15-	20-	25-	30-	35-	40-	45-	50-	55-	60-	65-	70-	75-	80-	85- AND OVER	ALL AGES	AGE UNKNOWN	ALL AGES (cases)	INTER-NATIONAL LIST No.	RATE PER CASE IN PERIOD
140	0.0	0.0	0.0	0.0	0.0	0.0	0.0	1.0	0.0	0.0	0.0	1.6	0.0	0.0	0.0	16.1	40.2	0.0	0.4	0	6	140	
141	0.0	0.0	0.0	0.0	0.0	0.7	0.0	0.0	0.0	0.0	2.8	0.0	2.0	5.3	7.8	24.2	20.1	0.0	0.7	0	12	141	
142	0.0	0.0	0.0	0.6	0.0	0.0	0.0	1.0	0.0	1.3	0.0	0.0	0.0	0.0	3.9	0.0	0.0	0.0	0.2	0	4	142	
143-4	0.0	0.0	0.4	0.0	0.0	0.0	0.0	0.0	0.0	1.3	1.4	1.6	4.1	5.3	3.9	0.0	0.0	0.0	0.5	0	8	143-4	
146	0.0	0.0	0.0	0.0	0.7	0.0	0.0	0.0	2.4	1.3	0.0	0.0	4.1	0.0	3.9	8.1	0.0	0.0	0.5	0	9	146	
145,147-8	0.0	0.0	0.0	0.0	0.0	0.7	0.7	0.0	0.0	0.0	0.0	0.0	2.0	2.6	3.9	0.0	0.0	0.0	0.2	0	4	145,147-8	
150	0.0	0.0	0.0	0.0	0.0	0.0	0.7	0.0	4.8	10.3	21.0	42.3	69.4	103.0	101.5	80.5	140.6	61.7	10.1	5	171	150	
151	0.0	0.5	0.0	1.9	4.4	7.8	12.4	22.8	64.7	132.5	178.1	280.1	394.0	636.6	651.8	692.4	542.2	432.1	73.3	0	1244	151	
152	0.0	0.0	0.0	0.0	2.2	0.0	0.0	1.0	0.0	1.3	1.4	0.0	0.0	0.0	0.0	0.0	0.0	0.0	0.1	0	2	152	
153	0.0	0.0	0.0	0.0	0.7	0.7	0.7	1.0	3.6	9.0	8.4	8.1	8.2	21.1	23.4	8.1	0.0	185.2	2.5	0	43	153	
154	0.0	0.0	0.0	0.6	0.0	0.7	0.0	1.9	6.0	3.9	9.8	16.3	18.4	31.7	35.1	40.3	40.2	0.0	3.9	0	66	154	
155	0.0	0.0	0.0	0.0	0.0	0.0	0.0	1.9	1.2	5.1	9.8	9.8	38.8	50.2	50.7	56.4	0.0	0.0	4.6	0	78	155	
156	0.0	0.0	0.0	0.0	0.0	1.4	0.0	1.9	2.4	9.0	19.6	22.8	34.7	71.3	78.1	104.7	140.6	0.0	7.4	0	125	156	
157	0.0	0.0	0.0	0.0	0.0	1.4	0.0	0.0	0.0	3.9	18.2	26.1	16.3	39.6	39.0	64.4	40.2	61.7	4.6	0	78	157	
160	0.0	0.0	0.0	0.0	0.0	0.0	0.0	1.9	7.2	3.9	2.8	6.5	6.1	26.4	7.8	16.1	40.2	0.0	2.1	0	36	160	
161	0.0	0.0	0.0	0.0	0.0	0.0	0.0	0.0	1.2	1.3	2.8	11.4	10.2	7.9	19.5	32.2	20.1	123.5	1.8	0	31	161	
162-3	0.0	0.0	0.0	0.6	0.7	0.7	0.0	2.9	7.2	11.6	14.0	53.7	71.5	95.1	144.4	104.7	20.1	0.0	11.0	0	186	162-3	
170	0.0	0.0	0.0	0.0	0.0	0.0	0.0	1.0	0.0	0.0	0.0	3.3	2.0	0.0	3.9	0.0	0.0	0.0	0.3	0	5	170	
177	0.0	0.0	0.0	0.0	0.0	0.0	0.0	0.0	0.0	0.0	4.2	6.5	20.4	31.7	42.9	32.2	20.1	61.7	2.7	0	46	177	
178	0.0	0.0	0.4	0.0	1.5	0.0	0.0	0.0	0.0	2.6	0.0	0.0	0.0	5.3	7.8	0.0	0.0	0.0	0.5	0	9	178	
179	0.0	0.0	0.0	0.6	0.0	0.0	0.0	0.0	0.0	2.6	0.0	6.5	0.0	0.0	11.7	0.0	0.0	0.0	0.6	0	10	179	
180	1.2	0.0	0.0	0.0	0.0	0.7	0.0	0.0	0.0	0.0	2.8	4.9	2.0	5.3	7.8	0.0	0.0	0.0	0.7	0	12	180	
181	0.0	0.0	0.0	0.0	0.7	0.0	0.0	1.0	1.2	1.3	4.2	8.1	18.4	15.8	42.9	24.2	20.1	185.2	2.7	0	45	181	
190	0.0	0.0	0.0	0.0	0.0	0.0	0.0	0.0	1.2	2.6	0.0	0.0	0.0	2.6	0.0	0.0	0.0	0.0	0.2	0	4	190	
191	3.0	0.0	0.0	0.0	0.0	1.4	0.0	1.9	2.4	0.0	0.0	4.9	4.1	5.3	7.8	24.2	40.2	0.0	1.2	0	20	191	
192	1.8	0.0	0.0	0.0	0.0	0.0	0.0	0.0	0.0	0.0	0.0	0.0	0.0	0.0	0.0	8.1	0.0	0.0	0.4	0	7	192	
193	0.0	0.0	0.0	0.0	0.7	0.7	0.0	0.0	0.0	0.0	0.0	4.9	2.0	0.0	0.0	0.0	0.0	0.0	0.3	0	5	193	
194	0.0	0.0	0.4	0.0	0.0	0.7	0.0	0.0	0.0	1.3	2.8	4.9	2.0	2.6	0.0	8.1	0.0	61.7	0.7	0	12	194	
195	0.0	0.5	0.0	0.0	0.0	0.7	0.0	0.0	0.0	0.0	0.0	1.6	0.0	0.0	0.0	0.0	0.0	0.0	0.1	0	2	195	
196	0.6	0.0	0.4	2.6	0.7	1.4	1.5	1.0	0.0	5.1	4.2	4.9	6.1	7.9	19.5	8.1	0.0	0.0	2.1	1	35	196	
197	0.6	0.0	0.0	0.0	0.7	0.0	0.0	1.9	0.0	0.0	0.0	0.0	0.0	0.0	15.6	0.0	20.1	0.0	0.1	0	1	197	
200	0.6	0.5	0.0	0.6	0.7	0.7	0.7	1.0	2.4	3.9	5.6	13.0	6.1	21.1	15.6	0.0	0.0	0.0	2.4	0	40	200	
201	0.0	0.5	0.4	0.0	0.0	0.0	0.7	0.0	0.0	1.3	1.4	4.9	0.0	2.6	0.0	0.0	20.1	61.7	0.6	0	11	201	
203	0.0	0.0	0.0	0.0	0.0	0.0	0.0	0.0	0.0	0.0	0.0	0.0	6.1	2.6	0.0	0.0	0.0	0.0	0.2	0	4	203	
204	5.4	3.4	1.8	2.6	2.2	3.6	2.2	1.9	2.4	5.1	2.8	4.9	2.0	2.6	11.7	0.0	40.2	61.7	3.3	0	56	204	
202,205	0.0	0.0	0.0	0.0	0.0	0.0	0.0	0.0	0.0	0.0	0.0	0.0	2.0	0.0	0.0	0.0	0.0	0.0	0.1	0	1	202,205	
OTHER	0.6	0.5	0.0	0.0	1.5	2.1	0.7	3.8	6.0	7.7	5.6	14.7	12.2	15.8	19.5	80.5	60.2	0.0	3.9	0	66	OTHER	
140-205	13.3	5.3	4.0	10.9	17.0	24.9	19.6	48.5	116.2	229.0	315.5	565.1	765.6	1217.6	1362.2	1433.2	1245.0	1296.3	147.0	6	2494	140-205	
RATE PER CASE IN PERIOD	0.60	0.48	0.45	0.64	0.74	0.71	0.73	0.95	1.20	1.29	1.40	1.63	2.04	2.64	3.90	8.05	20.08	61.73	0.06	-	-	RATE PER CASE IN PERIOD	

AVERAGE ANNUAL INCIDENCE PER 100,000 — AGE IN YEARS

NO. OF CASES IN WHOLE PERIOD

TABLE 18 C

JAPAN, MIYAGI PREFECTURE :

FEMALE INCIDENCE RATES, 1959 - 60.

INTER-NATIONAL LIST No.	AVERAGE ANNUAL INCIDENCE PER 100,000 — AGE IN YEARS 0-	5-	10-	15-	20-	25-	30-	35-	40-	45-	50-	55-	60-	65-	70-	75-	80-	85- AND OVER	ALL AGES	No. OF CASES IN WHOLE PERIOD AGE UNKNOWN	ALL AGES	INTER-NATIONAL LIST No.
140	0.0	0.0	0.0	0.0	0.0	0.0	0.0	0.0	0.0	0.0	0.0	0.0	0.0	0.0	0.0	0.0	0.0	0.0	0.0	0	0	140
141	0.0	0.0	0.0	0.0	0.0	0.0	0.7	0.8	0.0	1.1	1.3	1.6	1.9	0.0	3.1	5.1	0.0	0.0	0.4	0	8	141
142	0.0	0.0	0.0	0.0	0.0	0.0	0.0	0.8	1.0	0.0	0.0	1.6	5.8	0.0	3.1	0.0	0.0	0.0	0.4	0	7	142
143-4	0.0	0.0	0.0	0.0	0.0	0.0	0.0	0.8	0.0	0.0	0.0	0.0	3.9	0.0	3.1	0.0	0.0	0.0	0.2	0	4	143-4
146	0.0	0.0	0.0	0.0	0.0	0.0	0.0	0.0	0.0	0.0	0.0	0.0	0.0	2.4	0.0	0.0	0.0	0.0	0.1	0	1	146
145,147-8	0.0	0.0	0.0	0.0	0.0	0.0	0.0	0.0	0.0	0.0	0.0	1.6	0.0	0.0	0.0	5.1	9.9	0.0	0.2	0	3	145,147-8
150	0.0	0.0	0.0	0.0	0.0	1.3	0.0	1.6	1.0	4.4	9.3	12.7	29.2	36.0	68.8	81.0	79.1	0.0	5.6	0	100	150
151	0.0	0.0	0.0	0.0	1.3	4.0	13.2	28.7	47.4	61.5	102.2	125.2	196.6	283.2	284.4	253.0	395.3	309.3	41.0	0	733	151
152	0.0	0.0	0.0	0.0	0.0	0.0	0.0	0.8	0.0	1.1	0.0	1.6	1.9	0.0	3.1	5.1	0.0	0.0	0.3	0	6	152
153	0.0	0.0	0.0	0.0	0.7	0.0	2.8	1.6	4.0	2.2	2.7	6.3	15.6	19.2	34.4	50.6	0.0	128.9	3.4	0	61	153
154	0.0	0.5	0.0	0.0	0.7	0.0	2.1	1.6	2.0	7.7	6.6	14.3	11.7	21.6	46.9	40.5	19.8	0.0	3.9	0	70	154
155	0.0	0.0	0.0	0.0	0.0	0.0	0.7	2.5	4.0	6.6	2.7	15.8	29.2	26.4	46.9	25.3	69.2	25.8	4.0	0	72	155
156	0.0	0.0	0.5	0.0	0.0	0.0	1.4	0.8	1.0	4.4	8.0	22.2	25.3	43.2	46.9	81.0	138.3	25.8	5.9	0	106	156
157	0.0	0.0	0.0	0.0	0.0	0.0	0.7	0.8	1.0	1.1	9.3	7.9	23.4	14.4	18.8	35.4	19.8	0.0	2.7	0	49	157
160	0.0	0.0	0.0	0.0	0.0	1.3	0.0	2.5	3.0	6.6	6.6	4.8	5.8	4.8	9.4	10.1	9.9	0.0	1.8	0	33	160
161	0.0	0.0	0.0	0.0	0.0	0.7	0.0	0.0	0.0	6.6	1.3	3.2	1.9	12.0	0.0	0.0	9.9	0.0	0.6	0	11	161
162-3	0.0	0.0	0.0	0.0	2.0	0.0	1.4	2.5	0.0	5.5	18.6	15.8	19.5	36.0	28.1	45.5	9.9	25.8	4.7	0	84	162-3
170	0.0	0.0	0.5	0.6	0.7	4.6	9.8	22.1	34.3	48.3	39.8	26.9	25.3	19.2	28.1	20.2	19.8	25.8	12.0	2	215	170
171	0.0	0.0	0.0	0.0	0.0	1.3	13.2	24.6	42.3	41.7	65.1	99.8	74.0	88.8	62.5	30.4	19.8	0.0	19.4	1	347	171
172	0.0	0.0	0.0	0.0	0.0	0.7	0.0	0.8	3.0	3.3	6.6	7.9	9.7	4.8	15.6	0.0	0.0	0.0	1.7	0	30	172
173	0.0	0.0	0.0	0.0	2.6	4.0	5.6	3.3	2.0	7.7	1.3	1.6	0.0	2.4	0.0	0.0	9.9	0.0	1.9	0	34	173
174	0.0	0.0	0.0	0.0	2.0	0.0	0.7	3.3	7.1	13.2	17.3	19.0	35.0	31.2	34.4	35.4	59.3	0.0	6.0	0	107	174
175	0.0	0.0	0.5	0.6	0.7	2.0	2.1	2.5	1.0	6.6	6.6	1.6	7.8	12.0	0.0	5.1	0.0	0.0	2.0	0	35	175
176	0.0	0.0	0.0	0.0	0.0	0.0	0.0	0.0	0.0	2.2	2.7	1.6	1.9	2.4	3.1	10.1	0.0	0.0	0.4	0	8	176
180	2.5	0.5	0.0	0.0	0.0	0.7	0.0	0.0	0.0	2.2	0.0	6.3	0.0	7.2	0.0	0.0	0.0	0.0	0.8	0	15	180
181	0.0	0.0	0.0	0.0	0.5	0.7	0.0	0.8	0.0	2.2	4.0	4.8	15.6	4.8	12.5	15.2	0.0	0.0	1.5	0	27	181
190	0.6	0.0	0.0	0.0	0.0	0.0	0.0	0.0	0.0	1.1	0.0	0.0	1.9	0.0	6.3	0.0	0.0	0.0	0.2	0	3	190
191	1.3	0.5	0.0	0.0	0.0	0.0	0.7	0.8	0.0	0.0	0.0	6.3	1.9	2.4	6.3	0.0	0.0	0.0	0.7	0	12	191
192	1.3	0.0	0.0	0.0	0.0	2.6	0.0	0.0	0.0	0.0	1.3	0.0	0.0	0.0	0.0	0.0	9.9	0.0	0.2	0	3	192
193	1.3	0.0	0.0	0.0	0.0	0.0	0.0	0.8	0.0	3.3	6.6	0.0	0.0	0.0	0.0	5.1	0.0	0.0	0.4	0	7	193
194	0.0	0.0	0.0	0.0	2.6	1.3	1.4	4.1	0.0	2.2	6.6	11.1	9.7	7.2	12.5	5.1	0.0	25.8	2.3	0	41	194
195	0.0	0.5	0.0	0.0	0.0	0.0	0.7	0.0	0.0	0.0	1.3	0.0	0.0	0.0	0.0	0.0	0.0	0.0	0.1	0	1	195
196	0.6	0.0	0.9	0.0	0.0	0.0	0.7	0.0	1.0	2.2	5.3	3.2	5.8	2.4	6.3	5.1	0.0	0.0	1.1	0	20	196
197	0.6	0.0	0.5	0.0	0.0	0.0	0.7	0.0	0.0	0.0	0.0	3.2	0.0	0.0	6.3	5.1	0.0	0.0	0.3	0	5	197
200	0.0	0.0	0.0	0.0	0.0	2.6	0.0	1.6	0.0	0.0	1.3	0.0	0.0	0.0	9.4	5.1	9.9	0.0	0.7	0	12	200
201	0.0	0.0	0.0	0.0	0.0	0.0	0.0	0.0	0.0	1.1	0.0	0.0	0.0	0.0	3.1	0.0	0.0	0.0	0.1	0	2	201
203	0.0	0.0	0.0	0.0	0.0	0.0	0.0	0.0	0.0	0.0	0.0	1.6	0.0	0.0	0.0	0.0	0.0	0.0	0.1	0	1	203
204	1.9	3.5	1.9	2.5	2.6	2.6	2.8	4.9	2.0	3.3	2.7	4.8	1.9	2.4	3.1	0.0	0.0	0.0	2.7	0	49	204
202,205	1.3	0.0	0.0	0.0	0.0	0.0	0.0	0.0	0.0	0.0	0.0	0.0	0.0	0.0	0.0	0.0	0.0	0.0	0.1	0	2	202,205
OTHER	1.3	0.0	0.0	0.0	0.7	2.0	2.8	3.3	2.0	4.4	6.6	6.3	9.7	12.0	37.5	5.1	29.6	0.0	3.1	0	55	OTHER
140-205	11.4	5.5	4.6	4.4	16.5	29.7	63.4	118.9	161.3	245.0	337.2	437.3	572.2	696.1	815.6	774.3	909.1	541.2	133.0	3	2379	140-205
RATE PER CASE IN PERIOD	0.63	0.50	0.46	0.62	0.66	0.66	0.70	0.82	1.01	1.10	1.33	1.58	1.95	2.40	3.13	5.06	9.88	25.77	0.06	-	-	RATE PER CASE IN PERIOD

SINGAPORE, (CHINESE)

There is no cancer registry in Singapore. However, a central card index of all histologically diagnosed malignant disease is maintained in the Institute of Pathology. Virtually all histological material, biopsy or necropsy, emanating from the civil populace of Singapore, whether it be from Government or from private institutions is examined in the Institute, which houses both the Government and University Departments of Pathology.

This card index records name, age, sex, race, biopsy or necropsy number, hospital admission, out-patient or other identifying information, and histological diagnosis. Biopsy and necropsy reports are readily available if history or other information is needed. Particular care has been taken to eliminate duplicate examinations such as occur when diagnostic biopsy is followed by excision of the entire growth, when there is a recurrence or when biopsy is followed by necropsy.

Material submitted from Malaya and Borneo has been excluded from the tabulations. It is known that a few patients seek treatment abroad, either in the West, Australia or Hongkong. However, for most of these the initial diagnosis of cancer is likely to be made in Singapore.

Rates based on biopsies only have well known drawbacks. The less accessible sites are rarely biopsied and the biopsies taken may vary according to surgical intersts. There is, for example, intense surgical interest in hepatic and oesophageal cancer in Singapore, while during the period reviewed there were no specialised neuro-surgical units. However, the inclusion of necropsies which are usually biased in the reverse direction, with relatively more of the inaccessible tumours, tends to correct this distortion. Over the 12 years there has been a gradual increase in the willingness of the population to seek hospital care, and in the quality of that care. It is thus probable that the proportion of cancers with histological confirmation was higher in later years.

It is almost certain that many cancers in older persons are not examined histologically. Many of the elderly eschew orthodox treatment, and are thus very much less likely to have a biopsy taken, or come to necropsy. Although figures are not readily available for hospital admission or biopsy rates, by age, the proportion of all Singapore dead who are necropsied is known

Percentages of all Chinese dead necropsied in Singapore in 1954-1958 by sex, age groups, and death category											
Age group (years)	0-4		5-24		25-44		45-64		65+		All Ages	
Death category*	AC	NC	AC	NC	AC	NC	AC	NC	AC	NC	AC	NC
Males	42.6	41.1	53.3	25.0	36.1	20.2	21.1	15.2	9.3	6.8	28.9	22.4
Females	39.2	37.5	43.2	27.7	27.6	18.3	10.4	7.3	3.6	2.2	22.2	18.7

* AC = All causes, NC = Natural causes.   Source : Muir, C. S. (1964)

While 16.9 per cent of dead male Chinese aged 45 years and over were necropsied, only 9.3 per cent of those in the 65+ age group came to post-mortem. Comparable figures for Chinese females were even lower, 6.7 per cent and 3.6 per cent. There is thus a much greater chance that cancer will be missed in older persons. Many of the older Singapore Chinese were born in China. There is a tendency for some to return to the country of origin to die and a proportion of them will have cancer.

With a high proportion of children necropsied, it is likely that the data for children are fairly accurate.

The figures for leukaemia are falsely low, as patients diagnosed by blood film or marrow smear only are not included in our figures. The figures for List No. 173 pertain to choriocarcinoma and malignant mole (chorioadenoma destruens) only.

The strength of our data lies in the fact that the true rates cannot be less than the values given, and they are not influenced by the diagnostic errors inherent in clinical and other methods of diagnosis.

C. S. Muir,
K. Shanmugaratnam

Registry Title and Address : University Department of Pathology, Institute of Pathology, General Hospital, Singapore 3, Far East. Commenced 1st January, 1947. Supported financially by the University of Singapore and the Government of Singapore.

Registration. Cases are registered by medical staff from pathology departments. Registration is substantially incomplete for Malays, old people of all races, people in rural areas, and for some internal sites (for example, the brain).

Follow-up : No cases are followed up.

Physical Description. The Registry covers the Republic of Singapore which is low lying, part urban, part agricultural land and part mangrove swamp. The soil is poor, mainly laterite. It has a moist, hot, marine equatorial climate with an average temperature of $30^{\circ}C$. Relative humidity is 83%. Rainfall is 95 inches (240 cms). Singapore is close to Sumatra and is connected to the Federation of Malaya by a causeway. The total registration area is 581.5 square kilometres.

Demographic Description. Total population of area under survey 1,036,350. The main ethnic groups are Chinese 75 %, Malays 14 %, Indians and Pakistanis 9 %, other races 2 %. The main occupational composition (economically active male Chinese over 10 years) is industry 24 %, commerce 36 %, agriculture 8 % and personal service 10 %. Of the total population 70 % live in conurbations of more than 100,000.

Medical Services. Total number of hospital beds of all kinds 7,436 (1959). Total number of doctors in practice in registration area 670 (1959). 5 % or more of the population might abstain from, or unduly delay seeking, medical advice due to Malayan and Chinese cultural patterns and religious beliefs. Muslim Malays avoid biopsy, necropsy and operation. Cancer caused approximately 11.1 % of all deaths in 1961.

Publications. Ali and Muir (1965); Muir (1964, 1965); Muir and Shanmugaratnam (1965, 1966); Singapore Ministry of Culture (1966).

TABLE 19 A
SINGAPORE, CHINESE :
POPULATION (100,000s), MEAN 1950 - 61

AGE (in years)	MALES No.	MALES Per Cent	FEMALES No.	FEMALES Per Cent
0-	0.9438	17.79	0.8712	17.22
5-	0.8244	15.54	0.7676	15.17
10-	0.5554	10.47	0.5067	10.02
15-	0.5261	9.92	0.4910	9.70
20-	0.4109	7.75	0.4051	8.01
25-	0.3623	6.83	0.3661	7.24
30-	0.2956	5.57	0.2923	5.78
35-	0.2837	5.35	0.2781	5.50
40-	0.2919	5.50	0.2685	5.31
45-	0.2652	5.00	0.2326	4.60
50-	0.2117	3.99	0.1853	3.66
55-	0.1498	2.82	0.1393	2.75
60-	0.0918	1.73	0.1026	2.03
65-	0.0519	0.98	0.0721	1.43
70- and over	0.0396	0.75	0.0809	1.60
- -	-	-	-	-
- -	-	-	-	-
TOTAL	5.3041	100.00	5.0594	100.00

NOTES

TO TABLES 19 A, B and C

(I)   I. L. number 193 excludes benign and unspecified tumours of the central nervous system.

(II)   Carcinoma in situ excluded.

TABLE 19 B

SINGAPORE, CHINESE :

MALE INCIDENCE RATES, 1950 - 61.

INTER-NATIONAL LIST No.	AVERAGE ANNUAL INCIDENCE PER 100,000 — AGE IN YEARS																		ALL AGES	No. OF CASES IN WHOLE PERIOD — AGE UNKNOWN	No. OF CASES IN WHOLE PERIOD — ALL AGES	INTER-NATIONAL LIST No.
	0-	5-	10-	15-	20-	25-	30-	35-	40-	45-	50-	55-	60-	65-	70-	75-	80-	85- AND OVER				
140	0.0	0.0	0.0	0.0	0.0	0.0	0.0	0.3	0.0	0.3	0.8	0.0	0.0	0.0	2.1				0.1	0	5	140
141	0.0	0.0	0.0	0.0	0.2	0.2	0.0	0.9	0.9	2.8	2.8	1.7	3.6	4.8	14.7				0.7	1	42	141
142	0.0	0.0	0.0	0.2	0.2	0.0	0.0	0.0	0.6	0.3	0.4	0.6	0.9	0.0	0.0				0.1	0	8	142
143-4	0.0	0.0	0.0	0.0	0.0	0.2	1.1	0.0	1.1	1.9	3.5	5.0	6.4	12.8	6.3				0.8	2	53	143-4
146	0.0	0.0	0.0	2.1	5.7	5.8	15.2	27.0	38.5	34.3	46.1	38.4	32.7	27.3	10.5				11.1	9	709	146
145,147-8	0.0	0.0	0.0	0.2	0.2	0.0	0.6	4.4	0.6	2.5	3.9	4.5	17.2	14.5	14.7				1.1	1	68	145,147-8
150	0.0	0.0	0.3	0.0	0.6	1.4	2.5	7.0	9.1	20.1	30.7	48.4	53.6	56.2	42.1				6.3	4	404	150
151	0.0	0.0	0.0	0.0	0.6	1.4	2.5	7.0	14.6	22.0	40.9	42.3	69.9	54.6	40.0				7.5	1	476	151
152	0.0	0.0	0.0	0.0	0.0	0.7	0.0	0.0	0.3	0.3	0.4	0.0	0.0	0.0	0.0				0.0	0	3	152
153	0.0	0.0	0.0	0.0	0.0	0.0	0.8	2.3	2.0	3.8	6.7	7.8	7.3	19.3	12.6				1.4	0	91	153
154	0.2	0.1	0.0	0.2	0.6	2.1	1.7	3.5	4.3	5.0	13.0	11.1	19.1	28.9	31.6				2.5	1	157	154
155.0	0.0	0.0	0.3	0.6	0.0	0.0	5.4	6.2	13.4	18.9	31.1	24.5	23.6	32.1	16.8				5.5	3	348	155.0
155.1	0.0	0.0	0.0	0.0	0.2	0.0	0.0	0.3	0.0	0.0	2.0	1.7	5.4	4.8	2.1				0.3	0	19	155.1
156	0.0	0.0	0.0	0.0	0.2	0.0	0.8	0.9	2.6	0.9	3.1	5.6	5.4	4.8	2.1				0.8	1	48	156
157	0.0	0.0	0.0	0.0	0.4	0.2	0.3	0.6	0.9	2.2	1.2	1.1	4.5	1.6	2.1				0.4	0	25	157
160	0.0	0.0	0.0	0.0	0.0	0.0	0.3	0.3	0.9	2.8	4.3	6.1	10.0	8.0	8.4				1.0	2	61	160
161	0.1	0.0	0.2	0.2	0.4	0.2	0.0	0.9	2.0	4.4	11.8	15.0	17.2	20.9	12.6				1.9	2	121	161
162-3	0.0	0.1	0.0	0.0	0.4	0.2	1.7	3.8	9.4	17.3	27.2	36.7	74.4	53.0	48.4				6.2	8	395	162-3
170	0.0	0.0	0.0	0.0	0.0	0.0	0.0	0.0	0.0	0.9	0.0	1.1	0.9	0.0	0.0				0.1	0	6	170
177	0.0	0.0	0.0	0.0	0.2	0.0	0.0	0.1	0.0	0.0	0.4	1.1	7.3	0.0	14.7				0.3	0	18	177
178	0.2	0.0	0.0	0.0	0.0	0.9	0.8	1.2	1.4	0.6	0.4	1.1	0.0	1.6	0.0				0.4	0	28	178
179.0	0.0	0.0	0.0	0.0	0.2	0.2	0.0	1.5	2.0	1.3	2.8	6.1	1.8	14.5	6.3				0.8	1	50	179.0
180	0.4	0.0	0.0	0.2	0.2	0.5	0.8	0.6	1.7	0.6	2.0	2.8	4.5	8.0	4.2				0.7	1	44	180
181.0	0.0	0.0	0.0	0.0	0.2	0.0	0.3	0.3	1.1	1.9	2.8	3.9	12.7	8.0	16.8				0.8	1	54	181.0
190	0.0	0.0	0.0	0.3	0.2	0.5	0.3	0.0	0.3	1.3	2.0	0.0	2.7	0.0	4.2				0.3	0	21	190
191	0.0	0.1	0.0	0.2	0.4	0.5	1.7	2.3	3.7	5.3	9.1	16.7	19.1	27.3	46.3				2.5	0	162	191
192	0.0	0.0	0.2	1.6	0.6	0.0	0.3	0.3	0.6	0.3	0.8	2.2	0.9	1.6	0.0				0.4	0	23	192
193	1.1	1.3	0.9	0.3	0.4	0.7	1.1	1.5	0.6	2.5	2.0	2.2	2.7	3.2	2.1				1.3	0	85	193
194	1.4	0.1	0.0	0.0	0.0	0.2	0.0	0.0	0.9	1.3	2.0	0.0	0.9	0.0	4.2				0.3	0	21	194
195	0.0	0.1	0.0	0.0	0.0	0.0	0.0	0.0	0.3	0.0	0.4	0.0	0.0	0.0	0.0				0.1	0	5	195
196	0.2	0.0	0.6	0.3	1.0	0.9	0.3	0.6	0.3	0.9	0.4	0.6	0.0	0.0	2.1				0.4	1	26	196
197	0.1	0.6	0.2	0.2	0.6	0.5	0.3	0.6	1.1	0.6	2.8	2.8	2.7	1.6	4.2				0.5	1	29	197
200	0.3	0.7	0.9	0.5	0.8	1.2	1.1	1.2	0.9	3.1	2.8	0.6	2.7	0.0	2.1				1.0	1	63	200
201	0.1	0.0	0.3	0.2	0.4	1.2	0.3	0.6	1.1	0.3	0.4	0.6	0.9	0.0	0.0				0.5	1	34	201
203	0.0	0.0	0.0	0.2	0.2	0.0	0.0	0.0	0.0	0.6	0.8	0.0	0.9	0.0	0.0				0.1	0	7	203
204	1.0	1.1	0.9	1.0	1.4	0.0	0.6	0.3	2.0	0.3	1.6	2.2	1.8	0.0	0.0				1.0	0	62	204
OTHER	0.5	0.0	0.2	0.8	1.2	3.0	7.3	12.0	16.8	22.6	29.9	37.8	43.6	41.7	29.5				7.4	7	468	OTHER
140-205	5.7	4.4	4.7	9.0	16.2	21.2	48.2	81.4	135.9	184.1	291.7	329.3	459.3	451.2	404.0				66.6	48	4239	140-205
RATE PER CASE IN PERIOD	0.09	0.10	0.15	0.16	0.20	0.23	0.28	0.29	0.29	0.31	0.39	0.56	0.91	1.61	2.10				0.02	-	-	RATE PER CASE IN PERIOD

TABLE 19 C

SINGAPORE, CHINESE :

FEMALE INCIDENCE RATES, 1950 - 61.

INTER-NATIONAL LIST No.	No. OF CASES IN WHOLE PERIOD — AGE UNKNOWN	No. OF CASES IN WHOLE PERIOD — ALL AGES	ALL AGES	AVERAGE ANNUAL INCIDENCE PER 100,000 — AGE IN YEARS — 85- AND OVER	80-	75-	70-	65-	60-	55-	50-	45-	40-	35-	30-	25-	20-	15-	10-	5-	0-	INTER-NATIONAL LIST No.
140	0	1	0.0				1.0	0.0	0.0	0.0	0.0	0.0	0.0	0.0	0.0	0.0	0.0	0.0	0.0	0.0	0.0	140
141	0	16	0.3				0.0	1.2	0.8	0.6	1.3	0.4	0.9	0.0	0.3	0.5	0.0	0.0	0.0	0.0	0.0	141
142	0	16	0.3				0.0	0.0	1.6	0.6	1.3	1.1	0.9	0.0	0.3	0.0	0.2	0.0	0.2	0.0	0.1	142
143-4	0	17	0.3				4.1	2.3	0.0	1.2	0.9	1.1	0.0	0.3	0.6	0.2	0.0	0.0	0.0	0.0	0.0	143-4
146	1	265	4.4				5.2	9.2	10.6	10.2	16.6	15.8	14.9	10.2	6.8	4.3	2.1	0.2	0.7	0.0	0.0	146
145,147-8	0	19	0.3				0.0	2.3	2.4	1.2	0.4	0.4	2.2	0.0	0.3	0.5	0.2	0.0	0.2	0.0	0.0	145,147-8
150	0	73	1.2				6.2	18.5	4.1	9.0	4.9	3.6	2.2	0.0	0.0	0.0	0.0	0.0	0.0	0.0	0.0	150
151	2	140	2.3				5.2	9.2	14.6	16.8	9.4	3.6	4.3	4.5	2.6	1.4	0.6	0.2	0.0	0.0	0.0	151
152	1	4	0.1				0.0	0.0	0.0	0.0	0.0	0.4	0.3	0.3	0.0	0.0	0.0	0.0	0.0	0.0	0.0	152
153	0	84	1.4				6.2	12.7	10.6	6.0	7.6	3.2	1.9	2.1	0.0	0.5	0.2	0.2	0.2	0.2	0.0	153
154	0	103	1.7				8.2	15.0	7.3	9.6	7.2	4.7	5.6	1.8	0.6	0.2	0.2	0.0	0.0	0.0	0.0	154
155.0	0	45	0.7				1.0	1.2	3.2	1.8	2.2	5.4	1.6	0.6	1.1	0.5	0.2	0.0	0.0	0.1	155.0
155.1	0	14	0.2				3.1	3.5	1.6	1.8	0.0	0.7	1.6	0.3	0.0	0.0	0.0	0.0	0.0	0.0	0.0	155.1
156	0	19	0.3				0.0	1.2	1.6	3.0	0.9	1.1	0.9	0.0	0.9	0.0	0.0	0.0	0.0	0.0	0.0	156
157	1	11	0.2				1.0	1.2	0.8	1.2	0.4	0.4	0.6	0.3	0.0	0.0	0.0	0.0	0.0	0.0	0.0	157
160	1	32	0.5				2.1	2.3	2.4	1.8	3.1	1.8	0.9	0.6	0.6	0.0	0.0	0.2	0.0	0.1	0.0	160
161	0	9	0.1				0.0	2.3	0.0	0.0	1.3	1.1	0.0	0.3	0.0	0.5	0.0	0.0	0.0	0.0	0.0	161
162-3	2	112	1.8				5.2	11.6	13.8	15.6	7.6	3.9	4.3	1.2	1.1	0.9	0.0	0.0	0.0	0.0	0.0	162-3
170	4	317	5.2				9.3	22.0	21.9	24.5	22.5	23.3	14.3	10.5	4.3	4.3	0.4	0.0	0.0	0.0	0.0	170
171	10	886	14.6				23.7	35.8	43.0	56.8	59.8	65.5	51.5	36.1	14.0	0.2	0.6	0.0	0.0	0.0	0.0	171
172	2	160	2.6				7.2	6.9	14.6	17.9	16.2	11.5	5.9	2.4	0.3	2.7	0.0	0.2	0.0	0.0	0.0	172
173	0	68	1.1				0.0	0.0	0.0	0.0	0.0	3.2	2.8	4.2	3.1	1.4	2.5	0.7	0.7	0.2	0.0	173
175	2	129	2.1				5.2	8.1	8.1	7.8	9.4	6.8	3.7	2.4	2.9	0.5	1.2	0.2	0.0	0.0	0.0	175
176	0	46	0.8				1.0	4.6	4.1	3.6	4.9	2.1	0.3	2.4	0.6	0.7	0.0	0.2	0.0	0.2	0.8	176
180	0	40	0.7				0.0	4.6	1.6	4.2	0.9	0.7	0.6	0.6	0.3	0.2	0.2	0.2	0.0	0.5	0.8	180
181.0	0	21	0.3				0.0	2.3	3.2	2.4	1.8	1.1	0.3	0.3	0.3	0.5	0.2	0.0	0.0	0.0	0.0	181.0
190	1	17	0.3				2.1	1.2	0.8	2.4	0.9	0.0	0.3	0.6	0.3	0.2	0.0	0.0	0.2	0.0	190
191	2	94	1.5				22.7	12.7	4.9	5.4	3.1	6.4	3.1	0.0	1.7	0.2	0.0	0.2	0.2	0.5	1.0	191
192	0	19	0.3				1.0	0.0	0.0	0.0	0.4	0.0	0.3	1.8	0.0	1.1	0.6	0.0	0.5	0.8	1.1	192
193	2	60	1.0				0.0	1.2	1.6	1.2	1.8	1.4	0.9	1.2	0.9	0.7	0.2	0.3	0.2	0.2	0.0	193
194	1	37	0.6				1.0	2.3	2.4	1.2	2.2	0.0	0.0	0.6	0.0	0.0	0.0	0.0	0.0	0.3	0.3	194
195	0	8	0.1				0.0	0.0	0.0	0.0	0.0	1.1	0.0	0.3	0.6	0.2	0.2	0.0	0.5	0.0	0.1	195
196	0	19	0.3				1.0	1.2	0.8	0.0	0.9	0.4	0.3	0.3	0.0	0.2	0.4	0.3	0.2	0.2	0.4	196
197	0	18	0.3				1.0	1.2	0.0	1.8	0.9	1.8	1.2	1.2	0.3	0.7	0.4	0.0	1.0	0.2	0.0	197
200	0	46	0.8				3.1	3.5	2.4	1.2	3.1	0.4	0.3	0.6	0.3	0.5	0.2	0.0	0.3	0.1	0.1	200
201	0	12	0.2				0.0	0.0	0.0	0.0	0.0	0.0	0.0	0.0	0.0	0.0	0.2	0.0	0.0	0.0	0.0	201
203	0	4	0.1				0.0	0.0	0.0	0.6	0.0	1.1	0.0	0.0	0.0	0.5	0.0	0.0	0.0	0.0	0.0	203
204	0	30	0.5				1.0	2.3	0.0	0.6	0.9	0.0	0.9	0.0	0.3	0.0	0.0	0.3	0.8	0.7	0.5	204
OTHER	1	290	4.8				11.3	17.3	25.2	30.5	19.3	14.3	12.1	6.9	3.7	2.0	0.6	0.5	0.0	0.3	0.5	OTHER
140-205	35	3301	54.4				139.1	220.8	210.4	242.3	215.0	191.7	141.5	96.2	49.9	25.9	11.5	3.7	5.4	3.8	4.9	140-205
RATE PER CASE IN PERIOD	-	-	0.02				1.03	1.16	0.81	0.60	0.45	0.36	0.31	0.30	0.29	0.23	0.21	0.17	0.16	0.11	0.10	RATE PER CASE IN PERIOD

DENMARK

Registry Title and Address : The Danish Cancer Registry under the National Anti-Cancer League, The Finsen Institute, Strandboulevard 49, Copenhagen, Denmark. Commenced 5th May, 1942. Supported financially by Landsforeningen til Kraeftens Bekaempelse.

Registration. Cases are registered by physicians from hospital in-patients and out-patients, from radiotherapy and pathology departments, and from death certificates.

Follow-up. Follow-up is by therapeutic units, except for special studies.

Physical Description. The Registry covers the Kingdom of Denmark except for the Faroe Isles and Greenland; that is the peninsular of Jutland and islands in the entrance to the Baltic. It lies between latitudes 54°34' and 57°45' north and longitudes 8°5' and 15°12' east. The total registration area is 42,932 square kilometres.

Demographic Description. Total population of area under survey 4,433,850. The main occupational composition is industry 30 %; commerce 15 %; agriculture 25 %; personal service 10 %. Of the total population 25 % live in conurbations of more than 100,000.

Medical Services. Total number of hospital beds of all kinds 26,420 (1950). Total number of doctors in practice in registration area 5,500 (1957).

Publications. Clemmesen (1955, 1965).

TABLE 20 A
DENMARK :
POPULATION (100,000s), MEAN 1953 - 57

AGE (In years)	MALES		FEMALES	
	No.	Per Cent	No.	Per Cent
0-	1.9310	8.78	1.8318	8.20
5-	2.1241	9.66	2.0273	9.07
10-	1.9612	8.92	1.8816	8.42
15-	1.5842	7.20	1.5347	6.87
20-	1.4391	6.54	1.4287	6.39
25-	1.4449	6.57	1.4708	6.58
30-	1.5399	7.00	1.5807	7.07
35-	1.5187	6.91	1.5464	6.92
40-	1.5385	7.00	1.5647	7.00
45-	1.4769	6.72	1.5153	6.78
50-	1.3078	5.95	1.3777	6.17
55-	1.1427	5.20	1.2406	5.55
60-	0.9484	4.31	1.0438	4.67
65-	0.7723	3.51	0.8647	3.87
70-	0.5897	2.68	0.6634	2.97
75-	0.3912	1.78	0.4356	1.95
80- and over	0.2825	1.28	0.3376	1.51
-	-	-	-	-
TOTAL	21.9931	100.00	22.3454	100.00

NOTES

TO TABLES 20 A, B and C

(I) I.L. numbers 140-191 exclude all sarcomas; corresponding incidence rates for sarcomas of these sites are as follows :

Age in years	Male	Female	Age in years	Male	Female
0-4	0.6	0.5	45-49	3.4	5.3
5-9	0.7	0.5	50-54	6.0	5.7
10-14	0.7	0.4	55-59	8.1	9.2
15-19	0.9	1.2	60-64	10.3	10.9
20-24	1.3	0.7	65-69	10.1	8.5
25-29	1.4	1.8	70-74	10.8	12.3
30-34	1.4	2.7	75-79	16.4	10.6
35-39	1.8	2.7	80 and over	14.9	13.6
40-44	2.5	4.7	All ages	3.4	3.9

(II) I.L. number 160 includes malignant tumours of naso-pharynx and of lower jaw (I.L. numbers 146 and 196.1).

" " 155.0 includes malignant tumours of liver, secondary and unspecified (I.L. number 156).

" " 181.0 includes papilloma of bladder.

" " 193 includes benign and unspecified tumours of the central nervous system.

" " 196 excludes malignant tumour of lower jaw (I.L. number 196.1).

(III) Carcinoma in situ excluded.

TABLE 20 B
DENMARK :
MALE INCIDENCE RATES, 1953 - 57.

INTER-NATIONAL LIST No.	0-	5-	10-	15-	20-	25-	30-	35-	40-	45-	50-	55-	60-	65-	70-	75-	80-	85- AND OVER	ALL AGES	AGE UNKNOWN	ALL AGES (cases)	INTER-NATIONAL LIST No.
						AGE IN YEARS													AVG ANNUAL INCIDENCE PER 100,000	No. OF CASES IN WHOLE PERIOD		
140	0.1	0.0	0.0	0.0	0.3	0.4	1.7	2.5	4.0	7.9	10.7	16.3	19.4	22.3	24.1	25.1	41.8		5.9	0	647	140
141	0.0	0.0	0.1	0.0	0.0	0.0	0.4	0.4	0.5	0.5	0.8	2.3	2.5	4.7	3.4	6.6	7.8		0.9	0	99	141
142	0.0	0.0	0.1	0.3	0.8	0.4	0.9	1.3	0.6	1.8	1.7	2.1	2.5	3.9	3.7	5.1	3.5		1.1	0	123	142
143-4	0.0	0.0	0.0	0.0	0.0	0.0	0.4	0.4	0.1	0.5	0.9	2.1	3.2	2.8	5.8	10.2	9.9		1.0	0	106	143-4
145,147-8	0.0	0.0	0.1	0.0	0.0	0.0	0.0	0.1	0.3	0.5	0.9	2.1	3.2	4.4	6.4	7.7	7.1		0.9	0	102	145,147-8
150	0.0	0.0	0.0	0.0	0.0	0.0	0.1	0.5	1.2	1.1	4.7	8.4	12.0	21.2	30.9	49.6	57.3		4.6	0	509	150
151	0.0	0.0	0.0	0.0	0.4	0.6	2.2	4.2	9.4	21.8	39.0	65.5	122.5	194.5	276.1	360.9	501.9		40.7	0	4479	151
152	0.0	0.0	0.0	0.1	0.1	0.1	0.1	0.0	0.8	0.4	1.3	1.2	1.9	3.4	3.7	4.6	5.0		0.7	0	76	152
153	0.0	0.1	0.0	0.1	0.7	1.2	1.6	5.0	6.1	9.3	13.2	32.2	53.4	80.3	120.4	151.3	244.2		18.3	0	2011	153
154	0.0	0.0	0.0	0.1	0.3	0.7	2.2	2.6	5.3	11.6	20.3	41.0	65.6	92.2	153.3	163.6	212.4		20.7	0	2278	154
155.0,156	0.3	0.0	0.0	0.0	0.0	0.0	0.4	0.1	0.9	1.1	4.4	5.3	9.7	16.3	20.3	34.8	42.5		3.4	0	378	155.0,156
155.1	0.0	0.0	0.0	0.0	0.0	0.3	0.3	0.7	0.6	0.8	2.0	3.3	5.5	10.4	11.9	15.3	18.4		1.8	0	203	155.1
157	0.0	0.0	0.2	0.3	0.3	0.1	0.4	0.9	1.2	6.2	9.0	18.2	24.9	39.9	47.8	54.2	58.8		7.5	0	830	157
160	0.0	0.0	0.0	0.0	0.0	0.4	0.4	0.3	1.2	1.1	2.6	1.1	4.4	6.0	6.1	10.7	9.9		1.4	0	154	160
161	0.0	0.0	0.0	0.1	0.4	0.7	0.3	0.3	0.6	3.4	3.7	5.3	7.0	8.5	4.7	6.6	8.5		1.8	0	196	161
162-3	0.0	0.0	0.0	0.1	0.4	0.7	1.9	3.6	10.3	29.8	71.9	108.3	128.6	138.8	119.4	102.8	96.3		29.8	0	3274	162-3
170	0.0	0.0	0.0	0.0	0.0	0.0	0.0	0.1	0.4	0.5	0.8	0.9	1.5	3.4	1.7	4.6	4.2		0.5	0	57	170
177	0.0	0.0	0.0	0.0	0.1	0.0	0.0	0.1	0.6	1.2	4.9	21.4	51.2	109.8	203.8	306.7	399.3		23.7	0	2602	177
178	0.4	0.0	0.2	1.5	5.8	8.4	10.7	7.8	8.3	4.7	3.5	3.0	2.5	2.6	1.4	3.1	3.5		4.0	0	438	178
179.0	0.0	0.0	0.0	0.0	0.1	0.0	0.5	0.9	1.0	1.4	1.5	2.5	3.8	4.4	7.8	10.7	9.2		1.3	0	146	179.0
180	2.1	0.8	0.1	0.0	0.0	0.4	0.8	2.0	3.4	6.0	8.6	10.9	20.9	27.5	46.1	31.2	45.3		6.4	0	708	180
181.0	0.0	0.1	0.0	0.3	0.4	0.4	0.6	3.4	4.7	10.3	22.6	29.4	46.6	63.7	75.3	87.9	109.0		13.5	0	1481	181.0
190	0.1	0.2	0.3	0.3	0.3	0.6	0.8	2.4	2.1	2.8	3.8	3.3	3.6	2.6	8.1	10.2	11.3		1.9	0	206	190
191	1.3	0.0	0.3	0.0	0.7	0.8	2.7	7.6	10.3	19.2	35.5	45.3	76.5	118.9	150.9	215.2	311.5		26.7	0	2936	191
192	3.5	0.2	0.1	0.0	0.1	0.3	0.1	0.4	0.6	0.9	1.2	2.3	3.0	4.4	4.4	2.6	5.0		1.0	0	111	192
193	0.0	2.0	2.3	2.9	2.1	3.5	4.7	6.7	8.2	12.1	16.8	19.6	20.7	14.5	6.8	10.2	2.8		7.3	0	803	193
194	0.2	0.1	0.0	0.0	0.1	0.1	0.1	0.4	0.6	0.9	0.3	0.9	2.7	3.9	2.0	3.1	0.0		0.6	0	70	194
195	0.3	0.6	0.0	0.9	0.1	0.0	0.1	0.0	0.1	0.4	1.1	1.4	1.3	1.3	0.7	0.0	5.0		0.3	0	36	195
196	0.2	0.2	1.2	0.8	1.0	0.4	0.9	1.4	1.3	0.5	0.7	0.9	2.3	1.3	2.4	2.6	5.7		1.0	0	109	196
197	0.4	0.3	0.3	0.4	1.0	0.3	0.4	1.6	1.4	1.8	1.7	1.9	3.4	3.9	8.8	5.1	13.5		1.4	0	154	197
200	0.0	0.5	0.5	0.4	0.7	0.6	1.4	2.5	1.9	3.0	2.3	5.4	6.1	9.1	8.8	13.3	2.1		2.4	0	265	200
201	0.0	0.0	0.6	2.5	4.9	3.5	3.1	0.9	3.5	2.3	5.4	3.5	4.2	2.1	8.1	5.6	9.2		2.7	0	299	201
203	0.0	0.0	0.0	0.0	0.0	0.0	0.4	0.9	0.9	1.6	3.2	4.9	9.7	10.1	19.0	12.3	9.2		2.3	0	256	203
204	8.3	4.3	3.4	2.9	2.4	2.6	2.2	3.3	4.2	5.8	9.8	15.8	22.1	37.3	37.6	62.4	43.2		9.4	0	1032	204
202,205	0.0	0.1	0.0	0.1	0.0	0.0	0.1	0.0	0.6	0.3	0.8	1.2	1.1	1.3	2.0	0.5	0.0		0.3	0	38	202,205
OTHER	0.7	0.1	0.2	0.1	0.3	0.7	2.3	1.4	3.2	5.7	9.0	11.9	25.5	30.3	41.4	58.3	82.8		7.6	0	832	OTHER
140-205	18.1	9.4	10.1	13.6	23.5	27.5	44.9	66.8	100.2	179.4	320.1	500.7	776.0	1101.6	1475.3	1854.8	2392.2		255.0	0	28044	140-205
RATE PER CASE IN PERIOD	0.10	0.09	0.10	0.13	0.14	0.14	0.13	0.13	0.13	0.14	0.15	0.18	0.21	0.26	0.34	0.51	0.71		0.01	-	-	RATE PER CASE IN PERIOD

TABLE 20 C

DENMARK :

FEMALE INCIDENCE RATES, 1953 - 57.

INTER-NATIONAL LIST No.	AVERAGE ANNUAL INCIDENCE PER 100,000 (AGE IN YEARS)																		ALL AGES	No. OF CASES IN WHOLE PERIOD AGE UN-KNOWN	No. OF CASES IN WHOLE PERIOD ALL AGES	INTER-NATIONAL LIST No.
	0-	5-	10-	15-	20-	25-	30-	35-	40-	45-	50-	55-	60-	65-	70-	75-	80-	85- AND OVER				
140	0.1	0.0	0.0	0.1	0.0	0.0	0.0	0.1	0.3	0.3	1.3	1.1	1.3	2.1	4.5	1.8	3.0		0.6	0	63	140
141	0.0	0.0	0.0	0.0	0.0	0.0	0.3	0.3	0.0	0.4	0.3	0.3	1.1	2.5	4.5	2.3	7.1		0.5	0	60	141
142	0.0	0.1	0.1	0.4	0.7	1.1	1.3	1.6	1.3	2.2	1.9	2.6	2.7	2.1	4.5	3.7	7.1		1.4	0	154	142
143-4	0.0	0.0	0.0	0.0	0.0	0.0	0.1	0.0	0.1	0.0	0.7	0.6	1.0	1.4	2.4	4.1	5.9		0.4	0	46	143-4
145,147-8	0.0	0.0	0.2	0.0	0.0	0.0	0.0	0.1	0.0	0.5	0.7	0.5	1.5	2.5	1.8	2.8	2.4		0.5	0	52	145,147-8
150	0.0	0.0	0.1	0.0	0.0	0.0	0.0	0.1	0.4	0.3	1.0	3.9	2.9	8.8	17.2	25.3	41.5		2.4	0	272	150
151	0.0	0.0	0.0	0.0	0.0	0.5	1.8	4.1	5.1	10.7	17.9	31.0	54.6	101.8	179.4	302.6	476.3		29.3	0	3269	151
152	0.0	0.0	0.0	0.0	0.0	0.0	0.1	0.0	0.6	0.3	1.0	1.3	2.7	2.1	1.8	3.2	7.1		0.6	0	71	152
153	0.0	0.1	0.3	0.0	0.3	1.0	2.4	7.0	6.9	14.1	24.2	38.7	50.2	77.5	120.3	185.0	258.9		22.3	0	2490	153
154	0.0	0.0	0.0	0.0	0.3	0.5	1.5	2.8	7.0	12.5	20.8	28.4	36.2	52.0	75.1	81.3	115.5		13.8	0	1544	154
155.0,156	0.1	0.0	0.0	0.0	0.0	0.3	0.9	0.8	0.6	1.5	1.6	6.3	8.2	13.0	19.9	37.6	65.2		3.9	0	439	155.0,156
155.1	0.0	0.0	0.0	0.0	0.0	0.0	0.0	0.1	1.0	1.7	3.2	8.5	13.6	22.2	25.3	32.1	35.0		4.3	0	477	155.1
157	0.1	0.1	0.0	0.3	0.0	0.1	0.3	0.6	1.4	2.9	6.8	10.8	16.3	26.6	36.5	40.9	32.0		5.5	0	619	157
160	0.0	0.1	0.0	0.0	0.0	0.0	0.1	0.4	0.5	0.1	0.6	1.3	0.8	1.6	1.2	1.4	1.2		0.4	0	45	160
161	0.0	0.0	0.0	0.0	0.0	0.0	0.1	0.0	0.1	0.5	0.3	0.3	0.4	0.9	1.5	2.8	2.4		0.3	0	31	161
162-3	0.0	0.0	0.0	0.0	0.1	0.5	0.4	1.6	3.8	3.8	8.6	13.1	22.2	24.7	29.2	25.3	39.7		5.9	0	661	162-3
170	0.0	0.0	0.0	0.1	1.0	4.1	10.2	37.9	66.2	105.2	105.5	115.1	148.3	176.7	203.5	225.0	273.1		56.7	0	6333	170
171	0.0	0.0	0.1	0.3	2.7	19.2	37.6	65.7	69.7	72.3	73.2	68.8	58.6	46.3	43.7	38.1	40.3		34.0	0	3794	171
172	0.0	0.0	0.0	0.0	0.3	0.4	1.0	3.5	7.8	19.4	35.6	50.9	52.1	50.2	38.6	32.1	22.5		13.7	0	1534	172
173	0.0	0.0	0.0	0.1	0.3	0.1	0.4	0.0	0.0	0.3	0.0	0.0	0.0	0.0	0.0	0.0	0.0		0.1	0	9	173
174	0.0	0.0	0.0	0.0	0.1	0.1	0.5	1.7	0.9	3.2	3.5	4.5	4.2	7.2	8.4	11.0	26.1		2.2	0	251	174
175	0.0	0.1	0.5	1.0	1.7	1.4	3.3	7.5	18.2	31.4	42.0	48.7	47.1	46.3	47.6	42.2	40.3		16.6	0	1855	175
176	0.0	0.0	0.0	0.1	0.1	0.1	1.0	1.7	2.8	3.2	4.4	6.9	8.6	10.4	19.6	17.9	23.7		3.4	0	377	176
180	1.3	0.5	0.1	0.1	0.0	0.1	0.6	1.0	1.4	3.4	6.1	11.0	15.9	24.5	23.8	31.7	23.7		5.0	0	558	180
181.0	0.0	0.0	0.0	0.1	0.0	0.0	0.3	1.2	1.7	2.2	4.9	8.1	13.8	21.3	25.9	37.6	43.2		4.8	0	531	181.0
190	0.0	0.4	0.2	0.3	1.0	1.6	3.0	4.3	3.5	4.1	4.9	4.4	3.8	5.1	8.4	6.0	7.1		2.7	0	298	190
191	0.1	0.1	0.0	0.0	0.4	1.1	3.0	3.8	9.2	13.7	22.9	30.0	41.2	63.4	94.1	138.2	194.3		18.0	0	2016	191
192	0.8	0.1	0.0	0.0	0.1	0.1	0.4	0.3	0.6	1.2	1.2	1.9	2.5	2.5	4.5	4.5	4.3		0.9	0	98	192
193	3.2	2.3	2.2	1.8	2.7	3.5	4.9	6.1	6.3	9.9	13.8	16.3	14.8	11.3	7.8	7.8	7.1		6.4	0	719	193
194	0.0	0.0	0.1	0.4	0.4	0.7	0.8	1.0	1.5	2.2	1.3	3.1	5.7	6.5	6.6	11.9	8.9		1.8	0	204	194
195	0.3	0.1	0.0	0.0	0.0	0.4	0.0	0.4	0.0	0.4	0.4	0.3	0.6	0.5	0.9	1.4	1.2		0.3	0	31	195
196	0.5	0.5	1.2	1.3	1.0	0.4	0.5	0.1	0.4	0.3	0.7	2.3	1.5	2.3	1.8	2.8	3.0		0.8	0	85	196
197	0.5	0.3	0.4	1.0	0.8	0.8	0.4	1.3	1.8	1.6	1.7	3.4	2.7	2.5	2.7	5.1	7.1		1.4	0	162	197
200	0.0	0.4	1.0	0.4	0.3	0.5	0.4	1.7	0.9	0.9	1.5	1.8	3.3	5.8	6.3	11.0	10.7		1.6	0	180	200
201	0.0	0.0	0.3	1.2	3.8	5.0	2.0	1.0	1.4	1.8	1.7	1.8	2.9	3.0	1.8	3.2	4.1		1.8	0	206	201
203	0.0	0.0	0.0	0.0	0.0	2.0	0.3	0.0	0.3	1.6	1.9	4.4	7.5	8.1	10.3	10.6	8.3		1.8	0	201	203
204	5.6	2.8	1.8	2.7	0.8	2.0	1.8	2.7	2.6	6.3	5.7	11.6	16.5	20.4	22.0	27.1	25.5		6.3	0	701	204
202,205	0.0	0.0	0.0	0.3	0.0	0.0	0.0	0.3	0.5	0.3	0.6	0.5	0.6	0.7	1.5	1.4	1.2		0.3	0	33	202,205
OTHER	0.7	0.0	0.2	0.0	0.0	0.8	1.4	1.4	2.8	6.6	12.3	19.2	33.9	53.2	67.8	109.7	149.9		12.9	0	1436	OTHER
140-205	12.8	7.8	8.8	12.2	19.0	46.8	82.5	164.3	229.8	343.3	436.4	563.3	701.9	909.9	1173.0	1527.1	2024.3		285.6	0	31905	140-205
RATE PER CASE IN PERIOD	0.11	0.10	0.11	0.13	0.14	0.14	0.13	0.13	0.13	0.13	0.15	0.16	0.19	0.23	0.30	0.46	0.59		0.01	-	-	RATE PER CASE IN PERIOD

ENGLAND AND WALES (4 REGIONS)

Cancer registration in England and Wales is a regional responsibility. Each of the 15 Regional Hospital Boards has set up its own scheme (apart from 3 which have voluntarily combined for this purpose) and each is responsible for the validity and completeness of the data it collects. Each region reports results to a national register, where duplication is eliminated and some analyses are undertaken. In this volume we have presented data for 4 regional registries, including the one which covers three Regional Hospital Board areas, and also for the 4 regions combined. The combined rates represent the experience of nearly 40 per cent of the population and are reasonably representative of the country as a whole. Information about the work of the individual registries is given only in relation to the Tables for the separate regions.

TABLE 21 A
ENGLAND and WALES (FOUR REGIONS) :
POPULATION (100,000s), CENSUS 1961

AGE (in years)	MALES		FEMALES	
	No.	Per Cent	No.	Per Cent
0 –	7.2295	8.10	6.9487	7.18
5 –	6.6707	7.47	6.3610	6.57
10 –	7.6664	8.59	7.3092	7.55
15 –	6.6332	7.43	6.4433	6.66
20 –	5.7624	6.46	5.7826	5.97
25 –	5.7098	6.40	5.5498	5.73
30 –	5.9402	6.66	5.9138	6.11
35 –	6.2885	7.05	6.4936	6.71
40 –	5.9335	6.65	6.2456	6.45
45 –	6.3369	7.10	6.6816	6.90
50 –	6.2492	7.00	6.6743	6.89
55 –	5.6215	6.30	6.1964	6.40
60 –	4.4087	4.94	5.6093	5.79
65 –	3.3850	3.79	4.8548	5.02
70 –	2.5078	2.81	4.0121	4.14
75 –	1.6421	1.84	2.9472	3.04
80 –	0.8756	0.98	1.7805	1.84
85 – and over	0.3955	0.44	0.9982	1.03
TOTAL	89.2565	100.00	96.8020	100.00

NOTES

TO TABLES 21 A, B and C

(I)   Data for 4 registries only, covering 6 of the 15 hospital regions in England and Wales.

(II)   Period of registration 1960-62 for Birmingham, South Metropolitan and South Western Regions, and 1959-63 for Liverpool Region.

(III)   I. L. number 193 includes benign and unspecified tumours of the central nervous system.

(IV)   Carcinoma in situ excluded.

TABLE 21 B

ENGLAND and WALES (FOUR REGIONS) :

MALE INCIDENCE RATES, 1960 - 62.

AVERAGE ANNUAL INCIDENCE PER 100,000 — AGE IN YEARS

INTER- NATIONAL LIST No.	0-	5-	10-	15-	20-	25-	30-	35-	40-	45-	50-	55-	60-	65-	70-	75-	80-	85- and over	ALL AGES	No. of cases Age unknown	No. of cases All ages
140	0.0	0.0	0.0	0.0	0.1	0.2	0.3	0.4	1.1	1.7	3.3	5.4	5.6	9.6	14.6	17.5	22.7	25.5	2.6	3	776
141	0.0	0.0	0.0	0.0	0.2	0.1	0.1	0.5	0.8	0.8	1.8	2.9	4.3	7.9	10.8	15.1	23.7	32.9	2.0	1	571
142	0.0	0.0	0.2	0.5	0.3	0.8	1.4	1.4	1.2	1.8	1.7	2.2	2.5	3.0	4.4	5.8	7.8	6.1	1.3	0	393
143-4	0.0	0.0	0.1	0.0	0.1	0.0	0.3	0.2	0.7	1.0	1.6	3.3	5.6	10.1	12.3	15.9	26.7	30.5	2.2	2	653
146	0.1	0.1	0.0	0.2	0.2	0.1	0.1	0.1	0.6	0.8	1.2	1.2	1.4	1.8	2.8	1.6	0.8	0.5	0.6	0	170
145,147-8	0.0	0.0	0.0	0.1	0.1	0.1	0.1	0.3	0.4	1.1	2.4	5.0	9.7	11.4	16.2	26.2	27.3	28.2	2.9	1	848
150	0.0	0.0	0.0	0.0	0.2	0.1	0.1	0.3	1.1	2.9	5.7	9.3	15.2	26.9	39.3	50.1	68.4	84.8	6.2	1	1817
151	0.1	0.0	0.0	0.1	0.4	0.7	2.5	4.0	11.5	20.0	43.4	67.3	106.9	148.8	185.5	223.5	228.4	229.1	33.5	11	10147
152	0.0	0.0	0.0	0.0	0.0	0.2	0.3	0.3	0.6	0.6	0.9	1.4	2.4	2.4	3.3	3.1	4.0	1.7	0.7	1	204
153	0.0	0.0	0.2	0.3	0.7	0.8	2.0	4.1	6.0	12.6	16.7	29.5	52.1	75.1	109.6	152.4	191.8	210.0	19.0	4	5717
154	0.0	0.0	0.0	0.1	0.3	0.3	1.6	2.1	4.8	9.5	15.0	35.6	54.8	79.7	99.3	132.4	161.3	147.7	17.8	7	5162
155	0.3	0.0	0.0	0.0	0.1	0.1	0.5	0.4	0.8	1.5	3.0	5.5	10.2	14.0	15.4	20.9	20.6	19.0	3.0	1	901
156	0.0	0.0	0.0	0.0	0.0	0.0	0.1	0.3	0.3	0.7	1.6	3.4	5.0	8.2	8.8	11.0	12.3	10.3	1.6	2	468
157	0.0	0.0	0.0	0.0	0.0	0.1	0.4	0.6	3.0	5.8	9.4	18.9	26.6	38.9	54.6	61.3	65.3	73.2	9.0	2	2650
160	0.0	0.0	0.0	0.0	0.0	0.0	0.1	0.7	0.4	0.7	1.0	2.3	3.2	3.1	5.6	4.3	7.8	5.2	1.0	2	289
161	0.0	0.0	0.0	0.1	0.0	0.1	0.4	0.8	1.4	3.4	7.5	12.3	17.6	21.9	23.6	22.5	25.4	17.9	4.8	1	1425
162-3	0.1	0.0	0.0	0.1	0.6	1.1	3.7	9.7	26.6	66.8	144.3	258.1	399.4	443.4	438.3	375.7	250.7	183.2	93.1	40	27554
170	0.0	0.0	0.0	0.0	0.0	0.0	0.0	0.2	0.2	0.6	0.7	1.5	2.0	2.4	3.4	4.1	6.9	5.2	0.7	0	195
177	0.1	0.0	0.0	0.0	0.0	0.0	0.0	0.1	0.4	1.4	5.5	16.2	38.1	88.1	175.3	286.6	411.5	433.7	23.0	15	6740
178	0.4	0.2	0.2	0.8	3.4	5.2	5.9	4.3	4.3	2.8	2.0	1.8	1.5	0.8	1.6	1.8	1.9	2.5	2.3	2	681
179.0	1.5	0.0	0.0	0.0	0.0	0.1	0.2	0.4	1.0	0.7	1.6	2.3	3.3	5.2	5.0	6.7	9.1	15.5	1.2	0	353
180	0.1	0.5	0.2	0.1	0.3	0.4	0.6	1.1	2.6	4.9	7.6	11.3	15.6	16.3	17.1	19.0	17.9	16.4	4.6	3	1333
181.0	0.1	0.0	0.0	0.1	0.2	0.8	0.9	2.2	3.5	8.9	16.1	29.6	49.8	71.9	104.2	117.9	134.8	133.0	16.4	6	4769
190	1.0	0.0	0.1	0.3	0.5	0.9	1.1	1.1	1.0	1.8	2.1	2.4	2.3	1.9	3.2	3.3	5.8	15.3	1.2	0	353
191	0.0	0.1	0.1	0.3	1.1	1.6	4.2	10.0	19.8	31.9	47.7	63.7	92.8	116.7	165.0	222.2	307.9	396.0	34.9	80	10293
192	1.0	0.1	0.1	0.0	0.1	0.1	0.2	0.4	0.7	0.9	0.7	1.0	1.6	1.5	1.5	1.9	1.9	1.7	0.6	2	180
193	3.5	2.5	1.8	2.2	2.1	3.0	4.1	6.2	6.5	8.9	13.5	16.0	17.4	15.3	9.2	5.1	2.6	1.0	6.7	3	1964
194	0.0	0.0	0.1	0.1	0.1	0.2	0.2	0.3	0.2	0.6	0.8	1.5	2.0	2.3	4.0	3.0	0.8	5.7	0.7	0	203
195	0.6	0.1	0.5	0.2	0.3	0.5	0.4	0.8	0.5	1.2	1.0	1.4	1.6	1.5	1.5	1.3	3.2	0.0	0.7	1	213
196	0.1	0.5	1.1	1.7	0.8	0.7	0.9	0.3	0.7	0.8	0.7	1.0	3.5	2.7	4.1	3.9	3.2	8.4	1.1	0	326
197	0.5	0.2	0.4	0.7	1.2	0.5	1.0	2.2	1.7	1.9	1.8	2.6	4.7	4.7	4.5	6.6	8.1	11.3	1.7	0	520
200	0.5	0.7	0.7	1.2	1.0	1.4	2.8	2.2	2.4	3.1	5.1	6.9	9.3	11.2	12.8	10.8	9.9	5.9	3.4	2	983
201	0.0	0.4	1.1	1.9	3.3	3.3	3.1	2.4	3.8	3.3	4.2	3.9	3.9	5.5	4.9	4.1	3.3	2.2	2.7	1	810
203	0.0	0.0	0.0	0.1	0.0	0.2	0.1	0.3	1.0	1.5	2.5	3.6	6.1	6.5	8.4	7.3	5.5	4.7	1.6	1	465
204	5.2	3.0	2.2	2.1	2.4	1.8	3.1	3.4	4.4	5.2	6.0	9.9	13.9	19.9	27.4	36.8	41.4	37.4	6.9	5	2026
202,205	0.2	0.0	0.2	0.5	0.4	0.5	0.7	0.8	0.9	1.3	1.1	1.7	1.9	1.8	4.2	2.8	3.1	3.4	1.0	0	275
OTHER	0.3	0.1	0.3	0.3	0.3	0.6	0.9	1.6	2.9	5.0	8.1	13.4	20.1	28.4	32.1	39.5	37.2	36.4	6.5	3	1885
140-205	14.6	8.8	9.7	13.8	20.5	26.6	42.8	66.6	119.9	218.4	389.5	655.3	1011.0	1310.8	1633.6	1924.0	2160.7	2241.4	319.1	201	94312
RATE PER CASE IN PERIOD	0.05	0.05	0.04	0.05	0.06	0.06	0.06	0.05	0.06	0.05	0.05	0.06	0.08	0.10	0.13	0.20	0.38	0.84	0.04	-	-

TABLE 21 C

ENGLAND and WALES (FOUR REGIONS) :

FEMALE INCIDENCE RATES, 1960 - 62.

AVERAGE ANNUAL INCIDENCE PER 100,000

INTER-NATIONAL LIST No.	0–	5–	10–	15–	20–	25–	30–	35–	40–	45–	50–	55–	60–	65–	70–	75–	80–	85– AND OVER	ALL AGES	AGE UN-KNOWN	ALL AGES	INTER-NATIONAL LIST No.
140	0.0	0.0	0.0	0.0	0.0	0.1	0.1	0.1	0.3	0.1	0.3	0.7	0.6	0.9	1.1	1.7	2.8	2.2	0.4	2	114	140
141	0.0	0.0	0.0	0.0	0.1	0.0	0.1	0.4	0.4	0.5	1.0	0.7	1.8	2.9	3.4	4.9	5.4	5.9	0.9	1	289	141
142	0.0	0.0	0.3	0.8	0.8	1.5	1.7	1.6	1.1	2.0	2.4	3.2	2.5	1.9	3.1	2.4	3.5	5.5	1.6	0	497	142
143-4	0.1	0.0	0.0	0.1	0.2	0.1	0.1	0.3	0.4	0.4	1.2	1.3	2.2	2.8	5.2	5.7	5.1	5.4	1.1	1	349	143-4
146	0.0	0.0	0.0	0.2	0.0	0.0	0.1	0.1	0.3	0.2	0.3	0.1	0.6	0.9	0.5	0.7	1.2	0.7	0.2	0	76	146
145,147-8	0.0	0.1	0.0	0.0	0.0	0.0	0.3	0.5	0.7	1.7	2.9	3.3	5.2	4.9	5.9	6.0	7.9	7.9	1.8	0	614	145,147-8
150	0.0	0.0	0.0	0.0	0.0	0.0	0.2	0.4	1.4	2.2	4.2	5.1	9.4	13.2	16.6	28.7	34.2	33.3	4.6	0	1509	150
151	0.0	0.1	0.0	0.1	0.3	0.8	1.3	2.5	4.2	7.4	14.8	24.6	41.0	66.4	89.0	130.1	170.7	177.1	22.1	24	7307	151
152	0.0	0.1	0.0	0.0	0.0	0.0	0.2	0.3	0.5	0.3	1.0	0.8	1.6	1.6	2.3	2.9	1.7	3.5	0.6	1	206	152
153	0.0	0.0	0.3	0.9	1.1	1.2	3.2	4.5	8.7	14.7	24.3	34.2	52.5	66.8	96.3	125.4	157.5	179.4	25.1	15	8182	153
154	0.0	0.0	0.0	0.1	0.2	0.4	1.3	2.7	4.8	8.6	12.8	19.5	27.4	41.8	51.8	68.4	77.9	86.8	13.6	7	4299	154
155	0.2	0.1	0.0	0.0	0.1	0.0	0.3	0.4	0.6	1.7	2.1	5.5	7.3	13.0	17.6	21.2	20.2	23.6	3.8	3	1207	155
156	0.0	0.0	0.0	0.1	0.0	0.0	0.1	0.3	0.3	0.9	1.5	2.5	3.4	4.4	7.4	6.6	10.6	9.2	1.6	3	510	156
157	0.0	0.1	0.0	0.0	0.1	0.1	0.5	0.4	1.5	2.8	5.2	8.3	16.4	22.5	33.3	38.2	49.8	61.1	7.4	1	2377	157
160	0.0	0.0	0.0	0.1	0.1	0.1	0.2	0.1	0.7	0.9	0.8	1.4	1.2	2.1	2.0	3.5	3.5	3.7	0.7	0	241	160
161	0.0	0.0	0.0	0.1	0.0	0.4	0.2	0.1	0.2	0.7	1.0	1.2	1.6	1.6	2.7	2.6	2.7	1.5	0.7	3	219	161
162-3	0.0	0.0	0.0	0.1	0.0	0.4	1.3	3.6	7.4	12.8	21.6	30.0	40.7	50.5	46.6	48.6	41.9	35.9	14.6	3	4670	162-3
170	0.0	0.0	0.0	0.2	1.1	4.7	18.6	43.0	78.7	116.7	117.1	129.9	145.0	154.9	174.0	188.9	198.0	236.3	69.2	38	21819	170
171	0.0	0.0	0.0	0.1	0.2	1.8	7.8	21.8	31.6	31.9	31.1	30.4	31.1	31.0	30.5	31.9	30.6	27.4	16.9	12	5432	171
172	0.0	0.0	0.0	0.1	0.1	0.3	0.5	4.0	7.0	14.3	28.7	41.4	40.4	39.6	33.1	30.6	29.1	26.9	13.8	7	4388	172
173,174	0.0	0.1	0.3	0.1	0.5	0.5	0.4	0.3	0.7	1.4	1.6	1.6	1.7	2.5	1.6	2.1	1.1	4.0	0.9	1	271	173,174
175	0.0	0.1	0.3	0.6	1.4	2.7	4.2	6.9	14.8	23.2	29.7	35.2	37.8	37.0	35.1	34.3	30.5	26.9	15.3	5	4840	175
176	0.0	0.0	0.0	0.1	0.1	0.5	0.8	0.9	1.3	2.3	2.5	4.4	7.9	10.3	15.4	16.6	24.7	29.1	3.7	1	1182	176
180	1.7	0.6	0.0	0.0	0.1	0.5	0.3	0.5	1.5	2.1	2.8	4.2	6.5	8.4	8.1	11.8	10.4	9.8	2.8	0	883	180
181.0	0.0	0.0	0.0	0.0	0.1	0.2	0.3	0.8	1.0	2.5	4.1	6.9	11.5	17.4	24.3	32.1	36.2	37.5	5.6	2	1799	181.0
190	0.0	0.0	0.1	0.4	1.2	1.7	2.5	3.3	3.8	4.0	3.4	3.3	3.6	4.4	4.2	6.3	5.5	6.5	2.5	2	791	190
191	0.0	0.2	0.1	0.3	0.7	2.0	3.8	8.1	12.9	20.7	28.2	35.3	50.0	66.5	91.1	113.0	156.2	192.4	25.9	53	8314	191
192	0.8	0.2	0.1	0.1	0.2	0.2	0.3	0.4	0.5	0.8	0.7	1.1	0.8	1.0	1.6	1.5	1.1	1.5	0.6	1	187	192
193	3.4	2.4	1.9	1.4	1.3	2.5	3.7	3.8	4.9	8.7	9.6	11.5	11.6	10.2	6.3	2.5	2.7	2.4	5.3	0	1665	193
194	0.0	0.0	0.1	0.2	0.2	1.1	0.9	1.1	1.3	1.8	2.4	2.2	3.6	4.6	6.1	6.8	8.6	6.9	1.9	0	605	194
195	0.5	0.2	0.1	0.1	0.3	0.3	0.4	0.5	0.8	1.0	1.0	0.9	0.7	0.9	1.0	0.3	0.2	0.0	0.5	0	171	195
196	0.2	0.5	1.1	0.8	0.4	0.7	0.3	0.3	0.3	0.3	0.6	1.0	0.8	1.5	1.1	2.3	4.2	4.3	0.8	1	250	196
197	0.4	0.2	0.5	0.6	1.0	0.7	1.4	1.2	1.2	1.5	1.7	2.1	3.4	3.4	3.9	5.3	6.1	4.3	1.7	2	540	197
200	0.3	0.2	0.3	0.8	0.6	0.7	0.8	1.3	1.4	2.0	2.8	4.5	6.2	6.8	10.1	10.7	9.0	4.7	2.7	0	852	200
201	0.0	0.3	0.5	1.5	2.7	2.2	2.1	1.6	1.1	1.2	1.5	1.5	2.6	2.9	3.9	2.9	2.2	3.3	1.6	1	528	201
203	0.0	0.0	0.0	0.0	0.0	0.1	0.1	0.2	0.7	1.3	2.6	3.8	5.2	4.9	6.0	6.6	5.2	2.1	1.7	0	533	203
204	3.8	2.4	2.0	1.5	1.6	1.5	2.4	2.1	3.2	3.5	6.3	7.7	10.8	10.9	18.1	18.7	17.6	17.7	5.5	1	1775	204
202,205	0.1	0.1	0.1	0.2	0.2	0.1	0.5	1.0	0.6	0.7	0.8	1.6	1.6	1.8	2.2	2.4	3.8	2.7	0.8	0	260	202,205
OTHER	0.3	0.1	0.5	0.1	0.2	0.3	1.0	2.0	3.0	5.0	7.8	11.6	14.7	19.9	28.1	32.5	35.1	37.7	7.2	2	2216	OTHER
140-205	12.2	7.4	8.4	11.5	16.9	29.5	64.2	123.2	205.8	304.9	384.4	484.6	612.8	738.9	890.3	1057.5	1214.6	1327.4	287.9	192	91967	140-205
RATE PER CASE IN PERIOD	0.05	0.05	0.05	0.05	0.06	0.06	0.06	0.05	0.05	0.05	0.05	0.05	0.06	0.07	0.08	0.11	0.19	0.33	0.03	–	–	RATE PER CASE IN PERIOD

ENGLAND AND WALES, BIRMINGHAM REGION

Cancer registration in the Birmingham Region dates back to 1936, since when records have been maintained continuously without a break. Based originally on a single hospital, its scope was rapidly extended until in 1957 it included the whole of the area of the Region which has a population of nearly five million people. Though its data originate with medical personnel, in case notes, doctors' letters, pathology reports, etc., they are collected and abstracted mainly by clerical staff, often ex-nurses. A comprehensive record is made of each case, which includes, in addition to identifying particulars such as name, age, sex, residence, hospital attended, names of consultants, etc., full details of history, examination, treatment and subsequent progress. The data are transferred to punch cards, and updated annually until death.

A variety of systems of cross-checking helps to ensure the high degree of registration efficiency now achieved, and the available evidence (to be published shortly suggests that fewer than 2% escape the record. A close association is maintained with the Regional Histological Collection, a library which receives duplicate sections of malignant tumours and copies of the pathology reports, from pathological laboratories throughout the Region. The library can thus furnish material for studies in which tumours of a particular site are reclassified, in ignorance of the original histological report, and related to their subsequent course by means of the records of the Registry.

The chief value of the Registry and its records lies in the field of research, and in studies of incidence and therapeutic efficacy. Because of the efficiency of its follow-up section it has always been much in demand to provide results for a review of an individual's series of cases, and it is still widely used for this purpose. But it is for studies of the natural history of the disease that it can now make its most useful contribution, and this is in fact the direction of much of its research today.

J. A. H. Waterhouse

Registry Title and Address : Birmingham Regional Cancer Registry, Queen Elizabeth Hospital, Birmingham 15, England. Originally commenced in 1936, reconstituted in 1957. Supported financially by the United Birmingham Hospitals, the Regional Hospital Board and the University of Birmingham.

Registration. Cases are registered, mainly by clerical staff, from hospital in-patients and out-patients, and from radiotherapy and pathology departments. Registrations are also obtained from doctors who attend cases at home and from coroners. Information received from death certificates leads to registration only if it is possible to obtain further information by enquiry to hospitals or general practitioners. There is a pathological library of malignant sections which is run in close association with the Registry.

Follow-up. Except for rodent ulcers all cases are followed up until death.

Physical Description. The Registry covers the five West Midland counties - Worcestershire, Warwickshire, Staffordshire, Shropshire and Herefordshire - in the central part of England. It includes not only some of the most highly industrialized sections of the country, but also large areas of farmland. It lies between latitudes 52°08' and 53° North and longitudes 1°10' and 3°3' West. The total registration area is 13,014 square kilometres.

Demographic Description. Total population of area under survey 4,757,360. The main occupational groups of the total employed population are : industry 63.0%, commerce 28.8%, agriculture 1.5%, personal service 6.7%. 41.7% of the population live in conurbations of more than 100,000.

Medical Services. Total number of hospital beds of all kinds 43,543. Total number of doctors in practice in registration area 3,765. Cancer causes approximately 19. 9. % of all deaths.

Publications. Annual reports.

References to scientific reports based on the Registry's data are available on request.

TABLE 22 A
ENGLAND and WALES, BIRMINGHAM REGION :
POPULATION (100, 000s), CENSUS 1961

AGE (in years)	MALES No.	MALES Per Cent	FEMALES No.	FEMALES Per Cent
0-	1.9750	8.40	1.8612	7.73
5-	1.7897	7.61	1.6960	7.05
10-	2.0228	8.60	1.9248	8.00
15-	1.8453	7.85	1.7474	7.26
20-	1.5643	6.65	1.5302	6.36
25-	1.5746	6.70	1.4800	6.15
30-	1.6844	7.16	1.5798	6.57
35-	1.7793	7.57	1.7273	7.18
40-	1.6504	7.02	1.6324	6.78
45-	1.7027	7.24	1.6553	6.88
50-	1.6070	6.84	1.5929	6.62
55-	1.4023	5.96	1.4423	5.99
60-	1.0561	4.49	1.2644	5.25
65-	0.7442	3.17	1.0355	4.30
70-	0.5272	2.24	0.8095	3.36
75-	0.3331	1.42	0.5785	2.40
80-	0.1780	0.76	0.3357	1.40
85- and over	0.0746	0.32	0.1694	0.70
TOTAL	23.5110	100.00	24.0626	100.00

NOTES

TO TABLES 22 A, B and C

(I)   I.L. number 193 includes benign and unspecified tu-
      mours of the central nervous system.

(II) Carcinoma in situ excluded.

TABLE 22 B
ENGLAND and WALES, BIRMINGHAM REGION :
MALE INCIDENCE RATES, 1960 - 62.

AVERAGE ANNUAL INCIDENCE PER 100,000 — AGE IN YEARS

INTER-NATIONAL LIST No.	0-	5-	10-	15-	20-	25-	30-	35-	40-	45-	50-	55-	60-	65-	70-	75-	80-	85- AND OVER	ALL AGES	AGE UNKNOWN	ALL AGES (cases)	INTER-NATIONAL LIST No.
140	0.0	0.0	0.0	0.0	0.0	0.0	0.4	0.9	1.2	2.5	2.7	5.0	3.8	6.7	17.1	20.0	28.1	17.9	2.2	0	153	140
141	0.2	0.0	0.0	0.0	0.2	0.0	0.0	1.1	1.2	1.6	1.5	3.1	5.4	10.7	12.0	17.0	33.7	58.1	2.1	1	151	141
142	0.0	0.0	0.2	0.7	0.2	0.8	1.8	2.1	1.6	1.2	1.9	3.3	2.8	4.5	4.4	6.0	5.6	0.0	1.4	0	102	142
143-4	0.0	0.2	0.0	0.0	0.0	0.0	0.0	0.2	0.8	1.6	1.7	3.8	7.9	9.0	12.6	15.0	15.0	40.2	1.9	0	135	143-4
146	0.3	0.0	0.0	0.4	0.0	0.0	0.2	0.0	0.4	0.4	1.9	1.7	2.2	1.8	3.2	4.0	0.0	0.0	0.6	0	45	146
145,147-8	0.0	0.0	0.0	0.0	0.0	0.0	0.2	0.0	0.4	1.2	2.7	4.0	9.8	12.1	17.1	30.0	26.2	40.2	2.5	0	177	145,147-8
150	0.0	0.0	0.0	0.0	0.2	0.2	0.0	0.2	1.6	2.3	5.4	7.8	16.7	30.5	44.9	50.0	61.8	89.4	5.3	0	377	150
151	0.0	0.0	0.0	0.0	1.1	0.8	4.6	5.4	18.6	21.7	61.6	78.7	128.1	163.9	175.8	262.2	204.1	281.5	33.7	3	2379	151
152	0.0	0.0	0.0	0.0	0.0	0.0	0.0	0.0	0.6	0.6	0.8	1.4	3.8	2.7	5.1	4.0	5.6	0.0	0.7	0	52	152
153	0.0	0.0	0.3	0.5	0.9	0.8	2.2	4.7	5.5	12.5	16.2	31.1	49.6	84.2	122.0	185.1	230.3	232.4	17.7	1	1248	153
154	0.0	0.0	0.2	0.0	0.2	0.0	0.8	2.1	5.5	11.9	18.5	42.8	65.3	98.1	128.4	171.1	181.6	174.3	18.6	2	1312	154
155.0	0.3	0.0	0.0	0.0	0.0	0.0	0.4	0.0	0.6	0.8	1.5	1.9	3.5	4.0	4.4	8.0	1.9	13.4	0.9	0	65	155.0
155.1	0.0	0.0	0.2	0.2	0.0	0.2	0.4	0.7	0.2	0.6	1.7	5.0	7.3	9.9	9.5	19.0	16.9	4.5	1.8	0	129	155.1
156	0.0	0.0	0.0	0.0	0.2	0.0	0.0	0.6	0.4	0.8	1.9	4.0	7.3	11.6	15.2	25.0	30.0	13.4	2.2	0	153	156
157	0.0	0.0	0.2	0.0	0.2	0.0	1.0	0.7	3.0	6.9	9.3	18.8	23.4	42.6	60.7	55.0	76.8	80.4	8.0	0	563	157
160	0.0	0.0	0.0	0.0	0.0	0.0	0.0	0.6	0.2	0.8	1.0	1.7	4.4	4.0	7.0	8.0	7.5	8.9	1.0	0	68	160
161	0.2	0.0	0.0	0.2	0.2	0.2	0.2	0.7	1.6	1.8	9.3	12.4	14.8	22.8	27.2	23.0	24.3	22.3	4.3	0	302	161
162-3	0.0	0.0	0.0	0.0	0.4	1.1	4.6	12.6	29.3	67.5	157.2	281.2	430.2	448.8	445.8	389.3	207.9	169.8	87.1	7	6143	162-3
170	0.0	0.0	0.0	0.0	0.6	0.0	0.0	0.0	0.4	0.2	0.4	2.6	2.2	0.9	2.5	4.0	9.4	4.5	0.6	0	39	170
177	0.0	0.0	0.0	0.0	0.0	0.0	0.0	4.5	4.6	1.8	5.4	19.5	48.0	94.1	184.0	296.2	464.4	478.1	20.2	3	1425	177
178	0.3	0.0	0.2	0.2	3.0	5.9	3.2	0.6	1.0	2.7	1.2	1.2	1.6	0.4	0.0	1.0	3.7	0.0	2.2	1	152	178
179.0	0.0	0.0	0.0	1.3	0.0	0.0	0.2	0.6	1.0	1.0	1.2	1.9	2.5	5.8	5.1	12.0	5.6	22.3	1.1	0	77	179.0
180	1.0	0.4	0.6	0.0	0.6	0.2	0.0	0.6	2.0	4.9	8.7	11.4	16.7	18.4	15.8	21.0	16.9	8.9	4.1	0	291	180
181.0	0.0	0.0	0.2	0.2	0.0	0.4	1.8	2.1	1.6	9.4	13.9	24.2	44.5	60.5	94.8	116.1	108.6	102.8	12.2	1	863	181.0
190	0.2	0.2	0.0	0.2	1.5	1.3	3.2	1.1	1.2	1.0	1.5	2.9	1.9	1.3	3.8	3.0	8.9	8.9	1.1	0	75	190
191	0.0	0.0	0.0	0.0	0.2	0.8	0.0	9.0	17.2	28.2	43.4	54.4	89.6	97.6	136.6	209.1	292.1	348.5	27.3	22	1926	191
192	0.3	0.2	0.0	0.0	0.2	0.0	0.0	0.2	0.4	1.2	0.0	1.9	1.9	0.9	1.3	1.0	5.6	0.0	0.6	1	39	192
193	4.7	2.0	2.1	2.2	2.1	3.8	4.6	5.6	7.3	9.8	14.9	13.1	16.4	13.4	5.7	3.0	1.9	0.0	6.4	1	454	193
194	0.0	0.0	0.2	0.0	0.6	0.2	0.6	0.4	0.2	1.0	1.0	1.2	2.2	1.3	3.8	6.0	1.9	0.0	0.6	0	44	194
195	0.0	0.0	0.2	0.2	0.6	0.2	0.4	0.7	0.6	0.8	1.2	1.4	2.5	2.2	2.5	2.0	0.0	8.9	0.7	0	50	195
196	0.3	0.0	1.0	1.3	0.0	1.1	1.0	0.4	2.6	1.8	0.6	1.0	0.9	3.6	3.8	4.0	0.0	8.9	0.9	0	62	196
197	0.3	0.2	0.5	1.1	1.1	0.2	1.0	3.0	2.6	2.3	4.4	2.1	3.2	4.5	5.1	7.0	11.2	13.4	1.7	0	118	197
200	0.5	0.6	0.8	1.1	1.1	1.9	1.4	1.9	4.0	3.5	2.7	8.1	10.4	12.1	8.9	15.0	15.0	4.5	3.2	0	224	200
201	0.0	0.2	0.8	2.3	3.8	4.7	2.4	2.4	0.8	1.2	2.3	5.5	3.2	7.6	3.2	5.0	1.9	0.0	2.8	0	198	201
203	0.0	0.0	0.0	0.0	0.0	0.2	0.2	0.2	0.8	1.2	2.3	3.1	7.9	4.0	5.1	9.0	0.0	0.0	1.2	0	88	203
204	4.4	3.2	1.6	2.7	2.3	1.7	2.0	4.5	3.6	6.1	5.6	7.8	12.0	9.9	25.3	30.0	33.7	40.2	5.5	1	388	204
202,205	0.3	0.0	0.5	0.7	0.6	0.2	1.6	0.7	1.6	2.0	1.0	1.7	1.6	1.3	3.8	4.0	1.9	8.9	1.1	0	76	202,205
OTHER	0.0	0.0	0.3	0.5	0.2	0.8	1.0	1.7	3.8	5.1	9.3	15.7	26.5	28.7	44.9	50.0	41.2	49.2	6.8	0	482	OTHER
140-205	13.2	6.9	9.1	15.2	21.1	27.7	41.0	72.7	128.7	221.4	417.8	688.4	1082.0	1336.6	1667.9	2090.5	2172.3	2345.8	292.4	44	20625	140-205
RATE PER CASE IN PERIOD	0.17	0.19	0.16	0.18	0.21	0.21	0.20	0.19	0.20	0.20	0.21	0.24	0.32	0.45	0.63	1.00	1.87	4.47	0.01	-	-	RATE PER CASE IN PERIOD

TABLE 22 C

ENGLAND and WALES, BIRMINGHAM REGION :

FEMALE INCIDENCE RATES, 1960 - 62.

INTER-NATIONAL LIST No.	0-	5-	10-	15-	20-	25-	30-	35-	40-	45-	50-	55-	60-	65-	70-	75-	80-	85- AND OVER	ALL AGES	AGE UNKNOWN	ALL AGES (cases)	INTER-NATIONAL LIST No.
									AVERAGE ANNUAL INCIDENCE PER 100,000 — AGE IN YEARS											No. OF CASES IN WHOLE PERIOD		
140	0.0	0.0	0.0	0.0	0.0	0.2	0.2	0.2	0.4	0.0	0.8	1.4	1.3	1.6	1.6	4.6	5.0	3.9	0.6	2	46	140
141	0.0	0.0	0.0	0.0	0.0	0.0	0.2	0.0	0.6	0.4	1.0	0.9	1.6	1.9	5.8	3.5	6.0	3.9	0.8	0	55	141
142	0.0	0.0	0.2	0.8	0.9	1.6	1.3	2.5	1.8	1.8	3.3	4.6	2.9	1.9	4.5	1.7	3.0	5.9	1.7	0	126	142
143-4	0.0	0.0	0.0	0.2	0.0	0.0	0.2	0.0	0.4	0.6	0.8	0.7	1.3	2.6	4.5	6.9	5.0	3.9	0.8	1	58	143-4
146	0.0	0.0	0.0	0.6	0.0	0.0	0.0	0.2	0.2	0.4	0.6	0.0	0.5	1.3	0.0	0.6	1.0	2.0	0.3	0	19	146
145,147-8	0.0	0.0	0.0	0.0	0.0	0.0	0.2	0.6	1.0	1.2	2.9	3.5	4.5	7.4	5.4	4.6	5.0	2.0	1.5	0	111	145,147-8
150	0.0	0.0	0.0	0.2	0.2	0.9	0.4	0.4	1.6	3.2	4.0	3.7	10.0	11.6	16.9	24.8	32.8	33.5	3.8	0	271	150
151	0.0	0.0	0.0	0.0	0.0	0.0	1.7	2.5	5.9	10.5	19.5	30.7	47.7	90.8	126.8	160.2	213.5	179.1	23.6	18	1707	151
152	0.0	0.0	0.0	0.0	0.0	0.0	0.0	0.4	0.6	0.2	1.0	0.9	1.8	1.3	4.5	2.9	5.0	2.0	0.7	0	48	152
153	0.2	0.0	0.2	1.0	1.1	0.9	2.7	3.9	7.1	16.3	25.3	38.8	50.4	75.6	107.9	152.1	208.5	238.1	24.1	2	1739	153
154	0.0	0.0	0.2	0.0	0.0	0.2	1.7	3.9	4.5	10.1	16.1	20.6	31.6	43.5	60.9	83.0	102.3	137.7	13.7	1	989	154
155.0	0.2	0.0	0.0	0.0	0.0	0.0	0.0	0.0	0.6	0.0	0.2	0.2	0.5	2.9	1.6	2.3	4.0	2.0	0.4	0	30	155.0
155.1	0.0	0.2	0.0	0.0	0.0	0.0	0.2	0.4	0.4	1.2	1.5	5.5	5.0	12.6	22.6	26.5	24.8	25.6	3.3	1	239	155.1
156	0.0	0.0	0.0	0.0	0.0	0.0	0.4	0.4	0.6	1.0	2.1	4.4	5.5	6.1	11.9	11.5	25.8	13.8	2.3	1	165	156
157	0.0	0.0	0.0	0.0	0.2	0.0	0.4	0.0	1.6	3.2	4.4	9.2	17.7	24.1	37.1	40.9	52.6	76.7	6.7	0	482	157
160	0.0	0.0	0.0	0.0	0.2	0.0	0.6	0.0	0.8	0.4	0.4	0.5	1.3	2.9	2.1	5.8	5.0	5.9	0.7	0	53	160
161	0.0	0.0	0.0	0.0	0.0	0.0	0.6	0.2	0.0	0.4	1.7	0.7	0.3	0.6	2.1	2.9	3.0	2.0	0.5	0	34	161
162-3	0.0	0.0	0.2	0.2	2.0	0.5	1.7	4.1	7.4	12.3	14.9	22.6	29.5	48.0	39.5	46.7	36.7	31.5	10.9	1	790	162-3
170	0.0	0.0	0.0	0.2	2.0	4.5	19.0	42.3	83.1	113.6	123.5	135.9	142.6	164.8	181.6	212.0	259.2	279.4	65.9	3	4756	170
171	0.0	0.0	0.0	0.0	0.0	1.6	8.4	22.6	31.4	30.2	28.5	34.2	34.3	34.1	41.6	37.5	36.7	41.3	16.8	2	1214	171
172	0.0	0.0	0.0	0.2	0.0	0.2	0.0	3.1	7.6	12.3	24.9	38.1	39.8	39.0	26.8	24.8	29.8	23.6	11.4	2	823	172
173	0.0	0.0	0.0	0.0	0.9	0.5	0.2	0.8	0.2	2.4	2.5	1.6	1.3	4.5	3.7	1.7	1.0	3.9	0.9	1	67	173
174	0.0	0.0	0.0	0.0	1.5	2.7	3.8	0.0	0.2	1.0	1.0	1.6	0.8	1.9	3.7	5.2	5.0	9.8	0.9	1	62	174
175	0.0	0.0	0.0	0.2	0.2	0.5	0.8	7.9	13.3	23.2	31.0	31.2	39.5	38.3	34.6	36.9	30.8	19.7	13.9	1	1001	175
176	0.0	0.0	0.0	0.0	0.0	0.7	0.8	0.6	1.2	2.8	3.3	5.5	10.3	12.9	15.2	16.7	28.8	37.4	3.6	0	263	176
180	1.6	0.6	0.0	0.2	0.0	0.0	0.0	0.4	1.2	2.6	2.3	4.9	7.4	6.4	9.5	12.7	10.9	15.7	2.5	0	182	180
181.0	0.0	0.0	0.0	0.2	0.0	0.0	0.2	0.0	0.2	2.6	4.0	5.8	7.1	12.6	21.8	25.9	41.7	27.5	3.9	0	280	181.0
190	0.2	0.0	0.2	0.6	1.5	1.6	1.1	3.9	3.3	3.6	1.7	2.5	2.9	1.6	3.7	5.2	5.0	9.8	1.9	0	139	190
191	0.0	0.2	0.3	0.6	1.3	2.5	4.0	8.3	13.5	20.7	28.9	25.1	45.1	70.8	91.0	129.6	150.9	210.5	22.9	17	1656	191
192	0.7	0.2	0.0	0.0	0.0	0.5	0.4	0.4	0.8	1.0	0.6	0.9	1.1	1.6	1.6	2.3	0.0	0.0	0.6	1	45	192
193	4.7	2.4	1.6	1.9	1.7	1.8	4.4	3.3	4.5	7.7	8.6	13.4	7.1	9.7	4.5	2.9	4.0	3.9	4.8	1	349	193
194	0.0	0.0	0.0	0.0	0.0	1.1	1.1	1.5	2.2	1.4	2.1	2.1	4.5	3.9	5.4	8.6	9.9	9.8	1.8	0	127	194
195	0.0	0.0	0.7	0.8	0.2	0.5	0.4	1.0	0.8	0.6	1.0	1.2	0.8	1.0	1.0	0.6	1.0	0.0	0.5	0	39	195
196	0.0	0.2	0.5	0.4	0.7	1.1	0.2	0.0	0.2	0.6	0.6	0.9	0.5	2.3	0.8	3.5	3.0	9.8	0.7	0	54	196
197	0.2	0.4	0.2	0.8	1.3	0.5	1.3	1.4	0.8	1.2	1.9	2.3	4.0	4.2	3.3	6.9	3.0	2.0	1.5	0	109	197
200	0.4	0.4	0.5	1.9	0.4	0.9	1.1	1.5	2.0	3.2	2.3	6.2	5.5	5.8	11.9	12.1	7.9	13.8	2.7	1	197	200
201	0.0	0.4	0.0	1.1	3.5	1.4	2.1	1.0	0.4	0.8	1.0	1.2	2.6	3.5	3.7	3.5	3.0	5.9	1.5	0	110	201
203	0.0	0.0	0.0	0.4	0.0	0.0	2.1	0.4	0.4	1.8	2.1	3.2	5.3	3.2	4.1	3.5	2.0	3.9	1.2	0	88	203
204	3.4	2.8	1.7	0.4	0.9	1.8	2.7	2.5	2.7	3.8	6.5	6.9	11.3	8.7	18.9	15.6	16.9	17.7	4.8	1	350	204
202,205	0.2	0.2	0.2	0.4	0.4	0.0	0.4	1.5	0.6	0.4	0.6	1.6	1.8	1.3	1.2	2.3	7.0	0.0	0.8	1	57	202,205
OTHER	0.5	0.2	0.2	0.2	0.4	0.0	0.6	2.1	2.7	6.2	10.3	11.1	16.9	23.2	32.1	35.7	43.7	61.0	7.1	0	514	OTHER
140-205	12.2	7.7	6.6	11.6	19.4	28.6	65.4	126.2	209.1	307.5	389.9	496.7	606.1	791.9	975.9	1187.0	1439.8	1576.2	269.4	55	19444	140-205
RATE PER CASE IN PERIOD	0.18	0.20	0.17	0.19	0.22	0.23	0.21	0.19	0.20	0.20	0.21	0.23	0.26	0.32	0.41	0.58	0.99	1.97	0.01	-	-	RATE PER CASE IN PERIOD

ENGLAND AND WALES, LIVERPOOL REGION

In 1946, the Liverpool Clinical Registry was formed with the primary object of registering all cases of malignancy occurring in the areas served by the Liverpool Radium Institute, these being roughly South and South West Lancashire, South Cheshire, North Wales and the Isle of Man.

In 1948, at the inception of the National Health Service, the areas served became more defined and since that time the Registry has been responsible for the registration of malignant cases in the area controlled by the Liverpool Regional Hospital Board, in the counties of Merionethshire, Caernarvonshire, Denbighshire and Flintshire in North Wales and in the Isle of Man. All hospitals in these areas co-operate by sending details to the Registry of malignant cases recorded by them and cases not seen in hospitals are reported by the general practitioners concerned. There is, therefore, virtually 100 % registration of cancer in this region. The Registry also receives from the Registrar General copies of death certificates of all patients in these areas certified as dying from cancer and this acts as a check on the completeness of registration.

Besides the initial registration of cases, the Registry also records treatment details and the subsequent progress of every patient, whether treated or not, by means of annual reports. From this information the Registrar General's abstract cards are completed and returned to Somerset House.

The Registry also co-operates with research and other medical workers in making available statistical and clinical information regarding cancer. In addition, a Pathological Registry is maintained under the direction of a Consultant Pathologist to whom are submitted histological slides of malignant conditions.

The full time staff consisting of 14 - of whom twelve are clerical workers and two are punch card operators - are for administrative purposes, under the control of the Senior Consultant in Administrative Charge of the Regional Radiotherapy Service. In general, hospitals forward case histories of malignant cases to the Registry where the relevant administrative and clinical information is extracted and punched on to Powers Samas cards; but a few large hospitals, where the number of cases is large, are visited regularly by a member of the Registry staff to do this work.

The Powers Samas system has been satisfactory in the past, but with the large numbers of cards now available, mechanical sorting has become too time consuming and the question of using a computer for this work is now under consideration.

M. A. Stewart

Registry Title and Address : The Liverpool Clinical and Pathological Registry, 36 Rodney Street, Liverpool 1, England. Commenced 1946. Supported financially by the Liverpool Regional Hospital Board.

Registration. Cases are registered from hospital in-patients and out-patients, and radiotherapy departments by clerical staff, from the Pathology Registry to which all hospital are requested to submit histological slides of malignant conditions, from death certificates from the Registrar General, by doctors attending cases at home, from private nursing homes by consultants, and from Coroners.

Follow-up. All cases are followed up annually for up to 15 years.

Physical Description. The Registry covers the area of the Liverpool Regional Hospital Board, including south and south west Lancashire, south Cheshire, the Isle of Man. and North Wales comprising the counties of Anglesey, Flint-

144

shire, Denbighshire, Caernarvonshire and Merionethshire. It is mainly coastal plain and hill country in North Wales and the Isle of Man, and has a cold humid climate. It lies between latitudes 52°33' and 53°43' North, and longitudes 3°35' and 4°47' West. The Isle of Man lies between latitudes 54°02' and 54°24' North and longitudes 4°18' and 4°45' West. The total registration area is 8,400 square kilometres.

Demographic Description. Total population of area under survey 2,752,080. The main occupational groups of the total employed population are : industry 54.8 %, commerce 36.6 %, agriculture 0.7 %, personal service 7.9 %. Of the total population 42 % live in conurbations of more than 100,000.

Medical Services. Total number of hospital beds of all kinds 34,935. Total number of doctors in practice in registration area 3,014. Cancer causes approximately 21 % of all deaths.

Publications. Annual reports.
Five-year results of malignant cases, registered 1944-56.

TABLE 23 A
ENGLAND and WALES, LIVERPOOL REGION,
(including N. WALES and ISLE OF MAN) :
POPULATION (100, 000s), CENSUS 1961

AGE (in years)	MALES No.	MALES Per Cent	FEMALES No.	FEMALES Per Cent
0-	1.1272	8.60	1.1569	8.03
5-	1.0977	8.37	1.0478	7.27
10-	1.2158	9.28	1.1573	8.03
15-	0.9771	7.45	0.9767	6.78
20-	0.8416	6.42	0.8865	6.15
25-	0.8549	6.52	0.8352	5.79
30-	0.8811	6.72	0.8820	6.12
35-	0.9072	6.92	0.9420	6.54
40-	0.8404	6.41	0.9032	6.27
45-	0.8963	6.84	0.9677	6.71
50-	0.8547	6.52	0.9664	6.70
55-	0.8014	6.11	0.8955	6.21
60-	0.6291	4.80	0.8113	5.63
65-	0.4748	3.62	0.6917	4.80
70-	0.3397	2.59	0.5543	3.85
75-	0.2133	1.63	0.3951	2.74
80-	0.1087	0.83	0.2316	1.61
85- and over	0.0461	0.35	0.1125	0.78
TOTAL	13.1071	100.00	14.4137	100.00

NOTES

TO TABLES 23 A, B and C

(I) I. L. number 193 includes benign and unspecified tumours of the central nervous system.

(II) Carcinoma in situ excluded.

TABLE 23 B

ENGLAND and WALES, LIVERPOOL REGION :
(including N. Wales and Isle of Man)
FEMALE INCIDENCE RATES, 1959 - 63.

AVERAGE ANNUAL INCIDENCE PER 100,000 — AGE IN YEARS

INTER-NATIONAL LIST No.	No. OF CASES IN WHOLE PERIOD: ALL AGES	AGE UN-KNOWN	ALL AGES (rate)	0-	5-	10-	15-	20-	25-	30-	35-	40-	45-	50-	55-	60-	65-	70-	75-	80-	85- AND OVER
140	228	0	3.5	0.0	0.0	0.0	0.0	0.2	0.2	0.5	0.2	1.7	2.0	4.2	8.0	10.2	14.3	22.4	28.1	20.2	52.1
141	122	0	1.9	0.0	0.0	0.0	0.0	0.2	0.0	0.2	0.2	0.2	0.7	1.6	2.7	3.8	8.0	8.8	17.8	31.3	65.1
142	80	0	1.2	0.0	0.0	0.3	0.2	0.5	0.9	1.6	0.7	0.7	0.7	1.4	2.7	3.8	3.8	4.7	2.8	7.4	8.7
143-4	170	0	2.6	0.0	0.2	0.2	0.0	0.2	0.2	0.9	0.2	0.7	0.7	2.8	4.7	7.9	11.4	18.8	15.9	31.3	30.4
146	32	0	0.5	0.0	0.2	0.2	0.2	0.0	0.0	0.2	0.2	1.0	0.7	0.2	1.0	0.3	3.8	1.2	2.8	0.0	4.3
145,147-8	191	0	2.9	0.0	0.0	0.0	0.2	0.2	0.2	0.2	0.0	0.7	1.1	2.8	5.7	7.6	13.5	19.4	25.3	38.6	39.0
150	421	0	6.4	0.0	0.0	0.2	0.2	0.2	1.9	0.2	0.2	1.0	3.1	4.9	8.7	14.6	29.5	47.7	63.8	97.5	112.8
151	2914	0	44.5	0.0	0.0	0.2	0.2	0.2	1.9	3.4	4.4	11.2	28.8	58.5	87.1	144.0	205.1	278.5	344.1	386.4	446.9
152	39	0	0.6	0.0	0.2	0.2	0.0	0.2	0.0	0.2	0.4	0.5	0.4	1.4	2.0	2.0	1.3	4.1	4.1	0.0	0.0
153	1575	0	24.0	0.0	0.2	0.2	0.4	1.0	0.5	2.5	6.6	8.1	16.5	24.1	36.7	73.4	103.6	155.4	206.3	263.1	269.0
154	986	0	15.0	0.0	0.0	0.0	0.5	0.2	1.2	2.0	2.0	5.2	9.8	15.9	27.0	46.7	68.2	84.8	128.5	171.1	160.5
155.0	129	0	2.0	0.2	0.0	0.0	0.0	0.0	0.0	0.2	0.4	1.2	0.9	2.1	6.2	7.9	10.5	11.2	9.4	5.5	0.0
155.1	130	0	2.0	0.0	0.0	0.2	0.2	0.0	0.0	0.0	0.0	1.2	2.0	0.9	3.5	7.6	8.8	13.5	15.9	12.9	26.0
156	97	0	1.5	0.0	0.0	0.0	0.0	0.0	0.0	0.0	0.0	0.7	0.9	0.9	2.2	6.4	6.7	11.8	9.4	16.6	8.7
157	625	0	9.5	0.0	0.0	0.0	0.0	0.2	0.0	0.2	0.9	1.7	4.5	11.5	20.0	35.3	42.5	64.8	70.3	81.0	99.8
160	75	0	1.1	0.0	0.0	0.0	0.0	0.2	0.2	0.2	1.1	0.7	1.1	1.4	3.5	3.2	5.1	4.1	4.7	7.4	8.7
161	320	0	4.9	0.0	0.0	0.0	0.4	0.2	0.0	0.5	0.7	1.0	3.3	7.3	13.7	19.1	24.4	27.1	16.9	38.6	30.4
162-3	6558	0	100.1	0.0	0.0	0.0	0.4	0.7	2.6	5.9	11.2	35.2	73.4	156.5	285.5	427.6	529.1	504.0	466.9	296.2	256.0
170	41	0	0.6	0.2	0.0	0.0	0.0	0.0	0.0	0.2	0.0	0.0	0.7	0.9	1.2	1.6	2.1	5.3	4.7	3.7	8.7
177	1459	0	22.3	0.2	0.2	0.0	0.0	0.2	0.0	0.0	0.2	1.0	1.6	5.4	14.2	32.4	82.6	168.4	309.4	625.6	481.6
178	146	0	2.2	0.2	0.0	0.0	0.4	3.3	3.7	6.4	4.9	4.0	2.0	2.6	3.5	2.2	0.8	1.8	0.0	0.0	0.0
179.0	77	0	1.2	1.1	0.2	0.0	0.0	0.0	0.5	0.5	0.4	1.2	1.1	1.4	2.5	3.2	5.1	6.5	6.6	5.5	17.4
180	281	0	4.3	0.0	0.2	0.0	0.0	0.2	0.7	0.9	1.1	3.6	4.2	8.7	10.0	14.3	12.2	20.0	22.5	18.4	39.0
181.0	967	0	14.8	0.2	0.0	0.0	0.2	0.5	1.2	0.5	1.1	2.4	7.8	14.5	26.5	47.1	73.7	97.1	118.1	169.3	164.9
190	53	0	0.8	0.2	0.0	0.0	0.2	0.5	0.7	0.5	0.7	0.5	0.9	0.7	2.2	1.0	2.1	2.9	1.9	3.7	8.7
191	2354	0	35.9	0.0	0.0	0.0	0.0	0.5	1.4	3.4	8.2	21.7	33.5	51.2	76.6	96.3	128.5	185.5	279.4	364.3	468.5
192	28	0	0.4	0.4	0.2	0.0	0.0	0.0	0.0	0.0	0.7	0.2	0.7	0.7	0.5	1.6	0.4	2.9	1.9	3.7	6.0
193	447	0	6.8	3.0	3.1	1.3	2.3	2.6	4.0	5.0	6.4	7.4	8.7	13.6	17.2	15.6	12.6	15.9	6.6	5.5	8.7
194	50	0	0.8	0.0	0.0	0.3	0.0	0.0	0.2	0.2	0.2	0.0	1.1	0.9	1.0	1.6	5.5	4.1	2.8	5.5	13.0
195	33	0	0.5	0.7	0.4	0.3	0.2	0.0	0.5	0.5	0.9	0.2	0.4	1.4	1.0	1.0	0.4	0.6	0.9	7.4	0.0
196	86	0	1.3	0.2	0.2	0.5	2.5	1.4	1.2	1.1	0.4	0.5	2.5	1.9	4.2	3.5	3.8	3.5	6.6	7.4	21.7
197	130	0	2.0	1.2	0.2	0.3	0.8	0.7	0.7	1.1	2.0	1.2	2.2	5.9	6.2	5.1	5.9	4.7	3.8	7.4	17.4
200	183	0	2.8	0.5	1.3	1.2	1.2	3.3	2.8	0.9	1.1	1.4	2.2	5.9	6.2	6.7	11.0	13.0	9.4	9.2	0.0
201	192	0	2.9	0.0	0.7	0.0	0.0	0.0	0.0	3.6	3.3	4.0	3.6	4.2	3.7	3.5	8.4	4.7	4.7	1.8	4.3
203	74	0	1.1	0.0	0.0	0.0	0.0	0.0	0.0	0.0	0.2	0.5	0.4	3.0	2.0	5.4	3.8	8.8	1.9	7.4	4.3
204	462	0	7.0	4.8	4.2	2.0	2.5	2.4	1.2	2.5	2.9	4.8	4.7	6.6	9.7	14.9	26.5	35.3	31.9	42.3	60.7
202,205	48	0	0.7	0.4	0.0	0.2	0.6	0.5	0.5	0.5	0.7	0.5	0.7	1.2	1.7	1.7	2.1	3.5	0.9	3.7	0.0
OTHER	365	0	5.6	0.5	0.0	0.0	0.0	1.0	0.2	0.9	1.8	3.1	5.1	7.5	12.0	18.1	23.2	21.2	43.1	42.3	52.1
140-205	22168	0	338.3	13.5	10.9	7.1	14.5	21.6	26.7	47.2	66.6	130.7	233.2	431.5	718.2	1096.5	1500.4	1888.1	2289.7	2829.8	2989.2
RATE PER CASE IN PERIOD	-	-	0.02	0.18	0.18	0.16	0.20	0.24	0.23	0.23	0.22	0.24	0.22	0.23	0.25	0.32	0.42	0.59	0.94	1.84	4.34

ENGLAND and WALES, LIVERPOOL REGION : (including N. Wales and Isle of Man)
MALE INCIDENCE RATES, 1959 - 63.

AVERAGE ANNUAL INCIDENCE PER 100,000 — AGE IN YEARS

INTER-NATIONAL LIST No.	0-	5-	10-	15-	20-	25-	30-	35-	40-	45-	50-	55-	60-	65-	70-	75-	80-	85- AND OVER	ALL AGES	AGE UNKNOWN	ALL AGES (cases)	INTER-NATIONAL LIST No.
140	0.0	0.0	0.0	0.2	0.0	0.0	0.0	0.2	0.0	0.2	0.0	0.2	0.5	0.6	1.1	1.5	4.3	1.8	0.3	0	20	140
141	0.0	0.0	0.0	0.0	0.2	0.0	0.0	0.4	0.7	0.2	1.0	0.4	1.2	3.2	2.5	6.1	4.3	5.3	0.8	0	57	141
142	0.0	0.0	0.2	1.0	1.1	1.7	1.6	1.3	0.9	3.3	1.9	3.8	2.2	2.0	3.6	3.5	5.2	1.8	1.6	0	117	142
143-4	0.0	0.0	0.0	0.0	0.5	0.5	0.0	0.0	0.2	0.2	1.4	1.8	3.0	4.0	6.1	6.1	8.6	12.4	1.3	0	93	143-4
146	0.2	0.0	0.2	0.0	0.0	0.2	0.7	0.0	0.7	0.4	1.0	0.4	1.0	0.6	0.7	0.0	1.7	0.0	0.3	0	25	146
145,147-8	0.2	0.0	0.0	0.0	0.0	0.0	0.7	1.1	1.3	4.1	5.0	5.1	7.6	6.7	10.5	11.1	10.4	5.3	2.8	0	202	145,147-8
150	0.0	0.0	0.0	0.0	0.0	0.0	0.0	0.8	1.8	2.9	5.0	6.9	10.6	19.1	21.3	40.0	41.5	40.9	5.5	0	399	150
151	0.0	0.0	0.0	0.0	0.5	1.2	0.5	1.9	4.7	10.5	18.4	38.4	62.1	93.4	140.4	185.5	300.5	341.3	30.8	0	2222	151
152	0.0	0.0	0.0	0.0	0.2	0.2	0.0	0.4	0.2	0.6	0.4	0.4	2.0	3.8	4.0	2.5	1.7	1.8	0.7	0	52	152
153	0.0	0.0	0.2	1.2	1.6	1.0	2.0	4.9	12.4	19.0	31.0	42.7	64.1	83.6	118.3	181.2	213.3	314.7	30.5	0	2198	153
154	0.0	0.0	0.0	0.2	0.0	0.0	0.2	2.8	3.3	7.6	13.0	20.1	24.2	32.4	52.0	69.3	82.0	112.0	12.1	0	869	154
155.0	0.0	0.0	0.0	0.0	0.2	0.0	0.0	0.2	0.0	0.2	0.2	0.9	1.2	2.6	1.8	4.0	5.2	1.8	0.6	0	42	155.0
155.1	0.0	0.0	0.0	0.0	0.2	0.0	0.0	0.2	0.0	0.6	0.8	5.6	9.1	11.9	15.9	16.2	16.4	44.4	3.2	0	232	155.1
156	0.0	0.0	0.2	0.0	0.0	0.0	0.2	0.4	0.4	0.4	0.6	0.9	2.5	3.2	9.0	9.6	16.4	19.6	1.5	0	108	156
157	0.0	0.0	0.0	0.0	0.2	0.5	0.2	0.0	1.3	3.7	6.6	9.6	16.3	28.6	31.0	43.0	54.4	106.7	7.8	0	563	157
160	0.0	0.0	0.2	0.0	0.0	0.2	0.0	0.0	0.4	1.7	1.2	1.8	1.5	2.6	2.5	1.5	5.2	3.6	0.8	0	58	160
161	0.2	0.0	0.0	0.0	0.2	0.5	1.4	0.2	0.4	0.8	0.6	1.8	2.7	2.9	5.4	3.5	5.2	1.8	1.0	0	69	161
162-3	0.2	0.0	0.2	0.2	0.2	0.5	1.4	4.0	9.3	15.3	23.8	32.2	42.2	50.3	45.8	58.2	63.0	42.7	15.1	0	1089	162-3
170	0.0	0.0	0.0	0.4	0.7	6.0	16.8	41.8	64.0	96.1	105.1	119.7	129.9	141.4	158.0	177.2	202.1	250.7	59.4	0	4278	170
171	0.0	0.0	0.0	0.0	0.0	1.2	6.8	22.3	36.5	42.6	39.1	40.0	33.5	30.6	34.3	40.0	26.8	26.7	18.6	0	1341	171
172	0.2	0.0	0.0	0.2	0.0	0.2	1.1	4.0	7.1	13.8	28.6	36.2	33.5	38.7	35.4	26.3	42.3	37.3	12.7	0	915	172
173	0.0	0.0	0.0	0.0	0.0	0.0	0.7	0.2	0.9	0.4	1.7	1.1	0.7	1.4	1.1	0.5	0.0	0.0	0.5	0	36	173
174	0.0	0.0	0.0	0.2	0.0	0.0	0.0	0.0	0.0	0.0	0.0	0.0	0.0	0.0	0.0	0.0	0.0	0.0	0.0	0	0	174
175	0.0	0.0	0.5	1.0	0.9	1.7	3.2	5.5	16.4	20.3	24.0	35.3	36.2	38.7	35.7	36.4	30.2	28.4	14.0	0	1008	175
176	0.0	0.0	0.0	0.0	0.0	0.0	0.7	0.6	1.8	2.3	2.3	5.6	6.4	12.1	15.5	21.3	30.2	30.2	3.7	0	266	176
180	1.6	0.6	0.0	0.0	0.0	0.0	0.7	0.2	1.8	3.1	3.3	4.9	7.1	10.7	7.6	13.2	11.2	7.1	2.9	0	208	180
181.0	0.2	0.0	0.0	0.2	0.0	0.0	0.2	0.2	1.1	2.9	5.6	8.0	12.3	15.3	26.3	37.0	42.3	42.7	5.7	0	408	181.0
190	0.0	0.0	0.0	0.4	0.9	1.2	2.3	2.8	2.2	2.7	3.9	2.9	3.2	3.8	2.9	5.1	6.0	7.1	2.0	0	144	190
191	1.2	0.0	0.0	0.6	0.9	1.0	3.9	9.1	10.6	20.9	25.7	41.8	57.2	65.3	103.6	161.0	191.7	279.1	27.3	0	1970	191
192	1.4	0.4	0.0	0.8	0.0	0.0	0.0	0.0	0.0	0.0	0.8	0.4	1.0	1.2	1.8	1.0	1.7	1.8	0.5	0	38	192
193	0.0	0.0	2.2	0.8	1.8	2.2	4.5	3.0	5.8	8.3	7.7	11.6	11.1	8.1	5.8	6.6	13.0	3.6	4.6	0	335	193
194	0.0	0.0	0.0	0.4	0.9	1.2	0.2	0.8	1.3	2.1	2.7	3.4	5.7	4.6	7.6	1.0	0.0	5.3	2.1	0	151	194
195	0.9	0.0	1.0	0.0	0.2	0.2	0.5	0.2	1.6	0.2	1.2	0.2	0.5	0.9	1.1	0.5	0.0	0.0	0.5	0	34	195
196	0.5	0.6	0.5	1.0	1.6	0.5	0.5	0.6	0.0	1.9	0.6	0.7	0.5	0.6	1.8	2.5	3.5	0.0	0.6	0	45	196
197	0.2	0.2	0.2	1.0	1.1	1.0	1.4	0.8	1.6	1.9	1.2	2.9	3.5	5.2	5.1	3.0	5.2	5.3	1.8	0	129	197
200	0.2	0.2	0.7	0.6	1.6	1.0	0.7	1.5	1.6	1.7	2.5	2.9	6.4	8.1	10.5	5.6	13.0	3.6	2.4	0	175	200
201	0.0	0.4	0.0	1.8	2.3	1.2	1.8	1.5	0.4	1.0	1.9	2.9	3.9	3.8	5.1	2.0	0.9	8.9	1.8	0	127	201
203	0.0	2.7	0.0	0.0	0.0	0.0	0.0	0.0	0.7	0.6	2.7	2.0	3.9	5.2	6.5	6.1	6.9	3.6	1.4	0	102	203
204	2.9	2.7	1.9	1.6	2.0	1.7	2.3	3.0	3.1	4.5	5.8	7.8	10.8	10.7	20.9	27.8	19.0	17.8	5.8	0	415	204
202,205	2.0	0.2	0.2	0.4	0.0	0.5	0.2	0.2	1.1	0.4	0.2	1.6	1.2	1.2	2.5	1.5	1.7	0.0	0.6	0	44	202,205
OTHER	0.0	0.2	0.3	0.6	0.2	0.2	0.9	1.1	2.0	3.3	6.8	8.5	10.1	10.7	20.2	24.8	31.1	23.1	4.8	0	345	OTHER
140-205	9.5	6.9	8.3	13.9	18.3	27.1	56.0	119.1	199.5	301.5	385.6	513.5	632.8	769.7	981.1	1243.7	1518.1	1840.0	290.4	0	20929	140-205
RATE PER CASE IN PERIOD	0.17	0.19	0.17	0.20	0.23	0.24	0.23	0.21	0.22	0.21	0.21	0.22	0.25	0.29	0.36	0.51	0.86	1.78	0.01	-	-	RATE PER CASE IN PERIOD

ENGLAND AND WALES, SOUTH METROPOLITAN REGION

Registry Title and Address. The South Metropolitan Cancer Registry, Clifton Avenue, Belmont Sutton, Surrey, England. Commenced 1st January, 1958. Supported financially by Royal Marsden Hospital; South-West Metropolitan Regional Hospital Board; South East Metropolitan Regional Hospital Board; Wessex Regional Hospital Board.

Registration. Cases are registered from hospital in-patients and out-patients, from radiotherapy and pathology departments, and from death certificates, mainly by field secretaries on the Registry's staff, but also to a less extent by hospital clerical staff. Cases are also registered by doctors attending patients at home, and from chest clinics and some mass X-ray units, again by field secretaries on Registry's staff. Registration is thought to be less than 90 % complete for skin cancers, probably also for private patients.

Follow-up. Follow-up is attempted for 20 years in all cases other them rodent ulcers, which are followed for only 2 years, unless they recur or unless other rodent ulcers develop.

Physical Description. The Registry covers an area of Southern and South Eastern England comprising the counties of Dorset, Hampshire, East and West Sussex, Surrey, Kent, approximately one half of greater London, and the South of Wiltshire. It is an rea of entirely sedimetary geology with no land higher than 1,000 feet above sea level, characterised by an east-west anticline exposing chalk. Bounded to the south and east by the English Channel and to the North by the mercantile part of the Thames and its estuary. The total registration area is 17,590 square kilometres.

Demographic Description. Total population of area under survey 8,218,270. Groups born outside the British Isles represent only negligible fractions of the population; for example in 1961 only 0.6 % were W. Indian born. The main occupational groups of the total employed population are : industry 39.9 %,commerce 46.2 %, agriculture 1.0 %, personal service 12.9 %. 51.1 % of the population live in conurbations of more than 100,000.

Medical Services. Total number of hospital beds of all kinds 104,000. Total number of doctors in practice in registration area 9,400. Cancer causes approximately 18.0 % of all deaths.

Publications. Annual reports (reports for 1958 and 1959 contain descriptions of the methods used).

Bulletins on special topics (morbidity and treatment of selected sites).

Payne (1964).

Many scientific reports have been published which have made use of the Registry's data; details are available on request.

TABLE 24 A

ENGLAND and WALES, SOUTH METROPOLITAN REGION : POPULATION (100,000s), CENSUS 1961

AGE (in years)	MALES No.	MALES Per Cent	FEMALES No.	FEMALES Per Cent
0 –	3.0433	7.84	2.8988	6.69
5 –	2.7700	7.13	2.6473	6.11
10 –	3.2613	8.40	3.1125	7.18
15 –	2.7756	7.15	2.7488	6.34
20 –	2.4811	6.39	2.5418	5.86
25 –	2.4402	6.28	2.4245	5.59
30 –	2.5044	6.45	2.5879	5.97
35 –	2.6658	6.87	2.8474	6.57
40 –	2.5640	6.60	2.7742	6.40
45 –	2.7837	7.17	3.0405	7.01
50 –	2.8164	7.25	3.0746	7.09
55 –	2.5294	6.51	2.8688	6.62
60 –	1.9908	5.13	2.6060	6.01
65 –	1.5718	4.05	2.3006	5.31
70 –	1.1974	3.08	1.9613	4.52
75 –	0.8034	2.07	1.4777	3.41
80 –	0.4297	1.11	0.9049	2.09
85 – and over	0.1995	0.51	0.5373	1.24
TOTAL	38.8278	100.00	43.3549	100.00

NOTES

TO TABLES 24 A, B and C

(I)   I. L. number 181.0 includes some papillomas of the bladder.
     "   "   193   includes benign and unspecified tumours of the central nervous system.

(II)   Carcinoma in situ excluded.

TABLE 24 B

ENGLAND and WALES, SOUTH METROPOLITAN REGION :

MALE INCIDENCE RATES, 1960 - 62.

INTER-NATIONAL LIST No.	No. OF CASES IN WHOLE PERIOD — ALL AGES	No. OF CASES IN WHOLE PERIOD — AGE UNKNOWN	ALL AGES	85- AND OVER	80-	75-	70-	65-	60-	55-	50-	45-	40-	35-	30-	25-	20-	15-	10-	5-	0-
140	197	2	1.7	13.4	13.2	8.3	9.5	7.0	3.9	3.4	1.7	1.3	0.7	0.1	0.3	0.0	0.1	0.0	0.0	0.0	0.0
141	221	0	1.9	23.4	17.8	14.9	10.6	6.8	3.7	2.9	2.0	0.7	0.8	0.3	0.1	0.1	0.1	0.0	0.0	0.0	0.0
142	150	0	1.3	8.4	7.0	6.2	3.6	2.5	2.2	1.4	1.8	2.3	1.3	1.3	1.1	0.8	0.1	0.2	0.1	0.0	0.0
143-4	274	2	2.4	31.7	33.4	17.4	11.1	10.6	4.4	2.9	1.2	1.0	0.8	0.4	0.3	0.0	0.0	0.0	0.1	0.0	0.0
146	69	0	0.6	0.0	0.8	0.8	3.1	1.3	1.5	1.1	1.2	0.7	0.7	0.3	0.1	0.3	0.3	0.1	0.0	0.1	0.1
145,147-8	352	1	3.0	25.1	28.7	23.2	16.1	11.2	9.4	5.0	2.1	0.8	0.5	0.6	0.1	0.0	0.3	0.1	0.0	0.0	0.0
150	773	1	6.6	91.9	67.5	49.8	35.4	26.7	14.6	10.0	6.4	3.5	0.8	0.3	0.3	0.0	0.0	0.2	0.0	0.0	0.0
151	3589	8	30.8	192.1	219.5	197.9	174.5	125.3	90.6	55.7	30.8	17.6	8.8	3.8	1.3	0.4	0.3	0.2	0.0	0.0	0.2
152	95	1	0.8	3.3	3.1	3.7	3.1	2.5	2.5	1.2	1.2	0.7	0.7	0.3	0.3	0.5	0.0	0.0	0.0	0.0	0.0
153	2117	3	18.2	202.2	169.9	132.8	97.7	64.7	45.2	26.1	14.9	11.7	6.1	3.8	2.0	1.0	0.7	0.1	0.1	0.0	0.0
154	2080	5	17.9	142.0	152.0	116.2	88.5	78.7	53.9	33.9	12.8	8.6	4.2	1.8	2.0	0.3	0.4	0.0	0.0	0.0	0.0
155.0	127	0	1.1	6.7	7.8	4.1	3.9	4.7	3.7	1.8	1.4	0.7	0.5	0.1	0.3	0.1	0.1	0.0	0.0	0.0	0.4
155.1	198	0	1.7	15.0	14.0	14.1	8.9	6.8	5.2	2.2	1.9	0.7	0.1	0.3	0.3	0.0	0.0	0.0	0.0	0.0	0.0
156	173	1	1.5	13.4	7.8	8.7	6.1	7.8	4.0	4.0	1.4	0.4	0.1	0.3	0.3	0.0	0.0	0.0	0.1	0.1	0.0	0.0
157	1106	2	9.5	76.9	62.8	64.7	50.1	37.5	25.1	19.0	13.2	5.6	3.6	0.6	0.3	0.1	0.0	0.0	0.1	0.1	0.0	0.0
160	117	2	1.0	3.3	7.8	3.7	7.0	2.5	2.5	2.4	0.7	0.6	0.5	0.9	0.1	0.1	0.0	0.1	0.0	0.0	0.1
161	619	1	5.3	18.4	27.9	24.5	23.9	21.6	18.8	12.4	5.7	4.1	1.8	0.9	0.5	0.1	0.0	0.1	0.0	0.0	0.0
162-3	11820	33	101.5	205.5	304.9	402.9	465.7	460.2	410.6	256.8	142.9	67.1	23.8	8.5	3.2	0.7	0.8	0.1	0.0	0.0	0.2
170	89	0	0.8	6.7	7.0	4.6	3.9	2.5	2.2	1.2	0.8	0.6	0.1	0.5	0.0	0.0	0.0	0.0	0.0	0.0	0.0
177	2736	12	23.5	407.7	346.8	273.8	169.8	83.1	33.8	14.4	5.3	1.2	0.5	0.0	0.0	0.0	0.1	0.0	0.1	0.0	0.1
178	292	1	2.5	3.3	1.6	2.1	2.2	1.1	1.3	1.6	1.8	3.0	4.6	4.0	7.9	5.7	3.9	0.5	0.0	0.2	0.5
179.0	139	0	1.2	15.0	9.3	4.6	5.0	4.5	4.0	2.5	1.4	0.4	0.9	0.3	0.0	0.1	0.0	0.1	0.1	0.0	0.0
180	568	2	4.9	18.4	17.8	18.3	16.1	16.1	16.2	11.7	7.6	5.3	2.9	1.3	0.5	0.1	0.3	0.1	0.0	0.6	1.6
181.0	2201	5	18.9	150.4	145.8	118.7	115.2	77.2	53.2	30.2	17.6	9.5	4.6	2.8	1.6	0.8	0.3	0.4	0.1	0.1	0.2
190	163	0	1.4	18.4	7.0	4.1	2.8	2.1	2.3	2.1	2.6	2.8	1.2	1.1	0.9	0.5	0.7	0.1	0.3	0.0	0.0
191	4356	58	37.4	387.6	277.7	207.5	155.4	120.5	93.3	64.4	47.2	33.2	21.3	10.6	5.5	2.2	1.2	0.0	0.2	0.0	0.0
192	90	1	0.8	1.7	1.6	1.2	1.4	2.5	1.5	0.8	1.3	0.6	1.0	0.4	0.4	0.3	0.1	0.0	0.0	0.2	1.5
193	771	1	6.6	0.0	3.1	5.8	9.7	15.5	17.4	15.6	12.4	8.0	6.0	6.6	3.6	2.0	1.9	2.6	1.3	2.6	3.3
194	80	1	0.7	5.0	3.1	2.1	4.7	1.5	2.2	1.6	0.7	0.2	0.3	0.4	0.0	0.4	0.1	0.1	0.1	0.0	0.0
195	104	0	0.9	0.0	1.6	1.2	1.9	1.7	2.0	1.6	0.5	1.6	0.5	1.0	0.5	0.8	0.9	0.2	0.8	0.4	0.8
196	126	1	1.1	5.0	3.9	2.9	3.9	2.1	1.3	0.8	0.4	0.5	0.9	0.4	1.2	0.4	1.1	1.6	1.7	0.7	0.0
197	212	0	1.8	13.4	7.0	8.7	4.8	4.7	3.5	2.4	2.5	1.7	2.0	2.0	0.7	0.7	0.9	0.7	0.3	0.4	0.3
200	396	2	3.4	5.0	6.2	8.3	14.8	9.8	8.9	5.5	5.4	3.0	2.6	3.0	1.6	1.6	1.1	1.0	0.8	0.2	0.4
201	323	1	2.8	3.3	3.9	2.9	5.6	4.0	4.2	3.6	5.7	3.7	3.3	2.4	2.9	2.7	3.0	1.7	1.3	0.2	0.1
203	224	1	1.9	5.0	7.0	7.5	10.3	7.2	6.0	4.5	2.6	1.8	1.2	0.3	0.1	0.3	0.0	0.1	0.0	0.0	0.0
204	887	4	7.6	38.4	51.2	40.2	27.3	20.1	15.9	10.7	6.6	4.7	4.4	2.6	4.4	1.9	2.0	1.9	2.9	2.5	5.6
202,205	115	0	1.0	3.3	4.7	2.1	5.0	2.1	2.2	2.1	0.8	1.3	0.8	0.4	0.5	0.7	0.1	0.5	0.0	0.0	0.2
OTHER	748	3	6.4	31.7	34.9	36.1	29.5	27.8	17.2	11.9	8.3	5.1	2.3	1.4	0.7	0.8	0.3	0.2	0.3	0.2	0.2
140-205	**38697**	**154**	**332.2**	**2192.1**	**2089.1**	**1846.7**	**1617.7**	**1284.5**	**990.4**	**632.3**	**373.4**	**216.1**	**117.0**	**65.1**	**45.8**	**26.9**	**20.2**	**12.9**	**11.0**	**8.5**	**16.1**
RATE PER CASE IN PERIOD	–	–	0.01	1.67	0.78	0.41	0.28	0.21	0.17	0.13	0.12	0.12	0.13	0.13	0.13	0.14	0.13	0.12	0.10	0.12	0.11

AVERAGE ANNUAL INCIDENCE PER 100,000 — AGE IN YEARS

TABLE 24 C

ENGLAND and WALES, SOUTH METROPOLITAN REGION :

FEMALE INCIDENCE RATES, 1960 - 62.

AVERAGE ANNUAL INCIDENCE PER 100,000 — AGE IN YEARS

INTER-NATIONAL LIST No.	0-	5-	10-	15-	20-	25-	30-	35-	40-	45-	50-	55-	60-	65-	70-	75-	80-	85- AND OVER	ALL AGES	AGE UNKNOWN (cases)	ALL AGES (cases)	INTER-NATIONAL LIST No.
140	0.0	0.0	0.0	0.0	0.0	0.0	0.0	0.0	0.4	0.1	0.0	0.7	0.4	0.9	0.7	0.7	1.8	2.5	0.3	0	35	140
141	0.0	0.0	0.0	0.0	0.1	0.0	0.0	0.6	0.1	0.7	1.1	0.6	1.7	3.3	2.9	5.4	4.8	5.6	1.0	1	128	141
142	0.0	0.0	0.4	1.0	0.5	1.4	1.8	1.5	0.6	1.5	2.2	2.4	2.3	1.7	2.2	2.7	2.6	6.8	1.4	0	186	142
143-4	0.0	0.0	0.0	0.0	0.3	0.0	0.0	0.5	0.5	0.3	1.2	1.5	2.7	2.6	4.9	6.1	4.4	5.0	1.2	0	152	143-4
146	0.1	0.0	0.0	0.0	0.0	0.0	0.1	0.0	0.4	0.1	0.0	0.1	0.5	0.4	0.7	0.9	1.5	0.6	0.2	0	27	146
145,147-8	0.0	0.1	0.1	0.0	0.0	0.0	0.3	0.4	0.2	1.2	1.8	2.3	5.2	3.8	3.9	5.0	8.8	9.9	1.6	1	210	145,147-8
150	0.0	0.0	0.0	0.0	0.0	0.8	0.3	0.5	1.4	1.5	3.7	4.6	8.4	11.9	14.6	25.0	35.7	32.9	4.6	0	601	150
151	0.0	0.1	0.0	0.0	0.1	0.0	1.4	3.0	3.4	5.8	12.4	19.3	34.3	53.0	71.0	114.1	138.9	172.5	20.2	5	2623	151
152	0.0	0.0	0.0	0.0	0.0	0.0	0.4	0.2	0.6	0.2	1.2	0.8	1.5	1.4	1.7	3.2	0.7	5.0	0.7	1	88	152
153	0.0	0.0	0.3	1.0	0.9	1.5	3.9	5.0	8.8	13.6	22.0	30.1	52.1	58.0	87.2	102.4	131.9	153.9	24.2	13	3154	153
154	0.1	0.0	0.3	0.1	0.4	0.4	1.3	2.5	5.4	7.8	11.5	19.3	27.5	45.1	51.3	62.0	71.5	78.2	14.3	5	1855	154
155.0	0.5	0.0	0.0	0.0	0.3	0.0	0.0	0.1	0.1	0.5	1.2	1.4	1.0	1.4	2.7	4.3	3.3	1.9	0.8	0	101	155.0
155.1	0.0	0.0	0.0	0.0	0.0	0.0	0.5	0.1	0.1	1.5	1.8	3.1	5.8	10.0	12.2	12.9	15.1	16.8	2.9	0	375	155.1
156	0.0	0.0	0.0	0.0	0.1	0.0	0.5	0.2	1.7	1.1	1.6	2.2	3.3	3.9	7.0	4.7	6.3	8.1	1.5	2	194	156
157	0.0	0.0	0.1	0.0	0.1	0.0	0.0	0.5	0.6	2.4	4.9	7.9	17.1	21.0	34.8	38.1	54.9	60.2	8.1	1	1058	157
160	0.0	0.0	0.0	0.1	0.1	0.0	0.0	0.1	0.6	0.7	0.9	2.0	0.9	2.2	2.4	3.4	3.3	3.7	0.8	0	106	160
161	0.1	0.0	0.0	0.1	0.0	0.1	0.0	0.0	0.4	0.9	0.9	1.3	2.2	1.6	2.2	2.7	2.9	1.9	0.7	0	96	161
162-3	0.0	0.0	0.0	0.0	0.8	0.3	1.3	0.7	8.1	13.3	25.2	35.1	48.6	55.1	53.5	53.0	45.7	40.9	17.4	2	2268	162-3
170	0.0	0.0	0.1	0.0	0.5	3.7	20.2	43.0	84.7	123.4	116.8	132.1	146.5	159.4	176.1	191.7	184.9	238.2	74.2	33	9653	170
171	0.0	0.0	0.0	0.0	0.5	2.3	7.3	20.5	27.2	27.6	28.9	26.1	30.7	29.8	26.7	29.3	32.0	29.2	16.1	10	2100	171
172	0.0	0.0	0.0	0.1	0.3	0.3	0.5	4.8	6.5	15.2	31.3	40.6	40.9	37.2	34.0	33.8	28.4	29.8	14.9	5	1937	172
173-4	0.0	0.0	0.0	0.0	0.3	0.3	0.1	0.1	0.5	0.3	0.2	0.1	1.2	0.4	0.5	0.0	0.6	0.6	0.3	0	34	173-4
175	0.1	0.0	0.1	0.5	1.6	3.0	4.6	6.4	15.6	23.1	29.7	36.9	39.7	38.1	35.7	32.5	33.2	31.6	16.4	4	2136	175
176	0.0	0.0	0.0	0.1	0.0	0.1	0.9	1.3	1.2	2.2	2.1	3.6	7.8	8.1	15.0	15.8	21.7	26.1	3.7	1	477	176
180	2.0	0.9	0.0	0.0	0.1	0.5	0.3	0.7	1.8	1.8	2.8	3.8	6.1	9.1	9.2	12.2	9.9	9.3	3.0	0	388	180
181.0	0.0	0.0	0.1	0.0	0.1	0.3	3.2	1.2	1.2	2.0	4.0	6.2	13.4	19.1	25.7	32.9	35.0	36.0	6.3	2	822	181.0
190	0.0	0.0	0.1	0.6	1.2	2.5	3.2	3.3	3.8	4.5	3.7	4.0	3.6	5.1	3.4	5.9	4.4	4.3	2.8	2	358	190
191	0.8	0.1	0.1	0.4	0.1	2.2	3.5	6.9	13.3	21.6	30.0	33.9	47.7	61.6	83.1	92.5	142.6	163.2	25.9	34	3365	191
192	3.1	2.8	2.4	1.3	0.7	3.2	3.2	0.7	0.6	0.9	0.4	1.5	0.9	0.9	1.7	1.1	1.5	1.2	0.6	0	82	192
193	0.6	0.0	0.2	0.2	0.4	1.0	1.0	3.7	4.4	8.2	10.0	10.9	12.3	12.0	7.5	2.5	2.9	2.5	5.5	1	712	193
194	0.2	0.1	0.2	0.2	0.4	0.3	0.5	1.2	1.0	1.8	2.5	2.2	2.7	5.2	6.1	6.3	5.5	5.6	1.9	0	241	194
195	0.5	0.8	0.3	0.8	0.5	1.0	0.3	0.6	0.5	1.3	1.3	1.3	0.6	0.7	0.7	0.2	0.0	5.6	0.6	0	76	195
196	0.3	0.3	0.6	0.6	0.8	0.3	1.4	0.5	0.4	0.3	0.4	0.9	0.9	1.4	0.8	1.8	4.4	3.7	0.8	1	109	196
197	0.5	0.3	1.4	0.8	0.8	1.0	1.4	1.1	1.7	1.8	1.3	2.1	4.0	3.2	4.1	5.2	8.1	4.3	1.8	2	238	197
200	0.3	0.0	0.6	0.7	0.5	0.4	0.5	0.9	1.1	1.4	2.8	4.0	5.4	6.2	8.7	11.1	8.5	3.1	2.5	0	329	200
201	0.0	0.3	0.4	1.2	2.4	2.5	1.8	2.0	1.7	1.6	1.5	1.3	2.0	2.2	3.2	2.9	2.6	1.9	1.6	0	210	201
203	0.0	0.0	0.0	1.2	2.0	0.1	0.1	0.1	0.6	1.2	2.4	3.8	5.6	5.5	5.3	8.6	7.0	1.2	1.9	1	247	203
204	4.4	2.3	1.8	1.2	1.2	1.5	0.5	2.1	3.2	3.3	6.6	7.9	11.4	12.8	17.0	18.7	20.6	20.5	5.9	0	772	204
202,205	0.2	0.0	0.0	0.1	0.3	0.1	0.5	1.2	0.6	1.1	1.4	1.6	1.8	2.5	2.7	2.5	2.2	5.0	1.0	0	132	202,205
OTHER	0.2	0.0	0.3	0.0	0.1	0.5	1.2	2.6	3.2	4.7	6.4	13.0	15.2	21.4	28.2	32.9	33.5	41.6	7.8	2	1021	OTHER
140-205	12.9	7.7	9.2	10.6	14.7	31.2	65.2	123.7	207.6	302.7	379.9	472.9	615.9	719.4	851.3	987.1	1123.5	1265.0	297.9	131	38696	140-205
RATE PER CASE IN PERIOD	0.11	0.13	0.11	0.12	0.13	0.14	0.13	0.12	0.12	0.11	0.11	0.12	0.13	0.14	0.17	0.23	0.37	0.62	0.01	-	-	RATE PER CASE IN PERIOD

ENGLAND AND WALES, SOUTH WESTERN REGION

Registry Title and Address : (Northern) S.W. Regional Cancer Records Bureau, U.T.F. House, 26 King Square, Bristol 2. (Southern) S.W. Regional Cancer Records Bureau, Plymouth General Hospital, Greenbank Road, Plymouth, Devon. Commenced 1945. Supported financially by the South Western Regional Hospital Board.

Registration. Cases are registered from hospital in-patients and out-patients, from radiotherapy and pathology departments, and from death certificates, by clerical staff. Special groups for which registration is thought to be less than 90 % complete are private patients and cases only attended at home, but both are probably largely picked up from death certificate registrations.

Follow-up. All cases are followed up for 15 years, except for skin cancers, other than malignant melanoma, which are followed for 5 years, and rodent ulcers which are not followed at all.

Physical Description. South West England covering the counties of Bristol, Somerset, Gloucestershire, part of Gloucester, part of Wiltshire, Bath, Plymouth, Exeter, Devon and Cornwall. It is a peninsula 200 miles long, bordered by the Bristol Channel on the north, and the English Channel on the south. It lies between latitudes $45^O55'$ and 52° North and longitudes $6^O21'$ and 2^O West. The total registration area is 18,900 square kilometres.

Demographic Description. Total population of area under survey 2,878,180. The main occupational groups of the total employed population are : industry 42.3 %, commerce 42.2 %, agriculture 4.1 % and personal service 11.4 %. Of the total population 22 % live in conurbations of more than 100,000.

Medical Services. Total number of hospital beds of all kinds 31,000. Total number of doctors in practice in registration area 1,600. Cancer causes approximatelly 18 % of all deaths.

Publications. Annual reports.
        Bailar, Thomas, Thomson, Eisenberg and Vick (1966);
Henderson and Curwen (1961); Price (1962); Vick (1960).

TABLE 25 A

ENGLAND and WALES, SOUTH WESTERN REGION : POPULATION (100, 000s), CENSUS 1961

AGE (in years)	MALES No.	MALES Per Cent	FEMALES No.	FEMALES Per Cent
0-	1.0840	7.85	1.0318	6.89
5-	1.0134	7.34	0.9700	6.48
10-	1.1665	8.45	1.1145	7.44
15-	1.0352	7.50	0.9704	6.48
20-	0.8754	6.34	0.8241	5.50
25-	0.8401	6.08	0.8100	5.41
30-	0.8703	6.30	0.8642	5.77
35-	0.9363	6.78	0.9769	6.53
40-	0.8787	6.36	0.9357	6.25
45-	0.9543	6.91	1.0180	6.80
50-	0.9711	7.03	1.0403	6.95
55-	0.8884	6.43	0.9898	6.61
60-	0.7327	5.31	0.9277	6.20
65-	0.5942	4.30	0.8270	5.52
70-	0.4435	3.21	0.6870	4.59
75-	0.2923	2.12	0.4960	3.31
80-	0.1593	1.15	0.3083	2.06
85- and over	0.0753	0.55	0.1791	1.20
TOTAL	13.8110	100.00	14.9708	100.00

NOTES

TO TABLES 25 A, B and C

(I)   Corresponding rates for 155.0 are available for 2 years (1960-61); they are as follows :

Age in years	Male	Female	Age in years	Male	Female
0-4	0.0	0.0	50-54	1.0	0.5
5-9	0.0	0.0	55-59	2.3	2.5
10-14	0.0	0.0	60-64	5.5	1.6
15-19	0.0	0.0	65-69	8.4	1.2
20-24	0.0	0.0	70-74	10.1	3.0
25-29	0.0	0.0	75-79	8.6	6.0
30-34	0.6	0.0	80-84	9.4	1.6
35-39	0.0	0.0	85 and over	0.0	2.8
40-44	0.0	0.0			
45-49	0.0	1.0	All ages	1.5	0.8

(II)   I. L. number 193 includes benign and unspecified tumours of the central nervous system.

(III)   Carcinoma in situ excluded.

TABLE 25 B
ENGLAND and WALES, SOUTH WESTERN REGION :
MALE INCIDENCE RATES, 1960 - 62.

AVERAGE ANNUAL INCIDENCE PER 100,000 — AGE IN YEARS

INTER-NATIONAL LIST No.	0-	5-	10-	15-	20-	25-	30-	35-	40-	45-	50-	55-	60-	65-	70-	75-	80-	85- AND OVER	ALL AGES	No. OF CASES — AGE UNKNOWN	No. OF CASES — ALL AGES	INTER-NATIONAL LIST No.
140	0.0	0.0	0.0	0.0	0.0	1.2	0.4	0.4	1.9	1.0	8.2	9.4	9.1	16.3	19.5	31.9	43.9	48.7	4.8	1	198	140
141	0.0	0.0	0.0	0.0	0.0	0.0	0.0	0.0	0.8	0.0	1.7	2.6	5.0	7.3	11.3	11.4	23.0	13.3	1.9	0	77	141
142	0.0	0.0	0.3	1.0	0.8	0.4	1.1	1.4	0.8	2.4	1.4	2.3	1.8	1.7	6.0	6.8	12.6	4.4	1.5	0	61	142
143-4	0.0	0.0	0.0	0.0	0.0	0.0	0.4	0.0	0.0	0.3	1.4	2.6	3.6	9.0	9.8	12.5	18.8	17.7	1.8	0	74	143-4
146	0.0	0.0	0.0	0.3	0.0	0.0	0.0	0.0	0.4	2.1	1.0	1.1	0.9	1.7	3.0	0.0	2.1	0.0	0.6	0	24	146
145,147-8	0.0	0.0	0.0	0.0	0.4	0.0	0.0	0.4	0.0	1.4	2.1	6.0	12.3	9.5	12.8	30.8	16.7	17.7	3.1	0	128	145,147-8
150	0.0	0.0	0.0	0.0	0.0	0.0	0.0	0.7	1.1	2.1	5.1	9.8	15.5	20.8	36.8	41.1	58.6	44.3	5.9	0	246	150
151	0.0	0.0	0.0	0.0	0.0	0.0	0.8	1.8	6.1	15.4	36.4	64.5	88.7	147.0	155.6	161.9	171.6	141.7	30.5	0	1265	151
152	0.0	0.0	0.0	0.0	0.0	0.0	0.8	0.0	0.0	0.7	0.3	1.1	0.9	2.8	1.5	0.0	0.0	0.0	0.4	0	18	152
153	0.0	0.0	0.0	0.0	0.0	0.4	1.1	1.4	4.6	11.9	16.1	30.0	56.0	68.4	91.7	130.0	159.0	172.6	18.8	0	777	153
154	0.0	0.3	0.0	0.0	0.4	0.0	1.5	3.2	5.3	7.7	14.8	36.8	48.7	68.4	105.2	135.7	156.9	128.4	18.9	0	784	154
155	0.0	0.0	0.3	0.0	0.0	0.0	0.4	0.7	0.0	0.7	2.1	3.8	8.6	16.8	17.3	18.2	20.9	8.9	3.0	0	123	155
156	0.0	0.0	0.0	0.0	0.0	0.0	0.0	0.0	0.0	1.4	2.4	1.9	3.2	6.2	6.0	2.3	2.1	0.0	1.1	0	45	156
157	0.0	0.0	0.0	0.0	0.0	0.0	0.0	0.0	2.3	5.9	5.1	18.0	27.8	34.8	51.9	52.5	48.1	39.8	8.6	0	356	157
160	0.0	0.0	0.0	0.0	0.0	0.0	0.0	0.0	0.0	0.3	1.4	2.3	3.2	1.7	1.5	1.1	8.4	4.4	0.7	0	29	160
161	0.0	0.0	0.0	0.0	0.0	0.0	0.4	1.1	0.4	4.5	6.9	10.5	17.3	19.6	15.8	20.5	10.5	4.4	4.4	0	184	161
162-3	0.0	0.0	0.0	0.0	0.0	0.8	1.5	6.1	21.6	58.3	116.0	200.4	300.3	323.7	305.1	219.0	121.4	93.0	73.2	0	3033	162-3
170	0.0	0.3	0.0	0.0	0.0	0.0	0.0	0.0	0.0	1.0	0.3	1.1	1.8	3.9	1.5	2.3	6.3	0.0	0.6	0	26	170
177	0.3	0.0	0.0	0.0	0.0	0.0	0.0	0.4	0.0	1.4	6.5	18.0	40.5	98.2	184.9	294.2	380.8	429.4	27.0	0	1120	177
178	0.0	0.0	0.9	1.0	2.7	4.0	5.0	4.3	3.4	3.1	2.4	1.9	2.7	0.6	1.8	3.4	2.1	8.9	2.2	0	91	178
179	0.0	1.0	0.0	0.0	0.0	0.0	0.8	0.4	1.1	0.7	3.1	1.9	2.7	6.7	3.6	6.8	14.6	4.4	1.4	0	60	179
180	2.2	0.7	0.3	0.3	0.0	1.2	1.5	1.4	1.9	4.2	5.1	10.9	13.2	17.4	18.8	16.0	18.8	4.4	4.7	1	193	180
181.0	0.0	0.0	0.0	0.3	0.4	1.6	1.1	1.8	4.9	7.7	16.5	39.4	50.5	70.7	90.9	117.5	110.9	97.4	17.8	0	738	181.0
190	0.0	0.3	0.0	0.6	0.4	1.2	0.4	1.4	0.8	1.4	3.1	2.6	4.1	1.7	3.8	2.3	10.5	17.7	1.5	0	62	190
191	0.0	0.0	0.0	1.3	0.4	1.6	3.4	12.1	18.6	33.2	51.1	64.5	92.8	121.2	181.9	236.1	368.3	420.5	40.0	0	1657	191
192	1.2	0.0	0.0	0.0	0.0	0.0	0.4	0.4	0.0	0.4	0.3	0.6	0.3	0.4	0.8	0.4	0.0	4.4	0.6	0	23	192
193	2.2	2.3	2.9	1.3	1.9	3.2	3.4	5.7	5.7	10.1	14.4	17.6	20.5	19.1	6.8	4.6	0.0	0.0	7.0	1	292	193
194	0.0	0.0	0.3	0.3	0.0	0.0	0.0	0.0	0.4	0.3	0.3	2.3	1.8	3.4	2.3	2.3	2.1	8.9	0.7	0	29	194
195	0.9	0.0	0.3	0.0	1.1	0.4	0.0	0.4	0.4	1.4	2.1	1.1	0.0	1.1	0.0	1.1	0.0	0.0	0.6	0	26	195
196	0.0	0.3	0.9	1.9	0.8	1.2	1.5	0.0	1.9	1.4	1.0	1.9	1.4	3.9	5.3	4.6	2.1	8.9	1.3	0	52	196
197	0.3	0.3	0.0	0.0	1.9	0.8	0.4	0.0	0.0	2.4	1.0	2.6	2.7	3.9	4.5	2.3	8.4	0.0	1.4	0	60	197
200	0.6	2.0	0.9	2.3	0.8	0.8	1.5	1.4	2.3	5.6	4.8	9.8	11.4	14.0	12.0	13.7	14.6	13.3	4.3	0	180	200
201	0.0	0.0	1.1	1.0	3.0	3.2	2.7	1.8	4.6	1.7	2.4	2.3	4.5	4.5	5.3	5.7	4.2	0.0	2.3	0	97	201
203	0.0	0.0	0.0	0.0	0.0	0.0	0.0	1.1	1.5	2.4	2.1	3.4	4.5	10.1	6.8	9.1	6.3	8.9	1.9	0	79	203
204	5.8	2.6	1.4	1.0	3.4	2.0	1.9	3.9	5.3	5.9	4.5	10.9	10.5	26.4	24.1	38.8	23.0	17.7	7.0	0	289	204
202,205	0.0	0.0	0.0	0.3	0.8	0.4	0.0	2.1	0.4	0.7	1.7	0.8	2.7	1.1	3.0	4.6	4.6	0.0	0.9	0	36	202,205
OTHER	0.6	0.3	0.3	0.3	0.0	0.0	1.1	1.8	2.3	4.2	5.8	15.4	20.5	33.7	32.3	34.2	35.6	26.6	7.0	0	290	OTHER
140-205	14.1	10.5	10.0	13.5	19.0	23.4	33.3	59.1	101.3	205.7	352.2	611.6	891.2	1196.0	1440.8	1679.8	1883.2	1810.5	309.5	3	12822	140-205
RATE PER CASE IN PERIOD	0.31	0.33	0.29	0.32	0.38	0.40	0.38	0.36	0.38	0.35	0.34	0.38	0.45	0.56	0.75	1.14	2.09	4.43	0.02	-	-	RATE PER CASE IN PERIOD

TABLE 25 C

ENGLAND and WALES, SOUTH WESTERN REGION :

FEMALE INCIDENCE RATES, 1960 - 62.

International List No.	AVERAGE ANNUAL INCIDENCE PER 100,000 — AGE IN YEARS																		All Ages	No. of Cases in Whole Period — Age Unknown	No. of Cases in Whole Period — All Ages	International List No.
	0-	5-	10-	15-	20-	25-	30-	35-	40-	45-	50-	55-	60-	65-	70-	75-	80-	85- and over				
140	0.0	0.0	0.0	0.0	0.0	0.0	0.0	0.0	0.4	0.0	0.6	0.3	0.4	0.4	1.5	1.3	2.2	0.0	0.3	0	13	140
141	0.0	0.0	0.0	0.0	0.0	0.0	0.0	0.3	0.7	0.7	1.0	0.7	2.9	2.8	2.9	4.0	7.6	9.3	1.1	0	49	141
142	0.0	0.0	0.0	0.0	1.2	1.2	2.3	0.3	1.4	2.6	2.2	2.7	2.5	2.0	3.4	1.3	5.4	3.7	1.5	0	68	142
143-4	0.0	0.0	0.0	0.0	0.0	0.4	0.0	0.3	0.4	0.7	1.6	1.3	1.4	2.4	5.8	2.7	4.3	3.7	1.0	0	46	143-4
146	0.0	0.0	0.0	0.0	0.0	0.0	0.0	0.3	0.0	0.0	0.0	0.0	0.7	0.4	0.5	0.7	0.0	0.0	0.1	0	5	146
145,147-8	0.0	0.0	0.0	0.0	0.0	0.0	0.0	0.0	1.1	1.6	3.8	4.0	4.0	3.6	8.7	6.7	6.5	9.3	2.0	0	91	145,147-8
150	0.0	0.0	0.0	0.0	0.8	0.0	1.2	0.0	0.7	2.0	5.4	6.7	10.4	14.1	18.0	34.9	25.9	29.8	5.3	1	238	150
151	0.0	0.0	0.0	0.0	0.0	0.0	0.0	1.7	3.6	4.3	11.2	18.9	32.0	50.8	54.3	98.1	120.0	85.6	16.8	0	755	151
152	0.0	0.0	0.0	0.0	0.0	0.0	0.0	0.3	0.0	0.3	0.6	1.0	1.1	0.8	0.0	2.7	1.1	1.9	0.4	0	18	152
153	0.0	0.0	0.3	0.0	1.2	0.8	3.5	3.4	7.8	11.5	23.1	31.7	46.4	66.1	90.7	118.3	135.1	115.4	24.3	1	1091	153
154	0.0	0.0	0.0	0.0	0.0	0.8	1.9	1.0	4.6	9.8	11.2	18.2	24.4	38.7	42.2	69.9	67.0	48.4	13.0	0	586	154
155	0.0	0.0	0.0	0.0	0.0	0.0	0.0	0.7	1.4	2.0	1.0	7.1	8.3	12.9	17.0	24.9	15.1	20.5	4.2	0	188	155
156	0.0	0.0	0.0	0.3	0.0	0.0	0.0	0.3	0.4	0.3	1.3	2.4	1.4	4.4	1.9	4.0	2.2	1.9	1.0	0	43	156
157	0.0	0.0	0.0	0.0	0.0	0.4	0.8	0.7	0.7	2.3	5.8	6.7	12.9	19.8	26.2	31.6	28.1	20.5	6.1	0	274	157
160	0.0	0.0	0.0	0.0	0.0	0.0	0.0	0.0	0.7	1.0	1.0	1.0	1.4	0.4	0.5	2.7	1.1	1.9	0.5	0	24	160
161	0.0	0.0	0.0	0.0	0.0	0.0	0.0	0.0	0.0	0.3	0.6	1.0	0.7	2.0	2.4	1.3	0.0	0.0	0.4	0	20	161
162-3	0.0	0.0	0.0	0.0	0.0	0.4	0.8	2.0	3.6	9.8	19.5	24.2	32.3	41.1	35.9	30.2	20.5	20.5	11.6	0	523	162-3
170	0.0	0.0	0.0	0.3	1.2	6.6	15.0	45.4	67.7	121.4	119.2	124.3	157.4	141.5	171.8	162.6	166.5	180.5	69.7	2	3132	170
171	0.0	0.0	0.0	0.0	0.0	1.2	8.9	23.9	40.3	37.0	34.0	28.3	25.5	30.6	25.2	26.9	22.7	9.3	17.3	0	777	171
172	0.0	0.0	0.0	0.3	0.8	0.4	0.4	3.1	7.5	15.1	26.9	53.2	46.0	47.6	35.9	30.9	20.5	14.9	15.9	0	713	172
173	0.0	0.0	0.0	0.0	0.0	1.2	0.8	0.3	1.4	1.0	0.0	0.0	0.7	0.4	0.5	0.7	0.0	0.0	0.5	0	21	173
174	0.0	0.0	0.0	0.0	0.0	0.0	0.0	0.3	0.4	1.3	2.6	3.4	2.9	4.0	0.5	3.4	0.0	7.4	1.1	0	51	174
175	0.0	0.3	0.9	1.4	1.2	2.5	4.6	7.5	13.2	26.2	33.3	36.0	31.6	30.6	33.5	34.9	22.7	18.6	15.5	0	695	175
176	0.0	0.0	0.0	0.0	0.0	0.0	0.4	0.7	1.4	2.0	2.6	4.0	6.1	11.7	16.5	15.5	24.9	29.8	3.9	0	176	176
180	1.6	0.0	0.0	0.3	0.0	0.0	0.0	0.7	1.1	1.6	3.2	3.4	5.7	6.9	3.9	8.7	10.8	7.4	2.3	0	105	180
181.0	0.0	0.0	0.0	0.0	0.0	0.4	1.2	1.0	1.8	3.3	3.2	9.4	11.5	20.2	21.8	32.9	29.2	48.4	6.4	0	289	181.0
190	0.0	0.0	0.0	0.3	1.2	1.6	3.5	3.1	6.1	4.6	4.8	2.7	4.7	6.4	8.2	10.1	7.6	9.3	3.3	0	150	190
191	0.6	0.0	0.0	0.0	0.8	0.0	4.6	10.2	12.8	17.7	24.4	33.7	56.8	75.8	103.8	116.3	175.2	208.4	29.5	2	1323	191
192	0.0	0.0	0.0	0.0	0.0	0.0	0.4	5.8	1.6	0.7	1.6	0.7	0.0	0.4	1.0	2.0	2.2	3.7	0.5	0	22	192
193	4.2	2.4	0.9	1.4	2.0	2.5	3.1	0.7	6.1	12.4	12.2	10.4	16.5	7.7	5.3	3.4	1.1	0.0	6.0	0	269	193
194	0.0	0.0	0.0	0.3	0.0	1.2	1.2	0.0	0.4	2.3	2.6	1.3	3.2	4.0	5.8	6.0	13.0	9.3	1.9	0	86	194
195	1.0	0.7	1.2	0.7	0.0	0.4	0.0	0.0	1.1	1.3	0.3	0.0	0.7	1.6	1.0	0.0	0.0	0.0	0.5	0	22	195
196	0.6	0.3	0.9	0.7	0.4	0.8	0.8	1.7	0.7	0.0	1.0	1.7	1.1	1.2	1.5	2.0	5.4	3.7	0.9	0	42	196
197	0.3	0.7	0.0	1.4	0.4	0.0	1.9	1.7	0.4	1.0	3.2	1.0	1.1	1.6	3.4	5.4	4.3	5.6	1.4	0	64	197
200	0.0	0.7	0.3	0.0	0.4	0.8	1.5	1.7	1.1	2.0	3.5	5.1	9.3	8.5	11.6	12.1	8.6	1.9	3.4	0	151	200
201	0.0	0.0	0.0	1.4	2.4	3.7	3.1	0.0	1.1	1.0	1.6	1.3	2.9	3.2	5.3	2.7	1.1	1.9	1.8	0	81	201
203	0.0	0.0	0.0	0.0	0.0	0.0	0.0	0.7	1.4	1.3	4.2	6.1	5.0	5.2	9.7	4.7	2.2	1.9	2.1	0	96	203
204	4.2	1.7	3.3	2.7	3.6	0.4	3.9	0.0	3.9	2.6	5.4	8.4	8.6	8.9	18.0	14.8	8.6	9.3	5.3	0	238	204
202,205	0.3	0.0	0.0	0.0	0.0	0.0	0.8	0.0	0.0	0.3	0.0	1.3	1.1	1.2	1.5	2.7	6.5	0.0	0.6	0	27	202,205
OTHER	0.3	0.0	1.5	0.0	0.0	0.0	1.2	1.0	3.9	5.2	9.0	11.1	14.0	19.3	29.6	33.6	33.5	13.0	7.5	0	336	OTHER
140-205	13.6	6.5	9.3	11.7	17.8	28.4	67.5	120.4	200.9	310.4	388.7	474.8	595.7	701.3	827.3	967.7	1008.8	956.6	287.2	6	12898	140-205
RATE PER CASE IN PERIOD	0.32	0.34	0.30	0.34	0.40	0.41	0.39	0.34	0.36	0.33	0.32	0.34	0.36	0.40	0.49	0.67	1.08	1.86	0.02	-	-	RATE PER CASE IN PERIOD

FINLAND

The Finnish Cancer Register was founded on the initiative of the Cancer Society of Finland in 1952, and data on newly diagnosed cases of cancer have been compiled since the beginning of 1953. The Register is headed by a committee of eight persons in which the State Medical Board, the Central Bureau of Statistics and the Cancer Society are represented.

All hospitals, pathological laboratories and private practitioners are urged to report to the Register all the new cases of cancer that come to their attention. The making of reports has been compulsory since the year 1961; earlier, such reporting was on a voluntary basis, although physicians were very co-operative in this respect.

In addition to this, the Register receives through the Central Bureau of Statistics a copy of every death certificate in which cancer is mentioned. All other death certificates are collated annually with the files of the Register, for determination of the number of deaths in which cancer has not been mentioned.

The Register employs 2 full-time statisticians, 2 part-time physicians, and 6 clerks.

In cases where knowledge originates from pathological laboratories or from a death certificate alone, the sender of the speciemn, or the one signing the death certificate, is asked to supply additional information. Nevertheless, a proportion of the cases remain as no more than a laboratory notification or death certificate only. The frequency of such cases, and the changes which have occurred since 1954, are shown below.

	1954	1959
Death certificates only	14 %	8 %
Laboratory notification only	5 %	4 %

The Notification Card includes questions in regard to the patient's name, sex, date of birth, marital status, occupation, residence, primary site of tumour, date of first diagnosis, stage at diagnosis, methods used in treatment, and type of tumour. The date of the first diagnosis is recorded as the onset. In cases where a death certificate is the sole source of information, the disease is generally recorded as being diagnosed in the year of death.

The classification of neoplasms according to the antomical location of the lesion, as suggested by WHO, is used in classifying the cases. All cases of carcinoma and sarcoma are grouped as malignant neoplasms, as are all intracerebral tumours independent of their nature. Carcinoma in situ cases have been grouped as malignant if subjected to cancer treatment. This applies also to so-called malignant polyps, malignant papillomas, and malignant adenomas, although these are kept separate by the employment of different code numbers for each. Basal cell carcinomas are coded as malignant neoplasms. Lymphosarcomas and reticulum cell sarcomas are classified as tumours of a given anatomical site if primary and so stated; otherwise they are grouped as malignant lymphomas.

The nomenclature of the American Cancer Society is used in the definition of histological types of cancer.

If a number of primary neoplasms are noted in one and the same person, each of them is recorded as a separate case, appart from skin tumours of the same histology within a limit of 20 years.

Two types of residence distribution are used, each of them administrative in nature; the first is by provinces, and the second by urbanization. The urban areas include cities, towns and townships, some of which contain no industrial plants, and the rural areas some communities with an appreciable amount of industry.

The age is given as the number of years attained by the patient at the time of diagnosis.

The information on incidence is relatively reliable, since the Register obtains notifications from several independent sources. It is thus possible to check neglect of the duty of notification.

Nevertheless, deficiencies may of course come into being by reason of diagnostic accuracy, etc. The reliability of the data can be regarded from several points of view, and thus depends on several factors. The Finnish Cancer Register is in a favourable position, as the population at risk is well defined; furthermore, there are good vital statistics with respect to this population.

The Register has requested the notification of every case of cancer, regardless of whether somebody may already have made such notification or is going to do so. Thus the Register receives several reports on the same patient, and the paractice may lessen the possibility of the case not being reported all. The frequency of the reports naturally varies, dependent upon the nature of the case. For example, cases of cancer of the digestive system are more frequent than the average of those reported through a death certificate alone.

E. Saxén,
M. Hakama.

Registry Title and Address : Finnish Cancer Register, Liisankatu 21 B, Helsinki 17, Finland. Commenced 1952. Supported financially by the Cancer Society of Finland and by the State.

Registration. Cases are registered from hospital in-patients and out-patients, and from radiotherapy departments, by doctors, nurses and clerical staff; from pathology departments by laboratory staff; from death certificates by the Central Bureau of Statistics; by doctors attending cases at home; and all other practising physicians.

Follow-up. All cases are compared yearly with all death certificates of the population.

Physical Description. The Registry covers the whole of Finland which is bordered on the north by Norway, on the east by the USSR, on the west by Norway, Sweden and the Gulf of Bothnia, and on the south by the Gulf of Finland. The average altitude is 150 metres. It has 31,570 square kilometres of inland water and is a coniferous forest zone. The country lies between latitudes 60° and 70° north and longitudes 20° and 30° east. The total registration area is 337,113 square kilometres.

Demographic Description. Total population of area under survey 4,446,200. 93 % of the population are Lutherans. Ethnic groups are Nordic and East Baltic. The main occupational groups are industry 20 %, commerce 9 %, agriculture, forestry and fishing 32 %, personal service 11 %. Of the total population 16.7 % live in three conurbations each of more than 100,000.

Medical Services. Total number of hospital beds of all kinds is 13.0 beds per 1,000 inhabitants, i.e., approximately 58,000. Total number of doctors in practice in registration area is one per 1,500 i.e., approximately 3,000. Cancer causes approximately 16 % of all deaths (1962).

Publications. Annual reports from 1953 (cancer incidence in Finland).
Saxén and Hakama (1964).
A list of scientific reports based on Registry data is available on request.

TABLE 26 A
FINLAND
POPULATION (100, 000s), MEAN 1959 - 61

AGE (in years)	MALES		FEMALES	
	No.	Per Cent	No.	Per Cent
0-	2.1070	9.85	2.0210	8.76
5-	2.2600	10.56	2.1740	9.42
10-	2.4780	11.58	2.3810	10.32
15-	1.8350	8.58	1.7670	7.66
20-	1.6420	7.68	1.5930	6.91
25-	1.5150	7.08	1.4760	6.40
30-	1.5510	7.25	1.5510	6.72
35-	1.3850	6.47	1.5480	6.71
40-	1.1750	5.49	1.3910	6.03
45-	1.2780	5.97	1.4800	6.42
50-	1.2300	5.75	1.4390	6.24
55-	0.9900	4.63	1.2120	5.25
60-	0.7440	3.48	1.0140	4.40
65-	0.5180	2.42	0.7700	3.34
70-	0.3540	1.65	0.6010	2.61
75-	0.2010	0.94	0.3820	1.66
80-	0.0930	0.43	0.1890	0.82
85- and over	0.0360	0.17	0.0810	0.35
TOTAL	21.3920	100.00	23.0700	100.00

NOTES

TO TABLES 26 A, B and C

(I)   I.L. number 193 includes benign and unspecified tumours of the central nervous system.

(II)   Carcinoma in situ included.

TABLE 26 B
FINLAND
MALE INCIDENCE RATES, 1959 - 61.

AVERAGE ANNUAL INCIDENCE PER 100,000 — AGE IN YEARS

INTER-NATIONAL LIST No.	No. OF CASES IN WHOLE PERIOD — AGE UNKNOWN	No. OF CASES — ALL AGES	ALL AGES	85- AND OVER	80-	75-	70-	65-	60-	55-	50-	45-	40-	35-	30-	25-	20-	15-	10-	5-	0-
140	10	533	8.3	92.6	78.9	68.0	56.5	43.1	33.2	27.9	17.6	11.2	8.8	3.6	1.7	0.7	0.0	0.2	0.0	0.0	0.0
141	0	41	0.6	0.0	3.6	6.6	4.7	4.5	2.7	2.4	1.4	1.0	0.6	0.0	0.0	0.0	0.0	0.0	0.0	0.0	0.0
142	2	88	1.4	9.3	3.6	0.0	4.7	5.1	5.8	4.4	1.6	3.1	2.6	1.4	0.4	1.1	0.4	0.2	0.1	0.1	0.0
143-4	0	48	0.7	18.5	7.2	6.6	5.6	4.5	3.1	2.7	0.8	0.3	0.3	0.5	0.4	0.0	0.0	0.0	0.3	0.0	0.0
146	0	20	0.3	0.0	3.6	8.3	1.9	1.3	0.4	0.7	0.5	0.5	0.0	0.5	0.2	0.0	0.4	0.0	0.3	0.0	0.0
145,147-8	1	75	1.2	18.5	14.3	8.3	8.5	7.1	2.2	3.4	3.3	1.8	1.1	0.7	0.0	0.0	0.2	0.0	0.0	0.0	0.2
150	0	396	6.2	92.6	86.0	69.7	68.7	47.0	30.5	18.5	8.4	3.4	0.9	0.7	0.2	1.5	0.2	0.0	0.0	0.0	0.0
151	3	3040	47.4	509.3	598.6	542.3	463.3	335.3	236.6	134.3	77.0	35.0	16.7	8.9	5.6	1.5	0.2	0.0	0.0	0.0	0.0
152	0	41	0.6	9.3	10.8	1.7	3.8	2.6	2.2	2.0	0.3	1.8	0.6	0.2	0.4	0.2	0.0	0.2	0.1	0.1	0.0
153	0	351	5.5	64.8	43.0	74.6	52.7	31.5	23.7	15.5	7.9	3.7	3.7	2.6	1.9	0.9	0.2	0.4	0.0	0.0	0.0
154	0	355	5.5	64.8	78.9	71.3	48.0	48.9	22.4	12.5	6.8	5.5	3.4	1.0	1.1	0.4	0.0	0.0	0.0	0.0	0.0
155.0	0	79	1.2	27.8	7.2	11.6	8.5	5.1	7.2	4.7	2.2	1.0	1.1	0.7	0.0	0.0	0.0	0.2	0.0	0.0	0.0
155.1	0	41	0.6	18.5	3.6	0.0	3.8	6.4	3.1	2.7	1.9	0.3	0.3	0.0	0.0	0.0	0.0	0.0	0.0	0.0	0.2
156	0	93	1.4	27.8	7.2	18.2	17.9	8.4	5.4	5.1	3.0	1.0	0.0	0.5	0.0	0.9	0.6	0.0	0.0	0.0	0.2
157	0	464	7.2	74.1	75.3	49.8	66.9	48.3	43.9	22.9	13.0	6.0	3.1	1.7	0.4	0.2	0.2	0.0	0.0	0.0	0.0
160	0	85	1.3	9.3	3.6	10.0	8.5	9.7	7.2	7.1	1.9	0.8	0.0	0.2	0.4	0.2	0.2	0.0	0.1	0.0	0.0
161	1	428	6.7	9.3	39.4	29.9	23.5	31.5	26.0	27.9	20.1	12.5	9.4	5.8	0.0	0.0	0.4	0.4	0.1	0.0	0.0
162-3	1	3861	60.2	203.7	268.8	384.7	422.8	425.4	376.3	238.0	138.2	62.6	23.3	7.7	1.3	0.2	0.4	0.2	0.0	0.0	0.0
170	0	20	0.3	9.3	3.6	3.3	0.0	4.5	0.4	0.7	0.0	0.8	0.3	0.2	0.2	0.0	0.0	0.0	0.1	0.0	0.0
177	1	935	14.6	324.1	354.8	331.7	196.8	122.3	48.8	19.5	5.4	2.6	0.6	0.0	2.4	1.8	0.8	0.5	0.1	0.0	0.6
178	0	71	1.1	9.3	7.2	3.3	2.8	1.9	2.7	0.3	1.6	1.8	0.9	1.4	0.6	0.2	0.0	0.0	0.0	0.0	0.0
179-0	1	48	0.7	27.8	7.2	5.0	2.8	2.6	1.8	2.4	1.6	1.8	0.9	0.2	0.6	0.0	0.0	0.0	0.0	0.0	0.0
180	0	239	3.7	9.3	21.5	18.2	21.7	21.2	20.2	10.8	9.8	5.5	3.1	0.2	0.2	0.0	0.2	0.0	0.0	0.4	2.2
181-0	0	373	5.8	111.1	78.9	49.8	62.1	54.1	24.2	16.8	10.6	2.1	1.4	0.7	0.0	0.0	0.0	0.0	0.0	0.0	0.0
190	0	112	1.7	18.5	14.3	13.3	8.5	5.1	5.8	3.4	3.5	1.8	2.8	1.9	0.4	1.3	0.6	0.5	0.1	0.1	0.6
191	20	1209	18.8	268.5	175.6	215.6	148.8	117.1	65.9	49.2	33.9	20.6	17.0	10.6	3.4	2.9	1.4	0.4	0.3	0.1	1.7
192	0	66	1.0	9.3	0.0	5.6	2.8	4.5	1.8	3.0	1.9	1.6	0.9	1.0	0.4	0.4	0.0	0.3	0.0	1.7
193	1	354	5.5	9.3	0.0	6.0	7.5	5.1	11.2	16.5	14.1	12.0	7.1	3.4	5.6	2.6	2.0	3.3	3.2	2.1	2.7
194	0	48	0.7	0.0	10.8	1.7	0.0	5.1	1.8	1.7	1.9	1.8	1.4	0.2	0.4	0.9	0.2	0.0	0.0	0.0	0.6
195	1	39	0.6	0.0	0.0	0.0	0.0	1.3	0.9	1.3	1.6	1.3	1.1	0.7	1.1	1.5	1.4	2.4	1.2	0.4	0.2
196	0	146	2.3	18.5	3.6	10.0	5.6	9.7	7.6	5.1	4.3	2.6	1.7	1.7	0.4	1.5	0.6	0.7	0.4	0.1	0.8
197	1	88	1.4	0.0	3.6	6.6	5.6	3.9	4.0	3.0	1.9	1.0	2.0	2.2	1.1	1.5	0.8	0.2	0.1	1.0	0.6
200	1	137	2.1	18.5	3.6	13.3	12.2	11.6	6.3	7.1	2.4	2.9	1.7	1.2	1.1	1.5	1.4	1.5	0.7	0.4	0.0
201	2	160	2.5	0.0	0.0	10.0	3.8	9.0	4.9	6.7	4.3	2.3	5.7	2.6	3.0	2.2	1.4	1.5	0.7	0.4	0.0
203	0	75	1.2	0.0	3.6	10.0	7.5	9.7	5.4	3.7	3.0	1.3	0.9	0.5	0.0	0.2	0.0	0.0	0.0	0.0	0.0
204	1	416	6.5	18.5	35.8	36.5	33.9	31.5	18.8	11.8	10.0	5.7	4.5	2.9	2.8	1.8	1.6	4.2	2.4	3.1	6.5
202,205	0	14	0.2	0.0	3.6	1.7	0.9	0.6	0.9	0.7	0.8	0.3	0.0	0.0	0.0	0.2	0.0	0.0	0.0	0.0	0.2
OTHER	4	678	10.6	231.5	193.5	92.9	86.6	59.8	41.7	32.0	13.6	10.4	6.2	2.6	2.1	1.3	2.0	0.4	0.7	0.6	0.9
140-205	51	15267	237.9	2333.3	2254.5	2187.4	1880.4	1546.3	1107.1	728.3	433.1	231.9	135.9	71.0	38.9	27.1	15.2	15.8	10.9	9.0	17.9
RATE PER CASE IN PERIOD	-	-	0.02	9.26	3.58	1.66	0.94	0.64	0.45	0.34	0.27	0.26	0.28	0.24	0.21	0.22	0.20	0.18	0.13	0.15	0.16

TABLE 26 C
FINLAND
FEMALE INCIDENCE RATES, 1959 - 61.

AVERAGE ANNUAL INCIDENCE PER 100,000

INTER-NATIONAL LIST No.	0–	5–	10–	15–	20–	25–	30–	35–	40–	45–	50–	55–	60–	65–	70–	75–	80–	85– AND OVER	ALL AGES	No. OF CASES AGE UNKNOWN	No. OF CASES ALL AGES	INTER-NATIONAL LIST No.
140	0.0	0.0	0.0	0.0	0.0	0.2	0.0	0.4	0.0	0.7	0.7	1.7	2.3	3.5	2.8	10.5	5.3	12.3	0.8	0	53	140
141	0.0	0.0	0.0	0.0	0.0	0.5	0.0	0.2	0.7	0.2	1.9	1.4	1.6	3.0	2.8	3.5	0.0	4.1	0.6	1	43	141
142	0.0	0.0	0.1	0.2	0.8	0.5	2.6	2.6	2.2	2.9	2.5	5.2	3.3	5.6	5.0	0.9	7.1	4.1	1.7	0	117	142
143-4	0.0	0.0	0.0	0.2	0.2	0.2	0.4	0.4	0.2	0.7	0.9	1.7	2.3	2.6	5.0	3.5	5.3	4.1	0.7	0	50	143-4
146	0.0	0.0	0.0	0.2	0.0	0.2	0.0	0.0	0.0	0.7	0.7	0.3	0.7	0.4	2.2	1.7	0.0	8.2	0.2	0	17	146
145,147-8	0.0	0.0	0.0	0.2	0.0	0.5	0.4	0.4	1.0	0.9	1.6	2.2	2.3	2.6	5.0	5.2	7.1	8.2	0.9	0	61	145,147-8
150	0.0	0.0	0.1	0.2	0.0	0.0	0.4	0.4	1.7	2.0	4.2	9.1	19.1	38.1	59.9	89.0	93.5	94.7	7.3	0	503	150
151	0.0	0.0	0.1	0.2	0.6	1.6	4.3	8.0	12.9	23.4	27.1	57.8	98.6	179.7	255.7	363.9	432.1	485.6	36.3	1	2511	151
152	0.0	0.0	0.1	0.0	0.0	0.9	0.0	0.2	0.2	0.7	1.4	1.4	3.0	1.3	3.9	7.9	12.3	0.0	0.7	0	50	152
153	0.0	0.0	0.1	0.2	0.2	0.5	0.9	1.3	3.8	6.1	8.1	16.2	21.0	45.0	58.2	79.4	114.6	98.8	8.8	2	609	153
154	0.0	0.0	0.1	0.4	0.0	0.5	0.4	1.1	2.2	4.7	7.9	12.7	17.1	32.9	46.0	47.1	52.9	41.2	6.2	1	428	154
155.0	0.0	0.0	0.0	0.0	0.0	0.0	0.0	0.2	0.7	1.1	0.5	1.1	3.6	6.9	2.2	6.1	10.6	12.3	0.9	0	62	155.0
155.1	0.0	0.0	0.0	0.0	0.0	0.0	0.0	0.2	1.0	1.6	1.6	2.2	8.5	9.5	13.9	15.7	12.3	0.0	1.8	1	127	155.1
156	0.0	0.0	0.0	0.0	0.0	0.0	0.2	0.2	0.2	0.5	0.9	1.9	3.9	7.8	11.1	14.0	22.9	24.7	1.5	0	101	156
157	0.0	0.2	0.1	0.0	0.2	0.5	0.2	1.1	2.6	1.8	6.7	12.4	19.1	28.6	43.8	42.8	51.1	57.6	5.7	0	394	157
160	0.0	0.0	0.0	0.0	0.0	0.2	0.0	0.2	0.5	1.1	1.6	1.4	1.3	3.0	5.5	4.4	3.5	8.2	0.8	0	54	160
161	0.0	0.0	0.1	0.0	0.0	0.5	0.0	0.9	0.7	0.5	0.9	1.7	0.3	3.5	0.6	3.5	0.0	0.0	0.5	0	34	161
162-3	0.0	0.0	0.1	0.2	0.2	0.0	0.9	1.3	2.2	5.2	6.5	12.1	15.1	21.6	33.8	36.6	40.6	20.6	5.0	0	344	162-3
170	0.0	0.0	0.0	0.0	1.3	2.0	6.9	21.5	48.4	71.6	68.3	65.5	92.0	96.1	102.1	103.8	105.8	115.2	30.4	9	2102	170
171	0.0	0.0	0.0	0.0	0.2	3.2	14.0	30.8	38.8	39.6	53.7	41.5	34.5	42.4	36.1	25.3	24.7	28.8	18.3	3	1265	171
172	0.0	0.0	0.0	0.0	0.4	0.5	1.1	3.4	9.3	20.5	31.7	40.7	37.1	36.4	34.4	20.1	21.2	20.6	10.7	3	742	172
173	0.0	0.0	0.0	0.0	0.2	0.7	0.4	0.2	0.0	0.5	0.2	0.2	0.0	0.0	0.0	0.0	0.0	0.0	0.1	0	10	173
174	0.0	0.0	0.0	0.0	0.0	0.5	0.4	1.5	1.9	5.0	8.1	5.2	8.9	6.5	7.8	12.2	8.8	20.6	2.5	0	175	174
175	0.0	0.2	1.1	1.7	1.9	2.3	4.5	5.4	10.1	17.6	24.1	30.3	30.9	42.4	31.1	33.2	28.2	8.2	10.4	1	722	175
176	0.2	0.0	0.0	0.0	0.8	0.2	0.4	0.4	0.7	2.9	4.9	4.1	7.2	16.0	14.4	20.9	28.2	28.8	2.8	2	192	176
180	3.0	0.8	0.0	0.2	0.0	0.2	0.9	1.7	1.9	1.6	4.2	6.6	11.8	14.3	16.1	27.1	24.7	0.0	3.5	1	242	180
181.0	0.2	0.0	0.3	0.4	0.0	0.2	0.0	0.6	0.5	0.9	1.6	2.2	6.9	5.2	10.0	21.8	19.4	12.3	1.7	1	117	181.0
190	0.0	0.0	0.3	0.8	1.0	1.8	1.7	3.0	3.4	3.8	3.7	6.6	4.6	4.8	6.1	5.2	8.8	12.3	2.3	1	161	190
191	0.2	0.2	0.3	0.2	2.1	1.6	3.4	4.3	12.0	18.2	27.3	43.5	62.1	90.5	123.7	144.9	192.2	279.8	21.0	22	1454	191
192	0.3	0.2	0.3	2.1	0.4	0.5	0.6	0.4	1.2	1.6	1.6	0.8	1.3	3.5	1.7	1.7	7.1	4.1	0.9	0	59	192
193	1.6	2.1	2.1	0.2	2.1	4.7	5.2	6.7	5.8	6.8	8.3	10.2	10.5	6.9	8.3	4.4	1.8	4.1	4.8	0	333	193
194	0.3	0.0	0.1	0.2	1.0	1.8	1.9	1.5	3.1	5.4	4.4	5.0	8.5	7.4	10.0	13.1	8.8	0.0	2.7	0	186	194
195	0.2	0.3	0.4	1.5	0.2	0.9	0.0	0.4	0.5	1.4	0.3	0.3	0.3	1.3	0.9	0.9	1.8	8.8	0.4	0	27	195
196	0.7	0.0	1.0	0.6	1.0	1.1	1.1	1.1	1.2	1.8	1.9	1.9	4.6	6.5	8.3	4.4	7.1	0.0	1.7	1	119	196
197	0.2	0.0	0.3	0.6	1.0	0.5	1.1	0.9	0.2	3.6	1.6	2.2	3.0	4.3	3.9	6.1	7.1	8.2	1.4	1	100	197
200	0.2	0.2	0.1	1.3	0.2	1.8	0.4	0.9	1.9	1.1	1.9	2.8	4.9	9.1	6.1	11.3	3.5	0.0	1.6	0	108	200
201	0.0	0.0	1.0	0.0	1.9	2.3	2.1	2.2	2.2	0.9	0.5	1.9	2.6	2.2	3.3	2.6	1.8	0.0	1.4	0	97	201
203	0.0	0.0	0.0	1.5	0.4	0.5	0.0	0.6	0.7	1.1	0.9	3.0	5.3	4.8	9.4	4.4	1.8	8.2	1.2	1	82	203
204	5.4	3.1	2.2	0.0	2.7	2.3	3.2	3.9	4.3	5.6	7.9	10.5	12.8	15.2	22.2	24.4	22.9	28.8	5.9	1	411	204
202,205	0.2	0.0	0.0	0.4	0.2	0.5	0.0	0.0	0.0	0.2	0.5	0.6	0.7	1.3	0.6	0.9	0.0	4.1	0.2	0	17	202,205
OTHER	0.8	0.0	0.3	0.4	0.2	1.1	0.9	2.6	4.1	6.5	11.4	16.0	21.4	37.7	67.7	115.2	179.9	214.0	10.8	3	747	OTHER
140-205	13.4	6.9	10.4	13.0	21.8	34.3	61.0	112.6	185.0	272.3	344.9	443.3	595.3	850.2	1077.6	1339.4	1576.7	1683.1	217.1	56	15026	140-205
RATE PER CASE IN PERIOD	0.16	0.15	0.14	0.19	0.21	0.23	0.21	0.22	0.24	0.23	0.23	0.28	0.33	0.43	0.55	0.87	1.76	4.12	0.01	–	–	RATE PER CASE IN PERIOD

GERMANY, FEDERAL REPUBLIC, HAMBURG

Registry Title and Address : Hamburg Cancer Statistical Survey, Statistisches Landesamt, City of Hamburg, 2 Hamburg 11, Steckelhörn 12. West Germany. Commenced in 1927, but in its present form since 1954. Supported financially by the city of Hamburg.

Registration. Cases are registered from hospital in-patients and out-patients by house physicians, from radiotherapy and pathology departments by doctors in charge, and from the Registry Offices from death certificates issued by doctors. Registration is thought to be a hundred per cent.

Follow-up. All registrations are followed up for 5 years except for cases of disease of the female reproductive organs which are followed up for 10 years.

Physical Description. The limits of the area covered by the registry are the regional boundary of the city of Hamburg, which lies on the Elbe 120 kilometres from the estuary. The district is part of the north German lowland and lies between latitudes 53°24' and 53°44' morth and longitudes 9°44' and 10°19' east. The total registration area is 747 square kilometres.

Demographic Description. Total population of area under survey 1,835,340. The population comprises 76.6 % Protestant/Lutheran, 7.4 % Catholic, 14.2 % others. The main occupational composition of the working population is industry 38.7 %, commerce 18.9 %, agriculture 1.5 % and personal service 40.9 %.

Medical Services. Total number of hospital beds of all kinds 20,072 (1965). Total number of doctors in practice in registration area 4,003 (1965). Cancer causes approximately 21 % of all deaths, (1964).

Publications. Annual reports in Statistisches Jahrbuch der Freien und Hansestadt der Hamburg.

Mode of operation of the Registry is described in Hamburg in Zahlen, Heft 4, 1957.

TABLE 27 A
GERMANY, FEDERAL REPUBLIC, HAMBURG :
POPULATION (100,000s), MEAN 1960 - 62

AGE (in years)	MALES No.	MALES Per Cent	FEMALES No.	FEMALES Per Cent
0 –	3.6019	42.50	3.4824	35.25
30 –	0.5655	6.67	0.6088	6.16
35 –	0.5161	6.09	0.6939	7.02
40 –	0.4208	4.97	0.5788	5.86
45 –	0.5376	6.34	0.7010	7.10
50 –	0.6481	7.65	0.8123	8.22
55 –	0.6494	7.66	0.7596	7.69
60 –	0.5194	6.13	0.6968	7.05
65 –	0.3813	4.50	0.5985	6.06
70 –	0.3001	3.54	0.4428	4.48
75 –	0.1960	2.31	0.2829	2.86
80 –	0.0999	1.18	0.1536	1.55
85 – and over	0.0388	0.46	0.0671	0.68
TOTAL	8.4749	100.00	9.8785	100.00

NOTES

TO TABLES 27 A, B and C

(I)   I.L. numbers 142 to 148 grouped together.
     "   "   193 excludes benign and unspecified tu-
                 mours of the central nervous system.
     "   "   203 included with 202 and 205.

(II)   Carcinoma in situ excluded.

TABLE 27 B

GERMANY, FEDERAL REPUBLIC, HAMBURG :

MALE INCIDENCE RATES, 1960 - 62.

INTER-NATIONAL LIST No.	AVERAGE ANNUAL INCIDENCE PER 100,000 — AGE IN YEARS																		ALL AGES	No. OF CASES IN WHOLE PERIOD — AGE UNKNOWN	No. OF CASES IN WHOLE PERIOD — ALL AGES	INTER-NATIONAL LIST No.
	0-	5-	10-	15-	20-	25-	30-	35-	40-	45-	50-	55-	60-	65-	70-	75-	80-	85- AND OVER				
140							1.2	0.6	0.8	0.6	6.2	2.6	5.8	9.6	7.8	1.7	10.0	0.0	2.1	0	54	140
141							0.0	0.0	0.8	0.6	1.0	2.1	3.2	4.4	6.7	5.1	10.0	8.6	1.2	0	31	141
142-8							2.4	2.6	4.0	2.5	7.2	10.3	14.1	14.0	16.7	18.7	20.0	51.5	5.3	0	134	142-8
150							0.6	0.6	1.6	1.9	6.7	7.7	21.2	25.4	42.2	54.4	56.7	111.7	7.7	0	197	150
151							2.9	3.9	7.9	25.4	44.2	83.7	133.5	234.3	324.3	420.1	500.5	635.7	61.1	0	1554	151
152							0.0	0.0	0.0	0.0	1.0	1.5	3.2	0.9	1.1	1.7	3.3	17.2	0.6	0	16	152
153							2.4	2.6	3.2	8.1	10.3	19.0	36.6	58.6	97.7	158.2	190.2	240.5	18.9	0	480	153
154							0.6	0.6	2.4	6.2	12.3	20.5	36.6	57.7	104.4	139.5	176.8	171.8	17.7	0	451	154
155							0.6	0.6	3.2	2.5	6.7	21.0	37.2	43.7	82.2	86.7	96.8	146.0	13.5	0	343	155
156							0.0	0.6	1.6	0.0	2.1	3.6	6.4	4.4	15.6	8.5	16.7	43.0	2.3	0	59	156
157							0.0	2.6	6.3	9.9	8.7	12.3	30.2	44.6	55.5	62.9	76.7	111.7	11.4	0	291	157
160							0.0	0.0	0.0	1.2	0.5	2.1	1.9	4.4	3.3	1.7	6.7	8.6	0.9	0	22	160
161							0.0	0.0	3.2	5.0	10.8	12.8	25.7	22.7	27.8	23.8	23.4	25.8	6.9	0	175	161
162-3							1.8	5.8	10.3	45.3	106.5	204.3	335.0	444.1	435.4	340.1	260.3	197.6	95.6	0	2431	162-3
170							0.0	0.0	0.0	0.6	1.5	2.6	3.2	1.7	2.2	6.8	13.3	0.0	1.0	0	26	170
177							0.0	0.0	1.6	3.7	4.1	13.3	44.3	94.4	161.1	297.6	393.7	532.6	28.3	0	719	177
178							9.4	4.5	4.0	3.7	1.0	2.6	1.3	2.6	2.2	3.4	0.0	8.6	2.7	0	68	178
179							0.0	0.0	0.8	1.2	0.5	1.5	1.9	2.6	5.6	3.4	13.3	8.6	1.0	0	25	179
180-1							1.2	2.6	7.1	19.2	24.7	47.2	68.7	87.4	127.7	151.4	143.5	240.5	26.6	0	676	180-1
190-1							5.9	5.8	13.5	15.5	18.5	20.5	22.5	28.0	37.8	73.1	76.7	120.3	12.9	0	329	190-1
192							1.2	1.3	0.8	0.0	0.5	1.0	1.3	2.6	1.1	0.0	0.0	0.0	0.6	0	16	192
193							1.2	4.5	7.9	3.7	9.3	14.4	15.4	7.9	5.6	1.7	6.7	0.0	5.1	0	130	193
194							0.0	0.6	0.8	1.2	0.5	3.6	3.9	7.9	3.3	0.0	3.3	0.0	1.3	0	32	194
195							1.2	1.9	0.0	0.6	0.5	0.0	1.3	2.6	1.1	0.0	3.3	0.0	0.6	0	14	195
196							1.2	1.9	0.8	1.9	3.6	4.1	7.1	6.1	5.6	11.9	6.7	17.2	3.0	0	77	196
197							0.6	0.6	0.0	0.6	0.0	2.6	0.6	0.0	1.1	6.8	0.0	0.0	0.7	0	18	197
200							2.4	2.6	3.2	5.0	5.7	5.6	7.7	11.4	10.0	18.7	6.7	8.6	4.1	0	104	200
201							2.4	4.5	4.0	1.2	5.7	4.6	5.1	11.4	7.8	8.5	6.7	8.6	3.4	0	86	201
204							5.9	2.6	4.0	10.5	7.2	8.7	9.6	23.6	30.0	35.7	40.0	17.2	8.0	0	204	204
202,203-5							0.6	1.9	1.6	1.9	5.7	6.2	9.6	14.0	11.1	15.3	10.0	8.6	3.4	0	86	202,203-5
OTHER							2.9	1.3	3.2	11.2	11.8	15.9	28.9	40.2	48.9	64.6	90.1	120.3	12.0	0	304	OTHER
140-205							48.3	57.5	98.2	191.0	325.1	558.0	922.9	1313.1	1682.8	2022.1	2262.3	2852.2	360.0	0	9152	140-205
RATE PER CASE IN PERIOD							0.59	0.65	0.79	0.62	0.51	0.51	0.64	0.87	1.11	1.70	3.34	8.59	0.04	-	-	RATE PER CASE IN PERIOD

TABLE 27 C

GERMANY, FEDERAL REPUBLIC, HAMBURG :

FEMALE INCIDENCE RATES, 1960 - 62.

INTER-NATIONAL LIST No.	AVERAGE ANNUAL INCIDENCE PER 100,000 — AGE IN YEARS																		ALL AGES	No. OF CASES IN WHOLE PERIOD — AGE UNKNOWN	ALL AGES	INTER-NATIONAL LIST No.
	0-	5-	10-	15-	20-	25-	30-	35-	40-	45-	50-	55-	60-	65-	70-	75-	80-	85- AND OVER				
140							0.0	0.5	0.0	0.5	0.0	0.0	0.0	0.0	3.0	0.0	0.0	5.0	0.2	0	7	140
141							0.0	0.0	0.6	1.0	0.8	0.4	0.0	1.1	2.3	3.5	6.5	0.0	0.6	0	18	141
142-8							1.6	3.8	2.9	1.4	2.9	5.3	8.6	8.4	9.0	9.4	17.4	19.9	3.8	0	112	142-8
150							0.0	0.0	0.0	0.0	0.4	1.3	2.4	3.3	8.3	14.1	19.5	29.8	1.8	0	53	150
151							1.6	7.2	7.5	13.8	22.6	29.0	57.9	109.7	161.8	228.6	290.8	481.9	38.6	0	1144	151
152							0.0	0.0	0.6	0.5	0.4	0.9	2.4	3.9	3.0	2.4	6.5	5.0	0.9	0	28	152
153							1.1	2.4	3.5	9.0	12.3	24.6	50.2	64.0	110.7	126.1	191.0	193.7	24.4	0	724	153
154							1.6	1.4	5.2	9.5	10.3	17.1	32.1	31.7	49.7	69.5	78.1	99.4	13.7	0	406	154
155							0.5	0.5	1.7	6.2	11.9	19.3	34.0	49.6	88.8	107.2	125.9	154.0	18.5	0	549	155
156							0.0	0.5	1.2	1.0	1.2	2.6	2.4	5.0	7.5	9.4	8.7	9.9	1.8	0	53	156
157							0.0	0.5	1.2	3.3	5.3	11.8	22.0	26.7	39.1	44.8	43.4	54.6	8.9	0	265	157
160							0.0	0.5	0.0	1.4	0.8	1.3	0.5	1.7	3.8	3.5	4.3	0.0	0.8	0	25	160
161							0.0	0.5	0.6	0.0	1.2	3.1	2.4	1.1	2.3	1.2	2.2	5.0	0.8	0	25	161
162-3							0.5	1.9	5.8	11.9	14.4	22.4	34.0	41.2	51.2	58.9	49.9	54.6	14.3	0	423	162-3
170							16.4	29.8	73.7	109.8	84.9	92.6	119.6	133.7	152.8	149.6	193.1	273.2	62.1	0	1841	170
171							31.8	79.3	110.0	107.5	96.8	81.6	74.6	57.4	54.2	48.3	52.1	34.8	50.6	0	1501	171
172-4							4.4	5.8	13.2	28.5	42.7	43.9	44.5	51.2	61.0	40.1	30.4	54.6	21.6	0	639	172-4
175-6							7.7	9.1	19.6	35.7	47.2	49.6	65.1	75.2	65.5	87.2	89.0	59.6	29.6	0	876	175-6
180-1							0.0	1.9	1.2	5.2	7.0	11.4	24.4	26.7	21.8	37.7	56.4	54.6	9.2	0	273	180-1
190-1							5.5	5.3	11.5	9.5	20.1	11.4	16.3	13.9	21.8	29.5	21.7	44.7	9.5	0	283	190-1
192							0.5	0.0	0.0	0.0	0.0	0.4	1.4	0.0	0.8	2.4	2.2	5.0	0.4	0	11	192
193							2.2	1.9	2.9	2.9	8.6	6.6	7.7	6.7	3.8	2.4	4.3	0.0	3.4	0	101	193
194							0.5	1.0	0.0	2.4	1.6	1.3	3.3	2.2	4.5	9.4	2.2	14.9	1.6	0	46	194
195							0.0	0.0	0.6	0.5	0.8	0.0	1.0	1.1	1.5	0.0	0.0	0.0	0.4	0	11	195
196							0.0	1.0	0.6	1.4	1.6	4.8	3.3	3.3	7.5	9.4	8.7	14.9	2.1	0	61	196
197							0.5	0.5	1.7	0.0	1.6	2.2	2.4	1.7	2.3	2.4	0.0	0.0	0.9	0	27	197
200							0.0	1.0	3.5	0.5	0.8	4.8	6.2	5.6	6.0	11.8	10.9	9.9	2.5	0	73	200
201							1.6	3.4	2.3	2.4	2.5	2.6	2.4	4.5	6.8	8.2	6.5	14.9	2.6	0	77	201
204							2.7	1.0	5.2	4.8	4.5	8.3	9.6	17.3	23.3	15.3	32.6	14.9	6.3	0	188	204
202,203-5							0.5	0.0	0.0	0.5	1.2	3.1	3.8	3.9	9.0	9.4	13.0	14.9	2.0	0	59	202,203-5
OTHER							2.2	1.9	2.3	8.1	9.4	16.7	17.7	31.2	49.7	62.4	73.8	173.9	13.0	0	384	OTHER
140-205							84.3	162.4	278.7	379.0	416.1	482.7	652.0	783.1	1038.1	1204.2	1441.0	1897.7	347.0	0	10283	140-205
RATE PER CASE IN PERIOD							0.55	0.48	0.58	0.48	0.41	0.44	0.48	0.56	0.75	1.18	2.17	4.97	0.03	-	-	RATE PER CASE IN PERIOD

Note : Figures in column 30— relate to the years 0 to 34.

ICELAND

The Icelandic Cancer Registry started on 1st January 1954 as a voluntary organization under the auspices of the Icelandic Cancer Society.

The Registry's material is based on three main sources. In the first place the Registry receives reports from every hospital in Iceland, on all cases of cancer entering each hospital. In Iceland almost every cancer patient will sooner or later enter hospital for treatment or care. The doctors get a token payment of 50.00 Icelandic Kronur (approximately 8/2d) for each case notified for the first time, paid by the Icelandic Cancer Society. In the second place all cases histologically diagnosed at the Department of Pathology, University of Iceland, are notified and also every case of cancer found at autopsy (including forensic necropsies). The Department of Pathology is the only institute in Iceland where histo-pathologic examinations on human cancers are carried out and where practically all autopsies are done. Lastly all the death certificates received by the Statistical Bureau of Iceland are searched and cases of cancer collected and compared with the material received from the hospitals and the Pathology Department. A death certificate written by a doctor is now issued for every person dying in Iceland. In this way the Registry is supposed to receive reports on practically all cases of cancer diagnosed in Iceland.

The data recorded include : name of patient, date and place of birth, marital status, occupation, place of residence, name of hospital and hospital record number, date of admission and discharge, clinical and pathological diagnoses, treatment (surgery, radiation, other or none) dates of first symptoms and first visit to doctor, state on discharge, and, if dead, cause and date of death and result of postmortem examination.

Geography and demography of Iceland.

Iceland is an island situated in the Northern Atlantic close to the Arctic Circle. It comprises an area of 103,000 square kilometres. Hospitals are located in 6 places on the south east coast, 2 on the north east, 6 on the north and 2 on the west. In each place there is only one hospital located except in Reykjavik where 5 hospitals report to the Registry.

At the 1st December 1960 the population amounted to 177,892 (89,892 males and 88,000 females). At that time approximately 40 per cent of the population was living in Reykjavik the capital (35,417 males and 37,227 females). The remainder of the people was living in small coastal towns and villages and in rural areas. The distribution of the population by age and sex is given in Table 28A.

During 1960, 4,916 children were born alive and 1,167 persons died, including 131 males and 156 females from neoplastic diseases (Int. List numbers 140-205). The general death rate was 6.6. per 1,000 and the rate of live births 28.0. An autopsy was performed on 317 per 1,000 of those who died in the whole country during the year 1960. The infant mortality rate was 13.0. The expectation of life was 70.7 years for men and 75.0 for women based on the mortality statistics for the period 1951-60.

The registry material

The material includes all malignant neoplasms diagnosed for the first time during the nine years period 1955-63 among residents of Iceland. Papillomas of the urinary tract are also included, as are all neoplasms of the central nervous system, whether benign or malignant, diagnosed during the same period. The material registered during the first year (1954) is not included as it was assumed that among these cases were probably found some patients who actually were diagnosed for the first time in the preceding year or years.

168

The total number of new cases reported to have been diagnosed during the nine years period was 3, 305 of which 1, 620 were males and 1, 685 females. The crude incidence per 100, 000 population per year was 200. 2 for males and 212. 5 for females. In these calculations the census figures for the year 1960 are taken as the mean.

The whole material is arranged according to site and age in two tables of which Table 28B gives the male component and Table 28C the female component. From Appendix Tables 1 and 2 it is also to be seen that 73. 7 per cent of the cancers in males and 79. 9 per cent of the cancers in females had been verified by histological examination.

Appendix Tables 3 and 4 also show the number of cases notified on death certificates only and which have never been diagnosed in hospital. These comprise 5. 4 per cent of all the male and 4. 6 per cent of all the female cases.

All cases are classified in accordance with the International Statistical Classification of Diseases, Injuries and Causes of Death. The percentage distribution of the material by site groups is as follows :

International List No.	Site	Percentage	
		Males	Females
140-148	Lip, tongue, buccal cavity, pharynx	4.6	1.8
150-157	Digestive organs	49.7	33.4
160-163	Respiratory system	7.5	3.1
170-179	Breast and genital organs	9.7	37.4
180-181	Urinary organs	7.2	5.3
190-199	Other, and unspecified sites	13.3	14.9
200-205	Lymphatic and hemopoetic tissues	6.9	4.0

Conspicuous features are the high relative frequency rate of cancer of the digestive system in both sexes, but especially in the male, and the low rate of cancer of the respiratory system. If benign papillomas are excluded the percentage in the urinary organs will be 6.8 for males and 5.0 for females.

The percentage distribution by single organ sites is as follows :

Females				Males			
Hier-archical position	Site	Number of cases	per cent	Hier-archical position	Site	Number of cases	Per cent
1.	Breast	315	18.69	1.	Stomach	547	33.77
2.	Stomach	278	16.50	2.	Prostate	133	8.21
3.	Cervix uteri	124	7.36	3.	Carcinoma of skin	98	6.05
4.	Colon	116	6.88	4.	Lung	96	5.93
5.	Ovary, tube	98	5.82	5.	Colon	75	4.63
6.	Carcinoma of skin	72	4.27	6.	Kidney	69	4.26
7.	Corpus uteri	61	3.62	7.	Leukaemia	67	4.14
8.	Thyroid gland	60	3.56	8.	Nervous system	62	3.83
9.	ureter, Kidney	59	3.50	9.	Oesophagus	59	3.64
10.	Oesophagus	54	3.20	10.	Lip	50	3.29

The stomach is by far the most frequent site in the male, but takes the second place in the female preceded by the breast. Carcinoma of the lung is in the fourth place in the male, which certainly shows a remarkable rise in frequency. Comparable morbidity figures cannot be quoted for 20-30 years ago, but mortality figures show that lung cancer was an exceptionally rare diseare (Dungal, 1950). It is to be noted that the relatively high incidence rate of carcinoma of the skin includes also all basal-cell carcinomas of the skin.

Malignant tumours of lip, tongue, oral cavity and pharynx.

The malignant tumours in this region are relatively rare amounting to 4.6 per cent of the total in the male and 1.8 per cent of the total in the female. The male preponderance of carcinoma of the lip is especially conspicuous being 50:1. On the other hand the frequency of the other sites is similar in both sexes as can be seen from the figures below.

A few cases of doubtful malignancy of these sites have also been reported, 3 for males and 1 for females; these are not included in the figures presented.

Of the malignant tumours of the lip and buccal cavity 91 per cent were histologically confirmed in the male and 80 per cent in the female.

International List No.	Site	Males	Females
140	Lip	50	1
141	Tongue	5	6
142	Salivary glands	3	8
143-4	Other mouth	4	2
146	Nasopharynx	9	10
145, 147-8	Other pharynx	3	3

Malignant tumours of the digestive tract.

During the period 1955-63, a total of 1,368 new cases of the digestive organs were diagnosed in Iceland or 41.3 per cent of the whole material. For males the percentage was 49.7 per cent and for females 33.4 per cent. The distribution between different sites is as follows :

International List No.	Site	Males	Females
150	Oesophagus	59	54
151	Stomach	547	278
152	Duodenum, small intestine	8	5
153	Colon	75	116
154	Rectum	34	33
155	Biliary passages and liver primary	20	25
156	Liver secondary and unspecified	15	17
157	Pancreas	47	35

Cancer of the stomach is by far the most frequent form of cancer in males, accounting for 33.8 per cent of all cancers in males and 16.5 per cent of all cancers in females, exceeded in females only by cancer of the breast. During the nine years period the annual incidence of stomach cancer was 67.7 per 100,000 for men and 35.1 per 100,000 for women, the crude incidence for men being almost twice as high as for women.

Of the other digestive organs only the colon shows a noteworthy sex difference as 75 cancers occurred in the colon in males against 116 in females.

The percentage of histologically verified diagnoses for the digestive organs varies from 47 per cent for liver, secondary and unspecified, in women up to

100 per cent for duodenum in both sexes. The percentage of histologically verified stomach cancers was 67.8 per cent in men and 57.2 per cent in women, and colon cancers 70.6 per cent in men and 75.0 per cent in women.

Malignant tumours of respiratory system.

During the period 1955-63 new cases of cancer of the trachea, bronchus and lung primary were diagnosed in 96 males and 44 females which constitutes 5.9 per cent of all cancers in males and 2.6 per cent in females. The annual incidence was 11.9 per 100,000 for men and 5.6 per 100,000 for women.

Breast and genital organs.

Cancer of the breast is on the top of the list of relative frequency of cancer localizations in women, constituting 18.7 per cent of all cancers. Cancer of the uterine cervix is third in relative frequency accounting for 7.4 per cent of cases. The incidence of cervical cancer is fairly low in Iceland although it has increased somewhat during the last three decades (Bjarnason, 1963).

Of carcinoma of the breast 95.9 per cent have been verified by histological examination and of carcinoma of the cervix uteri 95.2 per cent. During this period 27 cases of carcinoma-in-situ were reported to the registry. That is, 3 cases of carcinoma-in-situ against 14 cases of invasive carcinoma per year. It should be pointed out that during the first years of this period carcinoma-in-situ was not reported although this diagnosis was made, so obviously the figure given above does not even represent the right number of diagnosed cases in the community during this time. The carcinoma-in-situ cases are not included in the figures for cancer of cervix presented in the tables. The carcinoma of cervix to carcinoma of corpus ratio was 2:1.

Cancer of the prostate comes next in frequency to gastric cancer in the male, being 8.2 per cent of the whole male cancer material. There were also reported 9 cases of doubtful malignancy of prostate during the same period.

Tumours of urinary organs.

Papillomas of the urinary tract are included in the figures given in the tables; the age and sex distribution of these cases is as follows :

	Age in years									
Sex	40-44	45-49	50-54	55-59	60-64	65-69	70-74	75-79	80-	All ages
M	0	1	1	2	1	0	0	2	0	7
F	1	0	1	1	1	1	0	0	0	5

Cancers of the urinary organs account for 117 cases in men, including 69 of the kidney, and 90 in women, including 59 of the kidney. Cancer of the kidney is the sixth most common type in men, constituting 4.3 per cent of all cancers, and the ninth most common type in women comprising 3.5 per cent of the total.

Malignant tumours of other and unspecified sites.

Malignant tumours of skin are third in the list of frequency according to site in men accounting for 6.1 per cent of all cancers, and sixth in the site frequency list for women making 4.3 per cent of all cancers.

The brain and other parts of the nervous system account for 62 tumours in men and 49 in women. In these figures are included both benign and malignant tumours of the central nervous system.

Of the endocrine glands the thyroid is the site of most of the malignant tumours. There were 14 cases of thyroid carcinoma in males and 60 in females, the male : female ratio being 1:4,3.

The leukaemias are the most common malignancies of the lymphatic and haemopoietic tissues, accounting for 67 cases in men and 37 cases in women. In the male 20 per cent of cases occur below the age of 10 years and in the female 19 per cent.

O. Bjarnason

Registry Title and Address : The Icelandic Cancer Registry, Department of Pathology, University of Iceland, P. O. Box 150, Reykjavik, Iceland. Commenced 1st January, 1954. Supported financially by the Icelandic Cancer Society.

Registration. Cases are registered by doctors from hospital in-patients and out-patients, from radiotherapy and pathology departments, and from death certificates by the Statistical Bureau of Iceland.

Follow-up. The Registry receives additional information on all patients registered whenever they enter hospital again. They are followed up until death.

Physical Description. The Registry covers the whole of Iceland which is an island in the North Atlantic near the Arctic Circle. It lies between latitudes 63°23' and 66°33' North and longitudes 13°22' and 24°35' West. The total registration area is 103,000 square kilometres.

Demographic Description. Total population of area under survey 177.880. The population is 100% Caucasian (mainly Nordic with some Celtic admixture). The religious groups are : Lutheran 97.7%, other Christian 1.18%, and others 1.12%. The main occupational composition is : industry 34.96%, commerce 19.19%, agriculture 33.02%, personal service 12.5% and other 0.33%, (1950).

Medical Services. Total number of hospital beds of all kinds 1,115 (1960). Total number of doctors in practice in registration area 221 (1960). Cancer caused approximately 20% of all deaths in 1964.

Publications. Annual reports in the Chief Medical Officer's annual reports on public health. Bjarnason (1963); Snaedal (1964).

TABLE 28 A
ICELAND :
POPULATION (100, 000s), CENSUS 1960

AGE (In years)	MALES		FEMALES	
	No.	Per Cent	No.	Per Cent
0 –	0.1194	13.28	0.1122	12.75
5 –	0.1058	11.77	0.1006	11.43
10 –	0.0943	10.49	0.0875	9.94
15 –	0.0743	8.27	0.0726	8.25
20 –	0.0591	6.57	0.0577	6.56
25 –	0.0610	6.79	0.0587	6.67
30 –	0.0612	6.81	0.0591	6.72
35 –	0.0564	6.27	0.0531	6.03
40 –	0.0499	5.55	0.0477	5.42
45 –	0.0446	4.96	0.0447	5.08
50 –	0.0407	4.53	0.0394	4.48
55 –	0.0363	4.04	0.0351	3.99
60 –	0.0308	3.43	0.0324	3.68
65 –	0.0269	2.99	0.0296	3.36
70 –	0.0174	1.94	0.0199	2.26
75 –	0.0110	1.22	0.0140	1.59
80 –	0.0063	0.70	0.0090	1.02
85 – and over	0.0035	0.39	0.0066	0.75
TOTAL	0.8989	100.00	0.8799	100.00

NOTES

TO TABLES 28 A, B and C

(I)   I.L. number 181.0 includes papilloma of bladder.
      "   "   193 includes benign and unspecified tu-
           mours of the central nervous system.

(II) Carcinoma in situ excluded.

TABLE 28 B
ICELAND :
MALE INCIDENCE RATES, 1955 - 63.

INTER-NATIONAL LIST No.	AVERAGE ANNUAL INCIDENCE PER 100,000 — AGE IN YEARS																		ALL AGES	No. OF CASES IN WHOLE PERIOD — AGE UNKNOWN	No. OF CASES IN WHOLE PERIOD — ALL AGES	INTER-NATIONAL LIST No.
	0-	5-	10-	15-	20-	25-	30-	35-	40-	45-	50-	55-	60-	65-	70-	75-	80-	85- and over				
140	0.0	0.0	0.0	0.0	0.0	0.0	0.0	0.0	0.0	7.5	13.7	18.4	28.9	28.9	51.1	50.5	88.2	95.2	6.2	0	50	140
141	0.0	0.0	0.0	0.0	0.0	0.0	1.8	2.0	0.0	0.0	0.0	3.1	0.0	0.0	6.4	0.0	0.0	31.7	0.6	0	5	141
142	0.0	0.0	0.0	0.0	0.0	0.0	1.8	0.0	0.0	0.0	0.0	0.0	3.6	4.1	0.0	0.0	0.0	0.0	0.4	0	3	142
143-4	0.0	0.0	0.0	0.0	0.0	0.0	0.0	0.0	0.0	0.0	0.0	0.0	3.6	0.0	6.4	0.0	35.3	0.0	0.5	0	4	143-4
146	0.0	0.0	0.0	0.0	0.0	0.0	1.8	0.0	0.0	0.0	5.5	3.1	3.6	4.1	6.4	0.0	17.6	31.7	1.1	0	9	146
145,147-8	0.0	0.0	0.0	0.0	0.0	0.0	0.0	0.0	4.5	7.5	5.5	0.0	3.6	4.1	0.0	10.1	0.0	0.0	0.4	1	3	145,147-8
150	0.0	0.0	0.0	0.0	0.0	0.0	3.6	9.9	26.7	54.8	158.3	122.2	25.3	33.0	44.7	50.5	158.7	349.2	7.3	1	59	150
151	0.0	0.0	0.0	0.0	0.0	0.0	0.0	2.0	2.2	0.0	2.7	162.2	295.8	351.1	549.2	727.3	687.8	952.4	67.6	1	547	151
152	0.0	0.0	0.0	0.0	1.9	0.0	0.0	0.0	2.2	0.0	0.0	0.0	7.2	4.1	0.0	0.0	0.0	0.0	1.0	0	8	152
153	0.0	0.0	0.0	1.5	0.0	0.0	1.8	0.0	2.2	7.5	10.9	15.3	28.8	37.2	89.4	111.1	194.0	158.7	9.3	2	75	153
154	0.0	0.0	0.0	0.0	0.0	0.0	0.0	0.0	2.2	2.5	16.4	12.2	18.0	12.4	38.3	40.4	35.3	63.5	4.2	0	34	154
155	0.0	0.0	1.2	0.0	0.0	0.0	0.0	0.0	2.2	2.5	2.7	3.1	14.4	16.5	19.2	20.2	17.6	31.7	2.5	0	20	155
156	0.0	0.0	0.0	0.0	0.0	0.0	0.0	0.0	0.0	0.0	2.7	6.1	0.0	12.4	31.9	0.0	0.0	127.0	1.9	0	15	156
157	0.0	0.0	0.0	0.0	0.0	1.8	0.0	0.0	2.2	2.5	5.5	15.3	18.0	28.9	57.5	111.1	105.8	31.7	5.8	0	47	157
160	0.0	0.0	0.0	0.0	0.0	0.0	0.0	0.0	0.0	2.5	0.0	3.1	3.6	4.1	6.4	0.0	52.9	31.7	1.2	0	10	160
161	0.0	0.0	0.0	0.0	0.0	1.8	0.0	0.0	0.0	0.0	5.5	3.1	10.8	8.3	12.8	10.1	35.3	0.0	1.6	0	13	161
162-3	0.0	0.0	0.0	0.0	1.9	1.8	0.0	3.9	8.9	14.9	54.6	58.2	50.5	53.7	38.3	80.8	17.6	31.7	12.0	1	97	162-3
170	0.0	0.0	0.0	0.0	0.0	0.0	0.0	0.0	0.0	0.0	0.0	0.0	0.0	4.1	0.0	0.0	0.0	0.0	0.1	2	1	170
177	0.0	0.0	0.0	0.0	0.0	7.3	0.0	0.0	2.2	2.5	5.5	18.4	36.1	78.5	159.6	282.8	458.6	412.7	16.4	1	133	177
178	0.0	0.0	0.0	0.0	3.8	0.0	0.0	5.9	2.2	2.5	2.7	3.1	0.0	0.0	0.0	10.1	0.0	31.7	1.9	0	15	178
179.0	0.0	0.0	0.0	0.0	0.0	0.0	0.0	0.0	0.0	0.0	0.0	0.0	0.0	8.3	12.8	20.2	17.6	31.7	1.0	0	8	179.0
180	1.9	0.0	1.2	0.0	0.0	0.0	0.0	2.0	4.5	27.4	21.8	24.5	21.6	53.7	31.9	50.5	70.5	95.2	8.5	0	69	180
181.0	0.9	0.0	0.0	0.0	0.0	0.0	0.0	0.0	10.9	14.9	10.9	12.2	18.0	33.0	44.7	60.6	105.8	31.7	5.9	2	48	181.0
190	0.0	0.0	0.0	0.0	0.0	0.0	0.0	0.0	0.0	0.0	0.0	0.0	0.0	4.1	12.8	30.3	0.0	0.0	0.7	0	6	190
191	0.9	0.0	0.0	0.0	1.9	1.8	0.0	9.9	13.4	7.5	10.9	21.4	64.9	37.2	70.2	141.4	158.7	254.0	12.1	0	98	191
192	0.9	1.1	0.0	0.0	0.0	0.0	0.0	0.0	2.2	0.0	0.0	0.0	7.2	7.2	7.2	0.0	0.0	31.7	0.7	0	6	192
193	1.9	2.1	5.9	1.5	3.8	3.6	9.1	7.9	4.5	12.5	16.4	33.7	18.0	12.4	19.2	20.2	35.3	31.7	7.7	0	62	193
194	0.0	0.0	0.0	1.5	0.0	0.0	0.0	0.0	0.0	2.5	2.7	0.0	10.8	8.3	19.2	10.1	17.6	31.7	1.7	0	14	194
195	0.0	0.0	0.0	0.0	0.0	1.8	0.0	0.0	0.0	0.0	0.0	6.1	3.6	4.1	0.0	0.0	0.0	0.0	0.6	0	5	195
196	0.0	0.0	1.2	3.0	1.9	1.8	1.8	0.0	0.0	0.0	5.5	3.1	7.2	8.3	0.0	10.1	17.6	0.0	1.6	0	13	196
197	0.0	2.1	0.0	0.0	0.0	1.8	0.0	0.0	2.2	0.0	0.0	3.1	7.2	4.1	6.4	30.3	0.0	63.5	1.5	2	12	197
200	0.0	0.0	0.0	3.0	3.8	1.8	3.6	0.0	4.5	5.0	8.2	9.2	3.6	8.3	0.0	0.0	0.0	31.7	2.8	0	23	200
201	0.0	0.0	0.0	0.0	0.0	1.8	1.8	2.0	0.0	0.0	0.0	0.0	0.0	8.3	0.0	0.0	31.7	0.0	1.4	0	11	201
203	0.0	0.0	0.0	0.0	0.0	0.0	0.0	0.0	0.0	0.0	0.0	0.0	7.2	8.3	19.2	0.0	0.0	0.0	1.0	1	8	203
204	10.2	3.2	3.5	1.5	7.5	0.0	3.6	3.9	6.7	12.5	5.5	12.2	28.9	33.0	25.5	30.3	70.5	0.0	8.3	0	67	204
202,205	0.9	0.0	0.0	0.0	0.0	0.0	0.0	0.0	0.0	0.0	0.0	3.1	0.0	0.0	0.0	0.0	0.0	0.0	0.2	0	2	202,205
OTHER	0.0	0.0	1.2	1.5	0.0	0.0	0.0	0.0	4.5	5.0	2.7	0.0	3.6	16.5	6.4	30.3	35.3	63.5	2.5	0	20	OTHER
140-205	16.8	8.4	14.1	13.5	26.3	23.7	30.9	49.3	98.0	196.8	376.7	465.3	754.0	929.4	1398.5	1959.6	2433.9	2952.4	200.2	13	1620	140-205
RATE PER CASE IN PERIOD	0.93	1.05	1.18	1.50	1.88	1.82	1.82	1.97	2.23	2.49	2.73	3.06	3.61	4.13	6.39	10.10	17.64	31.75	0.12	-	-	RATE PER CASE IN PERIOD

TABLE 28 C

ICELAND :

FEMALE INCIDENCE RATES, 1955 - 63.

AVERAGE ANNUAL INCIDENCE PER 100,000 — AGE IN YEARS

INTER-NATIONAL LIST No.	0-	5-	10-	15-	20-	25-	30-	35-	40-	45-	50-	55-	60-	65-	70-	75-	80-	85- AND OVER	ALL AGES	No. CASES AGE UNKNOWN	No. CASES ALL AGES	INTER-NATIONAL LIST No.
140	0.0	0.0	0.0	0.0	0.0	0.0	0.0	0.0	0.0	0.0	0.0	0.0	0.0	0.0	5.6	0.0	0.0	0.0	0.1	0	1	140
141	0.0	0.0	0.0	0.0	0.0	0.0	0.0	0.0	0.0	0.0	0.0	0.0	0.0	0.0	5.6	0.0	37.0	0.0	0.8	2	6	141
142	0.0	0.0	0.0	0.0	0.0	0.0	0.0	2.1	0.0	2.5	0.0	3.2	0.0	0.0	16.8	0.0	0.0	16.8	1.0	1	8	142
143-4	0.0	0.0	0.0	0.0	0.0	0.0	0.0	0.0	0.0	0.0	0.0	0.0	3.4	0.0	0.0	7.9	0.0	16.8	0.3	0	2	143-4
146	0.0	1.1	0.0	0.0	0.0	1.9	0.0	0.0	0.0	7.5	0.0	3.2	3.4	3.8	5.6	7.9	0.0	16.8	1.3	0	10	146
145,147-8	0.0	0.0	0.0	0.0	0.0	0.0	0.0	0.0	0.0	2.5	0.0	0.0	3.4	0.0	0.0	0.0	0.0	0.0	0.4	1	3	145,147-8
150	0.0	0.0	0.0	0.0	0.0	0.0	1.9	0.0	0.0	0.0	5.6	9.5	6.9	18.8	72.6	87.3	86.4	168.4	6.8	1	54	150
151	0.0	0.0	0.0	1.5	0.0	0.0	0.0	8.4	9.3	17.4	45.1	63.3	89.2	153.9	290.3	349.2	395.1	505.1	35.1	0	278	151
152	0.0	0.0	0.0	0.0	1.9	0.0	0.0	0.0	0.0	2.5	2.8	3.2	0.0	0.0	0.0	0.0	0.0	16.8	0.6	0	5	152
153	0.0	0.0	0.0	1.5	0.0	0.0	5.6	4.2	16.3	0.0	16.9	31.7	27.4	45.0	72.6	150.8	234.6	185.2	14.6	3	116	153
154	0.0	0.0	0.0	0.0	0.0	0.0	2.8	0.0	4.7	0.0	5.6	9.5	10.3	7.5	39.1	55.6	49.4	16.8	4.2	0	33	154
155	0.0	0.0	0.0	0.0	0.0	0.0	0.0	0.0	2.3	0.0	2.8	3.2	17.1	15.0	27.9	23.8	12.3	33.7	3.2	0	25	155
156	0.0	0.0	0.0	0.0	0.0	0.0	1.9	2.1	0.0	5.0	2.8	6.3	6.9	0.0	27.9	39.7	74.1	0.0	2.1	0	17	156
157	0.0	0.0	1.3	0.0	0.0	0.0	0.0	0.0	0.0	0.0	2.8	6.3	10.3	18.8	33.5	47.6	0.0	50.5	4.4	1	35	157
160	0.0	0.0	0.0	0.0	0.0	0.0	0.0	0.0	0.0	0.0	0.0	6.3	0.0	7.5	5.6	7.9	0.0	0.0	0.8	0	6	160
161	0.0	0.0	0.0	0.0	0.0	0.0	0.0	0.0	0.0	0.0	0.0	0.0	0.0	0.0	5.6	7.9	0.0	0.0	0.3	0	2	161
162-3	0.0	0.0	0.0	0.0	0.0	0.0	0.0	4.2	0.0	12.4	8.5	12.7	17.1	15.0	27.9	63.5	74.1	16.8	5.6	1	44	162-3
170	0.0	0.0	0.0	0.0	1.9	9.5	18.8	35.6	41.9	114.3	104.3	117.1	116.6	116.4	117.3	246.0	172.8	202.0	39.8	1	315	170
171	0.0	0.0	0.0	0.0	3.9	9.5	11.3	16.7	37.3	49.7	36.7	44.3	58.3	41.3	27.9	15.9	49.4	16.8	15.7	0	124	171
172	0.0	0.0	0.0	0.0	0.0	0.0	1.9	6.3	7.0	9.9	28.2	25.3	48.0	33.8	27.9	23.8	12.3	0.0	7.7	0	61	172
173	0.0	0.0	0.0	0.0	0.0	0.0	0.0	0.0	0.0	2.5	0.0	3.2	0.0	0.0	0.0	0.0	0.0	0.0	0.3	0	2	173
174	0.0	1.1	0.0	0.0	5.8	0.0	0.0	2.1	0.0	0.0	0.0	6.3	6.9	7.5	5.6	15.9	24.7	16.8	1.9	1	15	174
175	1.0	0.0	1.3	0.0	0.0	1.9	5.6	2.1	18.6	22.4	31.0	28.5	54.9	37.5	55.8	55.6	49.4	33.7	12.4	1	98	175
176	0.0	0.0	0.0	1.5	0.0	0.0	0.0	4.2	0.0	5.0	5.6	9.5	6.9	11.3	11.2	7.9	12.3	0.0	2.0	0	16	176
180	2.0	0.0	0.0	0.0	0.0	0.0	1.9	0.0	0.0	5.0	5.6	22.2	24.0	30.0	50.3	95.2	37.0	67.3	7.5	0	59	180
181.0	0.0	0.0	0.0	0.0	0.0	0.0	0.0	0.0	4.7	0.0	5.6	9.5	17.1	15.0	11.2	47.6	74.1	16.8	3.9	0	31	181.0
190	0.0	1.1	0.0	0.0	0.0	3.8	1.9	4.2	2.3	0.0	0.0	9.5	3.4	7.5	11.2	0.0	0.0	0.0	1.8	0	14	190
191	1.0	0.0	0.0	0.0	5.8	0.0	7.5	4.2	0.0	7.5	19.7	25.3	41.2	30.0	50.3	39.7	111.1	50.5	9.1	2	72	191
192	3.0	0.0	0.0	0.0	1.9	1.9	0.0	0.0	9.3	0.0	0.0	3.2	0.0	7.5	5.6	7.9	0.0	0.0	0.8	0	6	192
193	0.0	1.1	0.0	0.0	3.9	5.7	0.0	4.2	4.7	17.4	11.3	15.8	24.0	18.8	11.2	87.3	0.0	33.7	6.2	1	49	193
194	0.0	0.0	0.0	0.0	0.0	3.8	1.9	4.2	0.0	14.9	8.5	19.0	17.1	33.8	39.1	0.0	37.0	16.8	7.6	0	60	194
195	0.0	1.1	0.0	1.5	1.9	0.0	0.0	2.1	0.0	0.0	0.0	0.0	6.9	0.0	0.0	7.9	0.0	0.0	0.4	0	3	195
196	0.0	0.0	0.0	0.0	0.0	1.9	1.9	2.1	0.0	0.0	5.6	3.2	10.3	7.5	0.0	7.9	0.0	0.0	1.9	0	15	196
197	0.0	0.0	0.0	0.0	0.0	1.9	1.9	0.0	2.3	0.0	0.0	6.3	3.4	3.8	11.2	7.9	0.0	0.0	0.8	1	6	197
200	0.0	0.0	0.0	0.0	1.9	0.0	1.9	2.1	2.3	0.0	0.0	3.2	3.4	3.8	5.6	7.9	0.0	0.0	1.4	0	11	200
201	0.0	0.0	0.0	0.0	0.0	0.0	5.6	2.1	0.0	0.0	2.8	3.2	3.4	0.0	11.2	7.9	12.3	0.0	1.3	0	10	201
203	0.0	0.0	0.0	0.0	1.9	0.0	0.0	0.0	2.3	0.0	2.8	9.5	6.9	7.5	16.8	0.0	37.0	0.0	1.0	0	8	203
204	3.0	4.4	2.5	4.6	0.0	0.0	1.9	0.0	0.0	0.0	2.8	0.0	3.4	26.3	0.0	7.9	0.0	33.7	4.7	0	37	204
202,205	0.0	0.0	0.0	0.0	0.0	0.0	0.0	0.0	0.0	0.0	0.0	0.0	3.4	0.0	0.0	0.0	0.0	16.8	0.3	0	2	202,205
OTHER	1.0	0.0	0.0	0.0	0.0	0.0	0.0	2.1	0.0	0.0	2.8	9.5	20.6	11.3	27.9	7.9	49.4	16.8	3.3	0	26	OTHER
140-205	10.9	8.8	5.1	10.7	28.9	43.5	75.2	115.1	165.4	298.3	366.6	538.1	668.7	735.7	1133.4	1539.7	1654.3	1565.7	212.8	16	1685	140-205
RATE PER CASE IN PERIOD	0.99	1.10	1.27	1.53	1.93	1.89	1.88	2.09	2.33	2.49	2.82	3.17	3.43	3.75	5.58	7.94	12.35	16.84	0.13	-	-	RATE PER CASE IN PERIOD

NETHERLANDS (3 REGIONS)

Since its start in 1953 the Central Cancer Registry in the Netherlands has been building up an archive of cancer patients. One hundred and twenty of the 250 smaller and larger hospitals co-operate in this scheme, providing data of cancer patients admitted to these hospitals. Nearly all the large hospitals, among which are all cancer treatment centres, belong to this group of co-operating hospitals. An average of 20,000 new patients yearly have been registered and the data have been presented in W.H.O. Epidemiological and Vital Statistics Reports.

The collected data for each patient include name, date of birth, profession(s) and domicile and also duration of period of symptoms or complaints before calling for medical advice, diagnosis and method of confirmation, tumour-stage (T.N.M. system, if applicable and then in special surveys), the presence or absence of metastasis, and finally the method of treatment, if carried out. BULL.-punched cards also contain the histological diagnosis, if known.

This registry scheme of cancer patients is combined with the collection of follow-up information in hospitals or among general practitioners (depending on whether the patients are controlled by specialists or by general practitioners) and thus provide in 98% the requested information about the condition (with or without symptoms of the disease) or date and cause of death of the patients. This follow-up information is collected yearly in the frist five years after the diagnosis is made and afterwards after seven, ten and fifteen years, if the patients are alive.

The registry data are not supplemented by information from death certificates because of legal restrictions on their secrecy.

The registry project, which is parly financed by the government and partly by the Queen Wilhelmina Fund for the fight against cancer, is able to help in several ways the aims of the National Organization against Cancer in the Netherlands. First, the Central Cancer Registry is meant for measuring the incidence of cancer, since - as elsewhere - cancer mortality is failing to reflect the frequency of the disease when therapeutic results for some forms of cancer are improving. Secondly, data about the incidence of the disease are essential for geographical-pathological studies in respect of cancer, such as that in which a food survey was carried out in the period 1958-1961 among 340 patients with stomach cancer and 1,060 matched controls, among whom were 582 other cancer patients and 478 persons without apparent signs of cancer (Meinsma, 1964).

Since not all hospitals co-operate, we provided in some regions medico-administrative assistance, and in these regions (the province of Friesland and the cities of the Hague and Rotterdam) all cancer patients, admitted in the hospitals, are registered. Since practically all cancer patients or suspected cases are hospitalized or at least examined in poly-clinics, the data for these regions provide a reliable impression of the true incidence of cancer. The rates presented here are, therefore, limited to these regions.

A large survey (in which 2,000 of the 4,600 general practitioners in the Netherlands will participate) is being conducted to collect more information about the period of "after-care" of the cancer patient. With its results it will be possible to improve the relative significance of survival rates of cancer patients.

Finally it may be stated that the Central Cancer Registry provides important information for a cancer education programme aiming to diminish the fear of cancer.

L. Meinsma.

Registry Title and Adress : The Central Cancer Registry in the Netherlands, de Lairessestraat 33, Amsterdam, Netherlands. Commenced 1953. Supported principally by the National Organization Against Cancer, financed partly by Government Grant and the Queen Wilhelmina Fund for the Fight Against Cancer.

Registration. Cases are registered from hospital in-patients and from radio-therapy and pathology departments of 120 out of 250 of the larger and smaller hospitals including all those which are cancer treatment centres. Out-patients are registered from Poly-clinics. There are no registration from death cer-tificates as there are legal restrictions on their secrecy. Medico-adminis-trative assistance is sent by the Registry to collect information in the areas for which the present data are reported.

Follow-up. Ninety-eight per cent of registrations are followed annually for 5 years and then after 7, 10 and 15 years.

Physical Descriptions. The Registry covers the Netherlands which is in the north-western part of the continent of Europe and surrounded by Belgium and Germany. It lies between latitudes 50o46' and 53o34' north and longitudes 3o22' and 7o14' east. The national registration area is 33,433 square kilometres.

Demographic Description. Total population of selected area under survey 1,812,960 (Friesland, The Hague and Rotterdam). The national population is 40% Catholic, 38% Protestant, 3% other and 19% no religion. The main occupa-tional composition is : industry 29.9%, commerce 16.2%, agriculture 10.7% and personal service 43.2%. Of the national population 32%, and of the survey population 74%, live in conurbations of over 100,000.

Medical Services. Total number of hospital beds of all kinds 58,222. Total number of doctors in practice in whole registration area 9,000. Cancer causes approximately 24% of all deaths.

Publications. Annual reports (Jaarverslagen van de Stichting "Landelijke Orga-nisatie voor de Kankerbestrijding"). Meinsma (1963, 1964 and 1965)
World Health Organization (1950, 1952 and 1959).

TABLE 29 A
NETHERLANDS (THREE PROVINCES) :
POPULATION (100,000s), CENSUS 1960

AGE (in years)	MALES No.	MALES Per Cent	FEMALES No.	FEMALES Per Cent
0–	0.7071	7.98	0.6722	7.25
5–	0.7878	8.89	0.7492	8.09
10–	0.9277	10.47	0.8863	9.57
15–	0.6806	7.68	0.6571	7.09
20–	0.6116	6.90	0.5935	6.41
25–	0.5586	6.30	0.5530	5.97
30–	0.5583	6.30	0.5760	6.22
35–	0.5743	6.48	0.6239	6.73
40–	0.5463	6.16	0.5861	6.33
45–	0.5459	6.17	0.5998	6.47
50–	0.5352	6.04	0.5905	6.37
55–	0.4942	5.58	0.5544	5.98
60–	0.4176	4.71	0.4878	5.26
65–	0.3428	3.87	0.4104	4.43
70–	0.2604	2.94	0.3173	3.42
75–	0.1759	1.98	0.2187	2.36
80–	0.0939	1.06	0.1245	1.34
85– and over	0.0444	0.50	0.0652	0.70
TOTAL	8.8636	100.00	9.2660	100.00

NOTES

TO TABLES 29 A, B and C

(I) Data for Friesland, the Hague and Rotterdam only.

(II) I. L. number 193 includes benign tumours of the central nervous system, but excludes unspecified tumours.

       " " 205 included with other tumours.

(III) Carcinoma in situ included.

TABLE 29 B

NETHERLANDS (THREE PROVINCES):

MALE INCIDENCE RATES, 1960 - 62.

INTER-NATIONAL LIST No.	AVERAGE ANNUAL INCIDENCE PER 100,000 — AGE IN YEARS 0-	5-	10-	15-	20-	25-	30-	35-	40-	45-	50-	55-	60-	65-	70-	75-	80-	85- AND OVER	ALL AGES	No. OF CASES IN WHOLE PERIOD: AGE UN-KNOWN	ALL AGES	INTER-NATIONAL LIST No.
140	0.0	0.0	0.0	0.0	0.5	0.6	0.0	1.2	2.4	3.7	4.4	10.1	9.6	15.6	14.1	17.1	21.3	52.6	3.6	0	97	140
141	0.0	0.0	0.0	0.0	0.0	0.0	0.0	1.2	0.6	0.6	1.2	5.4	4.0	3.9	6.4	7.6	0.0	15.0	1.3	0	34	141
142	0.0	0.0	0.0	0.0	0.5	0.0	0.0	0.6	2.4	3.0	2.5	2.0	1.6	5.8	2.6	1.9	3.5	7.5	1.2	0	31	142
143-4	0.0	0.8	0.0	0.0	0.0	0.0	0.0	0.0	0.6	1.2	0.6	1.3	4.8	1.9	6.4	15.2	10.6	15.0	1.3	0	34	143-4
146	0.0	0.0	0.0	0.5	0.0	0.0	0.0	0.0	0.0	0.6	1.2	0.7	1.6	0.0	0.0	0.0	0.0	0.0	0.3	0	7	146
145,147-8	0.0	0.0	0.0	0.0	0.0	0.0	0.6	0.0	1.2	1.8	1.9	4.0	7.2	7.8	11.5	15.2	14.2	0.0	2.0	0	53	145,147-8
150	0.0	0.0	0.0	0.0	0.0	0.0	0.0	0.6	0.6	1.2	2.5	3.4	9.6	15.6	20.5	32.2	39.0	67.6	3.5	0	94	150
151	0.0	0.0	0.4	0.0	0.0	2.4	0.6	4.6	6.7	12.2	26.8	54.6	81.4	126.4	152.3	208.5	266.2	255.3	27.9	4	743	151
152	0.0	0.0	0.0	0.5	0.0	0.0	0.0	0.0	0.0	0.6	0.6	0.0	0.0	2.9	3.8	1.9	3.5	0.0	0.4	0	11	152
153	0.5	0.0	0.0	0.5	0.5	1.2	1.8	1.7	7.9	9.8	12.5	20.9	33.5	39.9	67.8	89.1	99.4	142.6	12.1	0	321	153
154	0.0	0.0	0.0	0.0	0.0	0.0	1.2	0.6	4.3	6.1	7.5	22.9	24.7	45.7	66.6	111.8	99.4	135.1	11.3	0	301	154
155.0	0.0	0.0	0.4	0.0	0.0	0.0	0.0	0.0	1.2	0.6	0.6	1.3	2.4	3.9	5.1	7.6	3.5	15.0	0.9	0	25	155.0
155.1	0.0	0.0	0.0	0.0	0.0	0.0	0.0	0.0	0.0	1.8	3.7	6.7	8.0	16.5	15.4	22.7	60.3	22.5	3.4	0	90	155.1
156	0.0	0.0	0.0	0.0	0.0	0.0	0.0	0.0	0.0	0.0	0.0	0.0	0.8	0.0	1.3	0.0	0.0	7.5	0.1	0	3	156
157	0.0	0.0	0.0	0.0	0.0	0.6	0.0	0.0	1.2	5.5	5.6	17.5	12.0	21.4	44.8	32.2	28.4	30.0	5.6	1	149	157
160	0.0	0.0	0.0	0.0	0.0	0.0	0.6	0.6	0.6	1.2	0.0	1.3	5.6	6.8	5.1	7.6	17.7	0.0	1.3	0	34	160
161	0.0	0.0	0.0	0.0	0.0	0.0	0.6	1.7	0.0	6.7	7.5	12.1	20.0	25.3	24.3	17.1	21.3	22.5	5.0	1	134	161
162-3	0.0	0.0	0.0	0.5	0.5	0.0	1.2	5.8	15.9	42.1	96.5	162.6	251.4	290.7	239.4	157.3	95.8	60.1	53.7	4	1428	162-3
170	0.0	0.0	0.0	0.0	0.0	0.0	0.0	0.0	1.2	1.2	2.5	1.3	0.8	4.9	2.6	5.7	3.5	0.0	0.8	0	22	170
177	0.0	0.0	0.0	0.0	0.0	0.0	0.6	0.6	0.0	1.2	2.5	13.5	39.1	91.4	206.1	242.6	411.8	510.5	24.2	0	644	177
178	0.9	0.4	0.0	0.0	3.8	4.8	5.4	6.4	7.3	4.9	1.9	2.7	2.4	1.9	3.8	5.7	3.5	0.0	2.9	0	77	178
179.0	0.0	0.0	0.0	0.0	0.0	0.0	0.0	1.2	0.6	0.0	1.2	1.3	1.6	2.9	5.1	17.1	7.1	7.5	1.1	0	28	179.0
180	2.8	0.4	0.0	0.0	0.0	0.6	1.2	4.1	1.8	4.3	6.9	6.7	19.2	20.4	15.4	26.5	28.4	0.0	4.8	1	128	180
181.0	0.0	0.0	0.0	0.0	0.0	0.0	0.0	0.6	1.8	4.3	11.8	22.3	31.9	47.6	62.7	64.4	124.2	127.6	10.8	0	287	181.0
190	0.5	0.4	0.0	0.0	0.5	0.0	1.2	4.1	1.2	4.3	2.5	1.3	1.6	4.9	3.8	3.8	17.7	0.0	1.7	0	44	190
191	0.0	0.4	0.7	0.0	1.1	0.6	4.8	8.7	15.3	20.1	26.2	45.9	75.8	98.2	139.5	221.7	298.2	427.9	28.8	6	766	191
192	0.9	0.0	0.0	0.0	0.0	0.0	0.0	0.6	0.6	0.0	0.0	0.7	0.8	1.0	0.0	5.7	0.0	0.0	0.4	0	10	192
193	2.4	3.0	0.4	2.4	1.1	1.8	4.2	3.5	8.5	8.5	10.0	16.9	14.4	13.6	5.1	3.8	7.1	0.0	5.5	1	146	193
194	0.0	0.0	0.0	0.0	0.5	0.6	0.0	0.6	0.6	0.6	1.9	2.7	0.8	1.9	2.6	5.7	3.5	7.5	0.8	0	22	194
195	0.0	0.4	0.0	0.5	0.5	0.0	0.0	0.0	1.2	1.8	0.6	0.7	0.8	1.0	1.3	0.0	0.0	0.0	0.5	0	13	195
196	0.0	0.4	2.2	2.4	0.5	0.6	0.0	1.2	0.6	1.2	0.0	0.7	2.4	2.9	3.8	1.9	0.0	0.0	1.1	0	30	196
197	0.5	0.0	0.0	0.5	1.1	0.0	0.0	2.9	1.2	0.6	1.2	1.3	1.6	7.8	6.4	5.7	3.5	0.0	1.3	0	35	197
200	0.5	0.0	0.4	1.0	0.5	0.6	1.8	1.2	0.0	0.6	4.4	1.3	2.4	1.9	9.0	5.7	3.5	0.0	1.4	0	37	200
201	0.0	0.4	1.1	4.4	3.8	2.4	2.4	3.5	3.1	4.3	3.1	1.3	3.2	1.9	1.3	11.4	7.1	0.0	2.6	0	68	201
202	0.0	0.4	0.0	0.5	0.0	0.6	0.0	1.7	1.2	0.6	1.9	2.0	2.4	1.0	2.6	1.9	0.0	22.5	0.9	0	25	202
203	0.0	0.0	0.0	0.0	0.0	0.0	0.0	0.0	0.6	1.8	1.9	3.4	5.6	8.8	14.1	5.7	10.6	15.0	1.8	0	47	203
204	0.5	0.8	0.0	2.0	0.0	0.6	1.2	2.9	1.8	3.7	8.1	8.8	10.4	14.6	10.2	20.8	42.6	7.4	4.1	0	110	204
OTHER	0.9	0.0	0.0	1.5	0.5	1.2	3.6	4.6	4.9	6.7	16.8	30.4	29.5	43.8	47.4	55.0	49.7	105.1	10.9	1	290	OTHER
140-205	10.4	8.0	5.4	17.1	16.4	19.1	32.8	66.7	99.5	169.4	280.9	492.4	724.8	1002.5	1230.2	1455.4	1806.9	2079.6	241.4	19	6418	140-205
RATE PER CASE IN PERIOD	0.47	0.42	0.36	0.49	0.55	0.60	0.60	0.58	0.61	0.61	0.62	0.67	0.80	0.97	1.28	1.90	3.55	7.51	0.04	-	-	RATE PER CASE IN PERIOD

TABLE 29 C

NETHERLANDS (THREE PROVINCES):

FEMALE INCIDENCE RATES, 1960 - 62.

INTER-NATIONAL LIST No.	0-	5-	10-	15-	20-	25-	30-	35-	40-	45-	50-	55-	60-	65-	70-	75-	80-	85- AND OVER	ALL AGES	Cases AGE UNKNOWN	Cases ALL AGES	INTER-NATIONAL LIST No.
140	0.0	0.0	0.0	0.0	0.0	0.0	0.0	0.0	0.0	0.0	0.0	0.0	0.0	0.8	0.0	1.5	2.7	5.1	0.1	0	4	140
141	0.0	0.0	0.0	0.5	0.0	0.0	0.0	0.0	0.0	0.0	0.0	1.2	3.4	1.6	6.3	3.0	10.7	15.3	0.9	0	25	141
142	0.0	0.4	0.4	0.5	0.6	1.2	0.0	0.5	1.7	2.2	1.1	2.4	6.2	3.2	3.2	1.5	0.0	0.0	1.3	0	37	142
143-4	0.0	0.0	0.0	0.0	0.0	0.0	0.0	0.0	0.0	0.6	0.6	1.2	0.7	0.8	1.1	3.0	2.7	5.1	0.4	0	11	143-4
146	0.0	0.0	0.0	0.0	0.0	0.0	0.6	0.0	0.0	0.0	0.0	0.6	0.0	0.0	2.1	0.0	2.7	5.1	0.2	0	5	146
145,147-8	0.0	0.0	0.0	0.0	0.0	0.0	0.0	0.5	0.6	0.0	0.0	0.6	1.4	2.4	3.2	4.6	2.7	5.1	0.6	0	16	145,147-8
150	0.5	0.0	0.0	0.0	0.0	0.6	0.0	0.5	0.0	0.6	0.6	3.0	2.7	2.4	12.6	9.1	13.4	5.1	1.4	0	39	150
151	0.0	0.0	0.0	0.0	0.0	0.0	0.6	1.6	4.0	8.9	7.3	20.4	36.2	51.2	69.3	115.8	104.3	127.8	14.3	0	398	151
152	0.0	0.0	0.0	0.0	0.0	0.0	0.6	0.5	0.0	0.0	0.0	1.2	2.7	1.6	4.2	1.5	0.0	0.0	0.5	1	15	152
153	0.0	0.0	0.0	1.5	0.0	1.2	2.9	4.8	10.2	11.7	18.6	27.7	39.6	60.1	83.0	89.9	107.0	107.4	16.9	0	470	153
154	0.5	0.0	0.0	0.0	0.6	0.0	0.0	1.1	4.5	3.9	6.8	16.8	25.3	26.8	39.9	48.8	42.8	86.9	8.3	1	232	154
155.0	0.0	0.0	0.0	0.0	0.0	0.0	0.0	0.0	0.0	0.6	0.6	0.6	1.4	0.8	1.1	0.0	0.0	5.1	0.3	0	8	155.0
155.1	0.5	0.0	0.0	0.0	0.0	0.0	0.6	0.0	0.6	1.1	2.8	4.2	14.4	19.5	48.3	56.4	34.8	30.7	5.9	1	165	155.1
156	0.0	0.0	0.0	0.0	0.0	0.0	0.0	0.0	0.0	0.0	0.0	0.0	0.7	0.0	1.1	0.0	0.0	0.0	0.1	0	2	156
157	0.0	0.0	0.0	0.0	0.0	0.0	0.6	0.5	0.0	1.1	2.3	3.6	8.9	17.1	22.1	29.0	26.8	30.7	3.7	0	104	157
160	0.0	0.0	0.0	0.0	0.0	0.0	0.0	0.5	0.0	0.6	0.0	0.6	0.0	3.2	1.1	0.0	2.7	0.0	0.4	0	10	160
161	0.0	0.0	0.0	0.0	0.0	0.0	0.0	0.5	1.1	0.6	0.0	1.2	0.0	0.8	2.1	1.5	0.0	5.1	0.4	1	12	161
162-3	0.0	0.0	0.0	0.0	0.0	0.0	1.2	1.1	1.1	2.2	8.5	6.6	15.0	9.7	15.8	16.8	13.4	0.0	3.7	1	102	162-3
170	0.0	0.0	0.0	0.0	0.6	3.0	11.0	29.9	77.3	110.6	112.3	123.9	150.3	165.7	203.8	236.2	219.4	260.7	62.3	6	1733	170
171	0.0	0.0	0.0	0.0	0.0	1.2	17.9	50.8	55.2	54.5	54.2	40.9	45.8	34.9	17.9	38.1	5.4	30.7	23.3	0	647	171
172	0.0	0.0	0.0	0.0	1.7	0.0	1.2	2.1	5.7	13.9	25.4	46.9	51.3	48.7	48.3	44.2	37.5	10.2	14.1	1	391	172
173	0.0	0.0	0.0	0.0	0.6	0.0	0.0	0.5	0.6	0.6	0.6	0.0	0.0	0.0	0.0	0.0	0.0	0.0	0.5	0	1	173
174	0.0	0.0	0.0	0.0	0.0	0.0	0.0	0.0	0.6	0.0	0.6	1.2	2.1	3.2	1.1	3.0	0.0	0.0	0.5	0	15	174
175	0.0	0.0	0.4	0.5	0.6	2.4	4.6	5.9	9.1	14.4	23.1	28.3	32.1	24.4	14.7	19.8	26.8	10.2	9.8	1	273	175
176	0.0	0.0	0.0	0.5	0.0	0.0	0.6	1.6	0.0	0.6	0.0	1.2	6.8	10.6	12.6	12.2	24.1	51.1	2.5	0	70	176
180	1.0	1.3	0.4	0.5	0.0	0.0	0.6	1.1	0.0	2.8	4.5	3.0	3.4	7.3	11.6	15.2	16.1	5.1	2.5	0	70	180
181.0	0.0	0.0	0.0	0.0	0.6	1.2	0.0	0.5	0.0	1.1	1.1	6.0	6.8	17.1	14.7	32.0	34.8	46.0	3.7	1	103	181.0
190	0.0	0.0	0.0	0.0	0.0	0.0	1.7	1.6	4.5	6.7	2.3	4.8	3.4	4.9	12.6	3.0	8.0	0.0	2.6	0	71	190
191	1.5	0.4	0.8	0.0	0.0	1.2	2.3	2.1	7.4	12.2	16.4	27.7	32.1	71.5	77.7	132.6	179.2	265.8	19.5	4	541	191
192	1.5	0.4	0.0	0.0	0.6	1.2	0.0	0.0	0.6	1.1	0.6	1.2	0.7	0.8	0.0	0.0	0.0	0.0	0.4	4	12	192
193	0.0	4.0	2.3	2.0	0.6	1.8	2.9	3.2	2.3	7.2	8.5	9.0	13.0	8.1	7.4	4.6	5.4	0.0	4.5	0	125	193
194	0.0	0.9	0.4	1.0	1.7	1.2	2.9	1.6	2.3	2.2	2.3	3.6	6.2	6.5	5.3	1.5	2.7	10.2	2.2	0	60	194
195	0.0	0.9	0.4	1.0	0.0	0.0	0.6	0.5	0.6	1.6	1.7	0.6	0.7	0.8	0.0	1.5	0.0	5.1	0.6	0	17	195
196	0.0	0.0	0.4	0.5	0.6	0.0	0.6	0.5	0.6	0.6	0.0	1.2	1.4	1.6	1.1	1.5	0.0	0.0	0.6	0	17	196
197	0.5	0.0	0.4	0.0	0.0	0.6	1.2	0.0	2.8	1.1	3.4	0.0	2.7	4.1	4.2	6.1	5.4	0.0	1.3	0	37	197
200	0.5	0.4	0.0	3.0	0.0	2.4	1.7	0.5	0.6	2.8	1.1	3.6	1.4	4.9	6.3	6.1	0.0	10.2	1.2	0	33	200
201	0.0	0.0	0.4	0.5	3.4	0.6	0.0	1.1	0.6	2.8	1.1	1.2	3.4	1.6	3.2	1.5	5.4	0.0	1.6	0	45	201
202	0.0	0.0	0.4	0.5	0.0	0.0	0.0	0.5	0.0	2.8	1.7	2.4	2.1	3.2	7.4	6.1	5.4	5.1	1.3	0	36	202
203	0.0	0.0	0.0	2.0	1.7	0.6	2.3	0.0	0.6	0.6	1.1	3.6	3.4	4.9	8.4	18.3	2.7	20.4	1.7	0	47	203
204	2.0	1.3	1.1	0.0	0.6	0.0	0.0	1.1	1.1	4.4	5.1	2.4	5.5	7.3	10.5	15.2	10.7	10.2	3.2	0	90	204
OTHER	1.0	0.0	0.0	0.0	0.6	0.0	0.0	1.6	5.1	9.4	11.3	15.6	31.4	34.9	47.3	65.5	53.5	61.3	10.4	2	289	OTHER
140-205	9.4	9.8	7.5	14.2	12.4	19.9	59.0	118.1	200.2	285.1	326.8	420.3	565.1	669.3	832.0	1047.1	1008.6	1232.1	229.4	20	6378	140-205
RATE PER CASE IN PERIOD	0.50	0.44	0.38	0.51	0.56	0.60	0.58	0.53	0.57	0.56	0.56	0.60	0.68	0.81	1.05	1.52	2.68	5.11	0.04	-	-	RATE PER CASE IN PERIOD

NORWAY

The Cancer Registry of Norway has been in operation since January 1, 1952. Based on compulsory notification, the registration scheme covers the whole of Norway and aims at a complete registration of all recognized cases of cancer among the total population of the country. All conditions are reportable which are classifiable under categories 140 through 205 of the International Statistical Classification of Diseases, Injuries, and Causes of Death, all kinds of neo-plasms of the central nervous system, "stage O" or "in situ" lesions of the uterine cervix, and papillomas of the urinary tract. Carcinoid tumors of the gastrointertinal tract are also registered, whether specified as malignant or not.

However, except for some types of tumors of the central nervous system, cases of questionable malignancy are not included in tabulations unless this is expressly stated.

According to rules laid down by the Ministry of Social Affairs, reports are required from (1) all hospital departments, (2) all institutes of pathology, and (3) all institutes of radiology.

Every new cancer patient is to be reported, whether treated or not, whe-ther occupying a hospital bed or seen only in outpatient departments. A new report is to be submitted every time a cancer patient is readmitted or re-exa-mined for his malignant disease. Records are to be filled in and signed by a physician. Instead of submitting ordinary reports, some hospitals prefer to send in the original records of cancer patients at regular intervals, for ab-stracting in the cancer Registry. Actually, the complete hospital records for approximately 30 per cent of all registered cancer patients in Norway are ab-stracted or reviewed by a phisician in the Registry.

As a consequence of the rules established for reporting cancer in Norway, most cases are reported repeatedly and from different institutions. Thus, more than 70 per cent of all cases (excluding skin cancer) are initially accounted for both from a clinician and a pathologist. Such independent reporting, besides increasing the probability that all cases will sooner or later be registered, in many instances also results in more accurate and complete information than the Registry would have received if records were submitted once and from one source only.

At regular intervals, all death certificates mentioning cancer or tumor are forwarded to the Cancer Registry from the Central Bureau of Statistics, to be matched against the file of registered cases. For every case that cannot be found in the Registry, a letter is mailed to the physician who signed the death certificate, asking him to assist in obtaining a complete report on the case. If necessary, the request is repeated.

The number of deaths queried per year has been gradually decreasing as registration has improved, but for the years 1959-61 approximetely 16 per cent of all death certificates mentioning cancer or tumor were the source of enquiries. Completed returns were received from physicians for over 90 per cent of the deaths queried. Depending on the information thus obtained, it was decided for each case whether it should be accepted for registration or rejected. As a result of this procedure less than 2 per cent of the cases registered as cancer in Nor-way are merely on the basis of the death certificate with no additional informa-tion.

Most of the cases that are first known from death certificates have never been hospitalized for malignant disease. In most of these, the diagnosis is based on an incomplete examination of patients in the terminal stage of the disease.

Organization, objectives and methodology of the Cancer Registry have been discussed in detail by Pedersen and Magnus (1959). Trends in cancer mortality in Norway after 1930, and cancer incidence figures for the years 1953-54 were also presented in the same report. Incidence figures for 1953-58 were published subsequently (Cancer Registry of Norway, 1961). Registry of Norway, 1961).

Since 1953 no major changes have been made in the registration system. The various checking procedures described in Monograph No. 1, on completeness of reporting and reliability of diagnoses, have been continued. Great care has been exercised in order to maintain uniformity in classification and coding of reported cases.

E. Pedersen

Registry Title and Address : The Cancer Registry of Norway, Montebello, Oslo 3, Norway. Commenced 1st January, 1952. Supported financially by the Norwegian Cancer Society, the Ministry of Social Affairs, and contracts with the U.S. National Institutes of Health for special studies.

Registration. Registrations are made by physicians in hospital or Registry from hospital in-patients and out-patients, radiotherapy and pathology departments, from death certificates by the Central Bureau of Statistics, and at the request of the Cancer Registry by doctors attending cases at home. Basal cell carcinoma of the skin is probably incompletely registered (less than 90%).

Follow-up. All registrations are followed up till death.

Physical Description. Whole of Norway which is bounded on the north by the Arctic Ocean, on the west and south by the North Sea and on the east by Finland, Sweden and the U.S.S.R. It lies between latitudes 58º and 71º north and longitudes 5º and 31º east. Total registration area is 324,000 square kilometres.

Demographic Description. Total population of area under survey 3,591,210. Percentages of principal groups in the population are Lapps approximately 0.5%, the rest are Caucasian. The principal religious group is Lutheran Protestants approximately 95%. The main occupational composition (males over 15 years) is industry 33%, commerce 10%, agriculture 20%, and personal service 5%. Of the total population 16.5% live in conurbations of more than 100,000.

Medical Services. Total number of hospital beds of all kinds 31,772, (1963). Total number of doctors in practice in registration area 4,621 (1963). Cancer causes approximately 18% of all deaths.

Publications. Cancer Registry of Norway (1961, 1964); Pedersen and Magnus (1959).

A list of other reports is available from the Registry on request.

TABLE 30 A
NORWAY :
POPULATION (100, 000s), 1960

AGE (in years)	MALES		FEMALES	
	No.	Per Cent	No.	Per Cent
0 -	1.5785	8.82	1.5037	8.35
5 -	1.5533	8.68	1.4745	8.18
10 -	1.6288	9.10	1.5427	8.56
15 -	1.3534	7.56	1.2886	7.15
20 -	1.0706	5.98	1.0250	5.69
25 -	1.0089	5.64	0.9757	5.42
30 -	1.1373	6.36	1.0966	6.09
35 -	1.2958	7.24	1.2682	7.04
40 -	1.2883	7.20	1.2855	7.13
45 -	1.2220	6.83	1.2141	6.74
50 -	1.1116	6.21	1.1392	6.32
55 -	0.9831	5.49	1.0556	5.86
60 -	0.8613	4.81	0.9556	5.30
65 -	0.6849	3.83	0.7723	4.29
70 -	0.4901	2.74	0.5946	3.30
75 -	0.3235	1.81	0.4170	2.31
80 -	0.1960	1.10	0.2574	1.43
85 - and over	0.1066	0.60	0.1518	0.84
TOTAL	17.8940	100.00	18.0181	100.00

NOTES

TO TABLES 30 A, B and C

(I) I.L. number 191 not used; skin cancers not registered.
     "   "   193 includes benign and unspecified tu-
     mours of the central nervous system.

(II) Carcinoma in situ excluded.

TABLE 30 B
NORWAY :
MALE INCIDENCE RATES, 1959 - 61.

AVERAGE ANNUAL INCIDENCE PER 100,000 — AGE IN YEARS

INTER-NATIONAL LIST No.	0–	5–	10–	15–	20–	25–	30–	35–	40–	45–	50–	55–	60–	65–	70–	75–	80–	85– and over	ALL AGES	AGE UNKNOWN	ALL AGES (cases)	INTER-NATIONAL LIST No.
140	0.0	0.0	0.0	0.0	0.0	1.3	0.6	0.0	2.1	3.5	3.0	9.2	12.4	19.5	28.6	40.2	49.3	50.0	4.9	0	262	140
141	0.0	0.0	0.0	0.0	0.0	0.0	0.3	0.3	0.8	0.8	0.6	2.4	1.9	7.3	5.4	8.2	8.5	6.3	1.1	0	60	141
142	0.0	0.0	0.0	0.0	0.0	0.0	0.3	0.3	0.3	0.5	0.9	1.4	0.4	3.9	3.4	2.1	6.8	0.0	0.6	0	32	142
143-4	0.0	0.0	0.0	0.0	0.0	0.0	0.3	0.0	0.3	1.1	1.8	3.7	7.7	9.2	7.5	10.3	8.5	21.9	1.8	0	95	143-4
146	0.0	0.0	0.0	0.0	0.0	0.0	0.0	0.0	0.0	0.3	1.2	1.0	2.3	1.0	2.7	0.0	1.7	0.0	0.4	0	22	146
145,147-8	0.0	0.0	0.0	0.0	0.0	0.0	0.3	0.0	0.0	0.5	1.2	2.0	5.4	7.3	11.6	5.2	8.5	15.6	1.4	0	74	145,147-8
150	0.0	0.0	0.0	0.0	0.0	0.0	0.3	0.0	0.5	0.8	5.4	7.1	14.3	18.0	34.0	31.9	42.5	71.9	4.6	0	247	150
151	0.0	0.0	0.0	0.0	0.3	0.3	3.2	3.9	11.9	18.3	41.7	64.8	130.8	208.8	302.0	346.2	479.6	531.6	46.0	0	2468	151
152	0.0	0.0	0.0	0.0	0.3	0.3	0.0	0.3	0.0	0.3	0.3	0.0	1.2	4.4	2.7	2.1	2.7	0.0	0.5	0	25	152
153	0.0	0.0	0.0	0.0	0.3	1.0	2.3	3.1	4.7	7.1	12.6	20.7	39.5	60.8	85.7	115.4	153.1	178.2	14.6	0	784	153
154	0.0	0.0	0.2	0.0	0.3	0.0	1.2	1.3	1.6	3.8	9.9	14.2	21.3	43.3	55.1	75.2	74.8	118.8	9.0	0	484	154
155.0	0.2	0.2	0.0	0.0	0.0	0.0	0.0	0.0	0.8	0.5	0.3	3.1	5.4	7.3	7.5	7.2	5.1	6.3	1.3	0	71	155.0
155.1	0.2	0.0	0.4	0.0	0.0	0.0	0.0	0.0	0.0	0.8	2.1	2.7	5.8	4.4	7.5	11.3	10.2	9.4	1.4	0	73	155.1
156	0.0	0.0	0.0	0.0	0.0	0.0	0.0	0.0	0.3	0.5	0.9	2.0	1.5	5.8	10.9	8.2	13.6	9.4	1.2	0	64	156
157	0.0	0.0	0.0	0.0	0.0	0.3	0.3	1.8	2.6	5.2	5.1	17.0	25.2	35.5	54.4	68.0	37.4	50.0	8.0	1	428	157
160	0.0	0.0	0.0	0.2	0.0	0.0	0.0	0.0	0.8	0.5	0.6	1.4	3.1	6.3	7.5	6.2	6.8	12.5	1.1	0	58	160
161	0.0	0.0	0.0	0.0	0.0	0.0	0.3	0.0	0.5	2.2	4.5	5.4	8.5	11.2	8.8	8.2	5.1	0.0	2.1	0	112	161
162-3	0.0	0.0	0.0	0.2	0.6	0.0	1.5	2.8	6.7	12.8	23.1	61.4	89.0	85.7	71.4	52.6	40.8	25.0	17.6	1	945	162-3
170	0.0	0.0	0.0	0.0	0.0	0.0	0.0	0.3	0.0	0.0	0.6	0.3	1.5	1.5	2.7	0.0	5.1	6.3	0.4	0	19	170
177	0.0	0.0	0.0	0.0	5.0	6.6	10.8	8.5	6.0	3.5	5.7	22.4	65.0	150.4	288.4	464.7	595.2	647.3	37.3	3	2002	177
178	0.6	0.2	0.0	1.0	5.0	0.3	0.0	0.0	0.3	3.5	3.3	3.1	1.5	1.9	2.7	2.1	11.9	3.1	3.5	0	186	178
179.0	0.0	0.0	0.0	0.2	0.0	0.3	0.0	0.0	0.3	0.5	0.9	1.7	2.7	3.9	8.2	5.2	5.2	6.3	1.0	0	53	179.0
180	3.0	0.4	0.2	0.0	0.3	0.3	0.3	1.3	2.1	4.4	9.3	14.2	26.3	26.3	34.0	46.4	37.4	40.7	7.0	0	375	180
181.0	0.0	0.0	0.0	1.0	0.0	0.0	0.0	0.5	1.8	3.8	6.3	14.9	22.4	26.3	34.0	55.6	64.6	71.9	6.8	0	365	181.0
190	0.0	0.0	0.2	0.0	0.9	1.7	3.5	5.7	4.9	3.5	5.7	4.4	6.6	7.8	9.5	10.3	10.2	15.6	3.3	0	178	190
192	1.3	0.0	0.0	0.0	0.3	0.0	0.0	0.5	1.6	3.5	0.9	1.7	1.9	3.4	4.8	7.2	3.4	0.0	1.0	0	56	192
193	3.6	4.7	4.1	3.0	3.7	3.3	6.2	7.7	8.5	8.7	15.0	19.3	20.5	25.3	10.9	6.2	6.8	3.1	8.3	0	448	193
194	0.0	0.0	0.0	0.0	0.0	0.3	0.9	0.8	0.5	1.4	1.5	2.4	3.5	5.4	6.1	8.2	6.8	3.1	1.3	0	68	194
195	0.8	0.2	0.0	1.7	0.0	0.3	0.3	0.0	0.0	0.0	0.3	0.0	0.0	0.5	1.4	0.0	1.7	0.0	0.2	0	13	195
196	0.2	0.4	0.4	1.2	1.6	0.7	0.3	1.0	0.5	0.3	0.6	0.0	1.2	1.9	0.7	4.1	0.0	0.0	0.7	0	35	196
197	0.0	0.0	0.0	1.5	0.3	0.3	0.0	1.0	1.4	1.1	1.8	1.4	3.1	4.9	3.4	4.1	13.6	15.6	1.2	0	67	197
200	0.2	1.5	1.0	1.5	1.2	0.7	2.1	1.8	2.8	3.0	2.4	3.4	10.4	14.1	17.7	17.5	13.6	6.3	3.5	0	188	200
201	0.0	0.6	0.2	0.0	3.4	4.3	2.9	3.6	2.3	3.0	5.4	3.1	5.4	6.3	8.2	7.2	8.5	9.4	3.0	0	159	201
203	0.0	0.0	0.0	3.7	0.0	0.0	0.0	0.0	1.0	1.9	3.9	7.5	12.0	19.5	30.6	23.7	42.5	21.9	4.0	0	217	203
204	5.7	6.0	3.7	1.5	2.8	1.7	2.1	2.3	2.8	3.5	9.9	11.9	20.9	28.7	55.1	44.3	42.5	34.4	9.0	0	483	204
202,205	0.0	0.2	0.0	1.5	0.0	2.6	0.0	0.8	1.8	1.9	3.0	2.4	3.9	4.4	4.8	7.2	5.1	6.3	1.6	0	87	202,205
OTHER	0.0	0.6	0.0	1.5	0.0	1.0	0.0	3.3	4.4	6.3	7.5	20.0	31.7	50.6	54.4	89.6	91.8	122.0	11.1	0	595	OTHER
140-205	15.8	15.2	10.4	18.2	21.2	27.1	39.9	52.0	75.3	109.4	199.1	353.3	616.5	922.8	1284.1	1602.3	1915.0	2120.1	221.6	5	11898	140-205
RATE PER CASE IN PERIOD	0.21	0.21	0.20	0.25	0.31	0.33	0.29	0.26	0.26	0.27	0.30	0.34	0.39	0.49	0.68	1.03	1.70	3.13	0.02	-	-	RATE PER CASE IN PERIOD

TABLE 30 C
NORWAY :
FEMALE INCIDENCE RATES, 1959 - 61.

AVERAGE ANNUAL INCIDENCE PER 100,000 — AGE IN YEARS

International List No.	Cases Age Unknown	Cases All Ages	Incidence All Ages	0-	5-	10-	15-	20-	25-	30-	35-	40-	45-	50-	55-	60-	65-	70-	75-	80-	85- and over
140	0	13	0.2	0.0	0.0	0.0	0.0	0.0	0.0	0.0	0.0	0.3	0.0	0.0	0.0	0.3	1.3	0.6	1.6	3.9	4.4
141	0	39	0.7	0.0	0.0	0.0	0.0	0.0	0.0	0.0	0.3	0.5	0.5	0.0	0.9	1.4	2.2	5.6	4.0	2.6	11.0
142	0	23	0.4	0.0	0.0	0.0	0.3	0.0	0.0	0.0	0.0	0.3	0.3	0.3	0.9	0.0	1.7	2.2	3.2	5.2	0.0
143-4	0	51	0.9	0.0	0.2	0.0	0.0	0.0	0.0	0.3	0.0	0.0	0.0	1.2	1.6	3.5	1.3	4.5	6.4	5.2	15.4
146	0	8	0.1	0.7	0.2	0.0	0.0	0.0	0.0	0.0	0.0	0.0	0.0	0.3	0.0	0.3	0.9	1.1	0.8	0.0	0.0
145,147-8	0	40	0.7	0.0	0.0	0.0	0.0	0.0	0.0	0.0	0.0	0.3	0.3	1.2	1.9	1.4	0.9	3.9	5.6	3.9	6.6
150	0	69	1.3	0.0	0.0	0.0	0.0	0.0	0.0	2.1	0.0	0.0	0.5	0.9	1.9	4.2	3.5	6.7	8.8	13.0	11.0
151	0	1707	31.6	0.0	0.0	0.0	0.0	0.3	0.0	2.1	6.0	8.6	14.0	16.1	40.4	61.0	113.1	134.0	242.2	316.0	408.4
152	1	20	0.4	0.0	0.0	0.0	0.0	0.0	0.0	0.0	0.5	0.0	0.3	0.6	0.0	0.7	1.7	1.1	4.0	1.3	0.0
153	1	884	16.4	0.0	0.0	0.0	0.0	0.3	0.7	0.9	3.9	5.4	8.8	12.9	22.1	42.6	56.1	76.2	100.7	146.3	149.3
154	0	360	6.7	0.0	0.0	0.0	0.0	0.3	0.0	0.6	1.3	2.3	4.1	4.7	12.3	14.0	24.6	37.0	38.4	46.6	59.3
155.0	0	37	0.7	0.7	0.2	0.0	0.0	0.0	0.0	0.0	0.3	0.0	0.3	0.9	0.9	0.7	3.5	2.2	4.4	3.9	8.8
155.1	0	144	2.7	0.0	0.0	0.0	0.0	0.0	0.0	0.0	0.3	0.3	0.5	2.3	2.8	7.7	12.5	15.7	19.2	24.6	17.6
156	0	74	1.4	0.0	0.0	0.0	0.0	0.0	0.7	0.3	0.3	2.9	2.2	2.0	0.6	2.4	2.6	5.6	10.4	22.0	8.8
157	0	323	6.0	0.0	0.0	0.0	0.0	0.0	0.3	0.3	0.3	2.9	2.2	4.4	6.0	18.1	23.7	35.3	36.0	42.7	39.5
160	0	33	0.6	0.0	0.0	0.0	0.0	0.0	0.0	0.0	0.0	0.0	1.1	0.6	0.9	1.0	1.7	2.2	3.2	3.9	8.8
161	0	4	0.1	1.8	0.2	0.0	0.0	0.0	0.7	0.0	0.0	0.8	0.0	0.0	0.3	0.0	0.4	0.6	0.8	0.0	0.0
162-3	0	228	4.2	0.0	0.0	0.2	0.0	0.0	0.7	0.0	0.5	0.8	2.5	5.3	11.1	14.0	15.4	20.2	19.2	19.4	15.4
170	4	2958	54.7	0.0	0.0	0.0	0.0	0.3	2.4	10.3	31.3	72.6	101.3	93.0	108.6	136.0	127.3	163.1	194.2	211.1	221.8
171	0	1044	19.3	0.0	0.0	0.0	0.0	0.3	4.8	21.0	35.5	41.7	37.3	36.6	40.4	37.0	27.2	26.9	21.6	28.5	19.8
172	0	579	10.7	0.0	0.0	0.0	0.0	0.0	0.3	0.9	2.4	7.5	12.1	29.3	36.9	36.3	31.9	27.5	22.4	22.0	8.8
173	0	10	0.2	0.0	0.0	0.0	0.0	0.0	1.4	0.3	0.5	0.5	0.3	0.0	0.0	0.0	0.0	0.0	0.0	0.0	0.0
174	1	76	1.4	0.0	0.0	0.0	0.0	0.0	0.0	0.0	0.0	0.5	2.2	1.8	2.5	4.2	3.9	4.5	3.2	15.5	13.2
175	0	834	15.4	0.0	0.0	0.6	1.6	2.9	2.7	6.1	7.6	14.8	25.0	32.2	37.6	40.5	47.0	44.8	35.2	29.8	22.0
176	0	199	3.7	0.0	0.2	0.0	0.0	0.0	0.0	0.6	2.4	1.6	2.5	5.9	5.4	10.5	11.7	15.7	16.8	20.7	30.7
180	0	272	5.0	1.8	0.2	0.0	0.3	0.0	0.0	0.3	0.8	1.8	1.6	5.9	11.7	12.6	23.3	17.9	32.0	22.0	19.8
181.0	0	182	3.4	0.0	0.0	0.0	0.0	0.7	2.0	0.0	0.3	0.5	1.4	2.0	3.5	5.9	10.8	20.7	29.6	25.9	43.9
190	0	180	3.3	0.0	0.0	0.0	1.0	0.0	2.0	3.0	4.7	6.5	3.8	4.4	4.4	4.5	6.0	10.7	5.6	19.4	8.8
192	0	50	0.9	1.3	0.0	0.0	0.0	0.7	0.0	0.0	0.5	1.3	1.1	1.2	2.5	1.0	2.2	3.9	3.2	3.9	2.2
193	0	395	7.3	2.4	2.7	1.7	4.4	2.0	5.1	6.1	5.8	7.8	8.2	15.8	18.6	12.9	16.0	13.5	6.4	3.9	4.4
194	0	152	2.8	0.0	0.2	0.4	0.0	1.0	1.4	1.8	1.6	2.9	2.2	4.1	4.4	4.9	8.6	10.7	11.2	15.5	8.8
195	0	9	0.2	0.4	1.4	0.2	0.0	0.0	0.0	0.3	0.0	0.0	0.0	0.3	0.3	0.0	0.0	0.0	0.0	2.6	2.2
196	0	33	0.6	0.4	0.2	1.7	1.0	0.7	1.0	0.6	0.8	0.3	0.5	0.0	0.0	1.0	0.9	0.0	0.8	2.6	0.0
197	0	59	1.1	0.0	0.0	0.9	0.3	0.7	0.3	0.3	0.8	1.6	0.3	0.9	1.6	3.5	1.7	2.8	3.2	3.9	4.4
200	0	120	2.2	0.0	0.0	0.0	0.3	1.6	2.7	0.6	0.5	1.0	1.6	3.2	4.4	5.6	8.2	7.8	13.6	10.4	2.2
201	0	103	1.9	0.0	0.0	0.4	2.3	1.6	0.3	0.0	1.3	2.3	2.5	1.2	1.3	3.8	3.5	6.7	4.0	5.2	2.2
203	0	109	2.0	0.0	0.0	0.0	0.0	0.0	2.0	2.1	0.3	0.5	0.3	2.9	3.8	4.9	10.4	12.9	8.0	7.8	11.0
204	1	394	7.3	5.3	4.7	1.3	1.6	1.3	1.0	0.0	3.4	4.1	4.1	7.3	10.4	14.7	20.3	31.4	32.0	28.5	22.0
202,205	0	65	1.2	0.0	0.0	0.0	0.3	0.0	1.0	0.0	0.8	1.0	0.5	2.0	2.8	2.8	3.5	3.9	6.4	1.3	2.2
OTHER	0	805	14.9	0.0	1.4	0.0	0.5	0.0	0.0	0.0	2.6	7.0	5.2	10.8	20.5	25.1	46.6	71.2	93.5	129.5	245.9
140-205	8	12685	234.7	12.4	12.0	7.6	13.7	13.3	31.4	60.2	116.7	199.4	250.1	314.3	426.6	541.0	678.9	851.6	1052.0	1266.5	1455.9
RATE PER CASE IN PERIOD	-	-	0.02	0.22	0.23	0.22	0.26	0.33	0.34	0.30	0.26	0.26	0.27	0.29	0.32	0.35	0.43	0.56	0.80	1.30	2.20

SWEDEN

Registry Title and Address : Medicinalstyrelsens Cancerregister, Fack, Stockholm 3, Sweden. Commenced 1958. Supported financially by the Government.

Registration. Cases are registered compulsorily from hospital in-patients and out-patients, and radiotherapy departments by physicians. Independent reports, also compulsory, are made from pathology departments on all biopsies and autopsies where cancer is found.

Follow up. There is no follow up.

Physical Description. The Registry covers the whole of Sweden. Bordered on the north and west by Norway, on the east by Finland, and on the east, south and west by the Baltic Sea, it lies between latitudes $55^{0}20'$ and $69^{0}4'$ north and between longitudes $10^{0}58'$ and $24^{0}10'$ east. The total registration area is 449.687 square kilometres.

Demographic Description. Total population of area under survey 7,480,400. Virtually the whole population is Caucasian and Protestant. The main occupational composition (of total male population) is industry 28.3%, commerce 11.4%, agriculture 10.9%, and personal service 6.2%. Of the total population 25.5% live in conurbation of more than 100,000.

Medical Services. Total number of hospital beds of all kinds 122,233 (1963). Total number of doctors in practice in registration area 8,520 (1965). Cancer causes approximately 19.9% of all deaths.

Publications. Annual reports (Ringertz, Törnberg, Sjöström and Swenson, 1962, 1963 and 1965).

TABLE 31 A
SWEDEN :
POPULATION (100,000s), 1960

AGE (in years)	MALES		FEMALES	
	No.	Per Cent	No.	Per Cent
0-	2.6830	7.19	2.5324	6.76
5-	2.7541	7.38	2.6041	6.95
10-	3.1616	8.47	3.0150	8.04
15-	2.9303	7.85	2.8182	7.52
20-	2.3217	6.22	2.2772	6.07
25-	2.2103	5.92	2.1768	5.81
30-	2.3909	6.41	2.3624	6.30
35-	2.7516	7.37	2.7041	7.21
40-	2.6594	7.13	2.6081	6.96
45-	2.7079	7.26	2.6586	7.09
50-	2.5903	6.94	2.5958	6.92
55-	2.2472	6.02	2.3366	6.23
60-	1.8818	5.04	2.0304	5.42
65-	1.4967	4.01	1.7079	4.56
70-	1.1473	3.07	1.3580	3.62
75-	0.7644	2.05	0.9206	2.46
80-	0.4250	1.14	0.5232	1.40
85- and over	0.1913	0.51	0.2598	0.69
TOTAL	37.3148	100.00	37.4892	100.00

NOTES

TO TABLES 31 A, B and C

(I) I.L. number 193 includes benign and unspecified tumours of the central nervous system.

(II) Carcinoma in situ excluded.

TABLE 31 B

SWEDEN :

MALE INCIDENCE RATES, 1959 - 61.

INTER-NATIONAL LIST No.	AVERAGE ANNUAL INCIDENCE PER 100,000 — AGE IN YEARS																		ALL AGES	No. OF CASES IN WHOLE PERIOD — ALL AGES	No. OF CASES IN WHOLE PERIOD — AGE UNKNOWN	INTER-NATIONAL LIST No.
	0-	5-	10-	15-	20-	25-	30-	35-	40-	45-	50-	55-	60-	65-	70-	75-	80-	85- AND OVER				
140	0.0	0.0	0.0	0.0	0.0	0.0	0.4	1.0	1.8	3.1	6.6	7.1	11.3	14.7	18.9	25.3	19.6	26.1	3.9	442	0	140
141	0.0	0.0	0.0	0.0	0.0	0.0	0.0	0.0	0.1	1.0	1.2	1.9	3.0	2.7	2.3	3.5	5.5	5.2	0.8	86	0	141
142	0.0	0.0	0.0	0.1	0.4	0.3	0.3	0.4	0.8	0.7	1.3	1.5	1.8	2.4	3.2	2.2	1.6	10.5	0.8	88	0	142
143-4	0.0	0.0	0.0	0.1	0.1	0.0	0.1	0.4	0.4	0.7	1.2	3.7	4.8	4.7	8.7	7.8	14.1	17.4	1.5	173	0	143-4
146	0.0	0.0	0.2	0.3	0.3	0.0	0.1	0.6	0.5	1.1	1.9	2.7	1.9	2.2	2.6	3.1	0.8	3.5	0.9	99	0	146
145,147-8	0.0	0.0	0.0	0.0	0.0	0.0	0.0	0.1	0.6	0.5	1.0	4.6	6.0	6.7	4.9	8.3	9.4	5.2	1.5	164	0	145,147-8
150	0.0	0.0	0.0	0.0	0.0	0.6	0.0	0.0	0.3	1.2	2.7	8.0	12.6	16.9	21.2	27.5	28.2	22.7	3.7	419	0	150
151	0.0	0.0	0.0	0.0	0.7	0.0	2.2	3.9	9.3	20.2	30.0	62.0	104.0	165.5	243.8	316.2	375.7	256.1	39.1	4466	0	151
152	0.0	0.0	0.0	0.0	0.0	0.0	0.6	0.4	0.4	1.5	1.7	0.9	2.5	4.7	5.2	9.2	7.1	3.5	1.1	126	0	152
153	0.0	0.0	0.0	1.1	1.1	1.7	2.4	4.1	6.9	8.2	15.1	27.7	48.9	79.1	111.6	154.8	196.9	156.8	19.8	2217	0	153
154	0.0	0.0	0.0	0.1	0.3	1.1	1.4	1.9	4.0	8.0	14.4	21.8	38.8	64.4	88.9	118.2	133.3	116.7	15.3	1714	0	154
155.0	0.5	0.0	0.0	0.1	0.0	0.2	0.0	0.0	0.4	0.4	1.3	6.1	7.8	12.7	15.1	16.6	22.0	17.4	2.6	292	0	155.0
155.1	0.0	0.0	0.0	0.0	0.1	0.2	0.3	0.2	0.5	1.0	1.4	3.4	6.0	12.9	15.7	14.4	23.5	22.7	2.4	273	0	155.1
156	0.0	0.0	0.0	0.0	0.0	0.0	0.1	0.0	0.1	0.5	1.3	0.9	3.0	4.9	6.7	3.1	3.1	8.7	0.9	105	0	156
157	0.0	0.0	0.0	0.1	0.1	0.0	0.8	1.0	1.9	4.3	10.2	17.9	31.7	43.9	57.5	65.8	75.3	61.0	10.0	1122	0	157
160	0.0	0.0	0.0	0.0	0.1	0.0	0.3	0.2	1.0	2.1	1.4	1.2	2.8	5.3	5.5	10.5	7.1	3.5	1.3	143	0	160
161	0.0	0.0	0.1	0.0	0.1	0.0	0.3	0.5	1.1	2.7	2.3	6.1	10.8	11.6	11.9	12.2	8.6	3.5	2.6	291	0	161
162-3	0.0	0.0	0.0	0.1	0.0	0.5	0.6	2.5	7.6	13.3	29.2	59.3	97.1	112.2	104.3	90.7	51.0	43.6	22.7	2537	0	162-3
170	0.0	0.0	0.0	0.0	0.3	0.2	0.0	0.2	0.3	0.2	0.9	0.6	1.2	3.8	2.6	3.1	3.9	3.5	0.6	65	0	170
177	0.0	0.0	0.0	0.0	0.1	0.0	0.3	0.2	0.3	2.3	9.4	28.6	78.6	173.9	323.4	462.2	554.5	496.6	41.8	4680	0	177
178	1.0	0.5	0.2	0.7	2.9	4.4	7.0	5.5	3.6	2.7	2.4	2.1	2.5	0.9	3.5	3.1	3.9	0.0	2.6	290	0	178
179.0	0.0	0.0	0.0	0.0	0.1	0.2	0.3	0.1	0.9	2.0	1.8	2.5	2.3	3.8	3.8	11.3	13.3	10.5	1.3	151	0	179.0
180	2.4	0.1	0.2	0.5	0.0	0.8	1.0	1.8	5.3	7.5	12.5	21.5	31.5	49.9	43.0	52.8	54.9	54.0	10.5	1170	0	180
181.0	0.2	0.0	0.0	0.3	0.6	0.3	1.5	2.3	3.5	6.0	12.1	23.1	37.7	54.3	66.0	74.6	78.4	71.4	12.2	1364	0	181.0
190	0.0	0.1	0.2	0.5	0.7	2.3	2.6	4.0	3.5	4.6	4.5	4.7	4.6	7.6	8.4	6.5	14.9	12.2	3.0	338	0	190
191	0.0	0.0	0.0	0.3	0.1	0.5	0.8	1.1	1.4	2.1	4.8	8.3	16.5	18.7	38.6	53.6	123.9	156.8	7.4	824	0	191
192	1.7	0.4	0.3	0.2	0.1	0.2	0.0	0.4	0.8	0.9	2.6	2.7	1.8	2.9	4.1	3.5	4.7	1.7	1.2	130	0	192
193	2.5	3.3	2.7	3.2	3.2	2.9	5.6	8.1	9.5	13.5	14.7	18.7	20.4	20.0	13.7	15.7	12.5	22.7	8.9	992	0	193
194	0.0	0.2	0.1	0.1	0.3	0.6	1.1	1.3	2.4	1.8	1.5	2.2	3.7	6.7	4.4	5.7	5.5	5.2	1.6	179	0	194
195	0.9	0.4	1.6	2.6	0.6	0.8	0.8	1.5	1.9	1.4	2.6	5.0	4.6	3.6	6.1	2.6	3.9	1.7	1.7	194	0	195
196	0.1	0.4	0.7	1.4	1.3	1.1	0.6	0.6	0.5	0.9	1.2	0.9	1.8	2.0	2.3	3.1	2.4	7.0	1.2	134	0	196
197	0.7	0.6	0.7	1.5	1.3	1.7	1.5	1.2	1.6	2.3	3.0	4.9	5.3	7.1	10.5	8.3	7.8	8.7	2.5	280	0	197
200	0.9	0.6	0.8	1.4	1.1	0.8	1.1	1.6	3.0	3.3	6.9	7.9	11.3	15.6	20.3	21.4	22.7	33.1	4.7	524	0	200
201	0.1	0.6	0.0	1.5	3.7	3.8	2.8	3.4	3.6	4.7	3.5	3.9	5.5	6.5	10.5	13.1	8.6	7.0	3.5	387	0	201
203	0.1	0.0	0.0	0.0	0.0	0.2	0.1	0.6	1.5	2.3	3.2	9.2	10.6	12.5	21.5	29.7	16.5	19.2	3.7	416	0	203
204	6.0	2.9	3.1	3.0	2.0	3.0	3.2	3.9	5.6	7.6	11.1	19.9	26.4	36.3	58.7	52.3	58.8	57.5	11.5	1285	0	204
202,205	0.0	0.0	0.0	0.1	0.1	0.3	0.7	0.1	0.6	0.4	0.1	1.0	0.9	1.1	0.6	1.3	1.6	3.5	0.4	45	0	202,205
OTHER	0.6	0.2	0.3	0.6	0.9	1.2	2.2	2.1	2.9	4.2	12.2	14.8	25.9	37.6	46.5	49.7	48.6	57.5	8.9	998	0	OTHER
140-205	17.8	9.9	11.4	17.7	23.0	29.1	42.9	57.2	89.9	141.3	235.0	419.5	688.0	1032.3	1416.4	1762.6	2027.5	1813.9	260.9	29203	0	140-205
RATE PER CASE IN PERIOD	0.12	0.12	0.11	0.11	0.14	0.15	0.14	0.12	0.13	0.12	0.13	0.15	0.18	0.22	0.29	0.44	0.78	1.74	0.01	-	-	RATE PER CASE IN PERIOD

TABLE 31 C
SWEDEN :
FEMALE INCIDENCE RATES, 1959 - 61.

AVERAGE ANNUAL INCIDENCE PER 100,000 — AGE IN YEARS

INTER-NATIONAL LIST No.	0-	5-	10-	15-	20-	25-	30-	35-	40-	45-	50-	55-	60-	65-	70-	75-	80-	85- AND OVER	ALL AGES	AGE UNKNOWN (cases)	ALL AGES (cases)	INTER-NATIONAL LIST No.
140	0.1	0.0	0.0	0.0	0.0	0.0	0.0	0.0	0.0	0.1	0.1	0.3	1.0	1.0	2.0	2.2	1.9	5.1	0.3	0	37	140
141	0.0	0.0	0.0	0.0	0.0	0.0	0.1	0.2	0.6	0.6	0.6	2.1	1.6	2.3	4.7	4.0	6.4	9.0	0.9	0	102	141
142	0.0	0.0	0.1	0.0	0.3	0.6	0.1	0.6	0.8	1.0	0.9	2.0	1.1	2.1	2.0	4.0	5.1	2.6	0.8	0	95	142
143-144	0.0	0.0	0.0	0.0	0.0	0.0	0.1	0.1	0.3	0.6	1.0	1.7	1.3	2.9	3.4	8.0	12.1	7.7	1.0	0	113	143-144
146	0.0	0.0	0.1	0.1	0.6	0.2	0.0	0.1	0.1	0.6	0.5	1.4	2.5	1.2	2.5	2.5	4.5	1.3	0.6	0	70	146
145,147-8	0.0	0.0	0.0	0.0	0.0	0.0	0.1	0.1	0.3	0.8	1.4	2.6	2.1	4.3	4.7	6.2	4.5	2.6	1.0	0	118	145,147-8
150	0.0	0.0	0.1	0.1	0.1	1.2	0.1	0.2	0.3	0.8	1.4	2.7	4.3	6.8	11.0	15.6	20.4	23.1	2.1	0	240	150
151	0.0	0.0	0.1	0.1	0.1	0.2	1.8	3.5	6.1	11.9	16.2	28.2	44.8	85.9	116.1	162.9	186.0	136.0	22.7	0	2553	151
152	0.0	0.0	0.0	0.0	0.1	0.2	0.0	0.5	0.1	0.5	0.8	1.0	2.5	4.5	4.2	6.5	6.4	6.4	1.0	0	112	152
153	0.0	0.0	0.1	0.7	1.3	2.0	1.7	5.1	6.9	15.7	18.7	28.4	53.4	67.7	100.9	130.0	134.4	132.2	21.0	0	2362	153
154	0.1	0.0	0.0	0.0	0.1	0.8	1.7	2.0	4.1	6.6	12.7	14.4	24.1	33.6	43.7	57.2	64.3	52.6	9.9	0	1117	154
155.0	0.4	0.0	0.0	0.0	0.3	0.2	0.3	0.1	0.1	0.4	1.5	1.4	1.6	5.1	5.6	11.9	10.2	10.2	1.3	0	149	155.0
155.1	0.0	0.0	0.0	0.0	0.0	0.0	0.0	0.1	0.8	2.1	4.2	5.8	13.0	19.5	29.9	34.0	32.5	38.5	5.1	0	574	155.1
156	0.1	0.0	0.0	0.0	0.1	0.2	0.1	0.6	0.3	0.5	0.6	2.3	3.4	2.7	4.9	7.2	3.2	5.1	1.0	0	115	156
157	0.0	0.1	0.0	0.0	0.1	0.3	0.7	0.2	1.4	3.1	4.9	10.3	19.4	29.9	36.1	47.1	54.2	41.1	7.3	0	824	157
160	0.1	0.0	0.0	0.1	0.1	0.0	0.1	0.2	0.1	0.8	1.2	1.6	2.5	2.7	4.2	4.0	6.4	6.4	0.9	0	106	160
161	0.0	0.0	0.0	0.0	0.0	0.0	0.0	0.1	0.1	0.3	0.1	0.1	1.3	0.8	1.0	1.1	0.6	2.6	0.3	0	35	161
162-3	0.1	0.0	0.0	0.0	0.0	0.2	0.8	1.5	2.2	4.9	7.4	9.4	17.1	22.8	31.7	32.9	27.4	15.4	6.2	0	696	162-3
170	0.0	0.0	0.2	0.0	0.7	2.9	11.1	30.7	70.7	109.0	117.2	121.1	164.2	181.3	214.8	226.3	248.5	220.7	66.9	0	7529	170
171	0.0	0.0	0.0	0.1	1.3	7.4	20.3	42.4	50.7	49.8	42.0	39.4	32.5	28.3	23.6	21.4	21.7	19.2	22.1	0	2490	171
172	0.0	0.0	0.0	0.0	0.0	0.8	0.4	2.0	6.4	19.4	39.4	47.5	51.2	57.6	47.6	51.1	35.7	32.1	16.8	0	1887	172
173	0.0	0.0	0.0	0.0	0.0	0.2	1.0	0.7	0.0	0.1	0.3	0.1	0.0	0.0	0.0	0.0	0.0	0.0	0.2	0	22	173
174	0.0	0.0	0.0	0.1	0.4	0.2	0.7	1.8	2.9	5.8	7.7	6.7	7.7	7.2	8.1	7.2	5.1	5.1	3.1	0	350	174
175	0.0	0.3	0.6	1.7	2.3	3.1	4.0	7.8	14.1	30.4	37.5	49.2	47.6	50.9	48.1	47.8	37.0	24.4	18.6	0	2097	175
176	0.3	0.0	0.0	0.1	0.3	0.3	0.1	1.2	1.0	1.8	3.9	6.3	8.2	10.9	14.5	17.4	22.3	20.5	3.4	0	378	176
180	1.7	0.6	0.0	0.1	0.1	0.2	0.8	0.7	3.6	4.3	8.9	14.0	19.2	23.4	30.9	33.7	28.7	24.4	7.0	0	782	180
181.0	0.0	0.0	0.0	0.1	1.8	0.3	0.6	0.4	1.2	1.9	5.0	8.0	11.5	18.2	22.3	31.9	21.7	33.4	4.7	0	532	181.0
190	0.0	0.1	0.4	0.9	0.0	1.7	2.5	4.1	5.0	6.0	6.0	5.4	5.6	6.4	8.8	8.7	10.2	10.3	3.6	0	410	190
191	0.0	0.0	0.2	0.2	0.0	0.3	1.0	0.9	2.0	2.0	2.8	4.4	7.6	9.4	20.9	27.2	49.7	79.5	4.4	0	490	191
192	1.2	0.1	0.0	0.1	0.0	0.6	0.4	0.7	1.0	0.9	1.5	2.7	1.8	3.1	4.4	1.4	5.7	1.3	1.1	0	129	192
193	3.0	3.2	2.0	1.9	2.2	3.8	5.8	5.3	9.5	12.2	13.5	20.5	20.2	13.9	15.5	19.2	21.0	10.3	8.7	0	977	193
194	0.4	0.1	0.6	0.9	2.5	2.3	2.8	3.3	4.6	4.0	5.8	4.0	7.7	10.1	14.5	13.0	19.8	10.3	4.2	0	467	194
195	0.3	0.1	0.1	0.2	0.6	0.6	1.6	1.8	2.2	2.1	4.4	3.1	2.8	2.9	4.7	2.9	3.2	2.6	1.7	0	196	195
196	0.8	0.3	1.0	1.4	1.5	0.3	0.4	0.5	0.9	0.6	0.9	1.1	1.1	2.0	0.7	1.4	2.5	1.3	0.9	0	99	196
197	0.4	0.5	0.2	1.5	1.2	0.9	0.7	1.6	2.0	2.0	2.8	3.3	4.1	3.9	6.9	5.4	7.6	3.8	2.1	0	235	197
200	0.4	0.1	0.8	0.7	0.3	0.9	1.1	1.0	2.3	2.5	5.0	5.8	10.7	11.5	17.7	23.9	18.5	16.7	4.1	0	466	200
201	0.0	0.1	0.3	1.5	2.2	2.9	1.1	2.5	2.0	2.8	1.9	2.4	3.4	6.4	5.6	6.9	10.2	6.4	2.4	0	266	201
203	4.1	0.0	2.3	1.5	0.0	0.2	0.1	0.1	0.8	2.0	3.1	4.9	8.5	11.5	17.2	15.6	17.2	12.8	3.1	0	344	203
204	0.1	4.0	0.0	0.0	1.5	2.5	3.2	3.0	4.0	5.6	10.3	12.4	17.2	22.2	35.6	29.7	41.4	21.8	8.4	0	940	204
202,205	1.1	0.1	0.0	0.0	0.0	0.2	0.1	0.0	0.3	0.9	0.8	1.3	0.7	2.1	0.7	1.4	1.3	1.3	0.5	0	53	202,205
OTHER	1.1	0.3	0.1	0.0	0.1	0.8	0.6	1.7	2.6	7.3	11.8	17.4	25.9	34.2	47.1	56.1	57.3	50.0	10.1	0	1136	OTHER
140-205	14.3	10.0	9.4	14.5	21.8	38.6	68.7	129.2	212.9	324.9	408.0	497.0	656.5	913.5	1018.7	1186.9	1266.6	1104.7	281.8	0	31693	140-205
RATE PER CASE IN PERIOD	0.13	0.13	0.11	0.12	0.15	0.15	0.14	0.12	0.13	0.13	0.13	0.14	0.16	0.20	0.25	0.36	0.64	1.28	0.01	-	-	RATE PER CASE IN PERIOD

YUGOSLAVIA, SLOVENIA

In 1949 nation-wide cancer registration, covering the population of Slovenia, was initiated by the Institute of Oncology in Ljubljana as one of its activities. In 1950, a decree providing compulsory cancer notification was issued by the Ministry of Health of the People's Republic of Slovenia, effective as of January 1st, 1950, by which the central Cancer Registry of Slovenia was also officially recognised.

From its inception until 1961 the Registry was financed by the University Hospital and the Medical Faculty of Ljubljana respectively. Later on means have been allocated from the Republic Ministry of Health on the basis of annual contracts with the Institute of Oncology.

In view of the steadily increasing amount of registered cases, and because of some deficiencies of the registration system, revealed during the first decade, an extensive revision of the Registry's operations has been carried out in 1959 and 1960, and the mechanical tabulation system was introduced. New standard report forms and a detailed code were designed and adjusted to the IBM punch card system. All the abstract cards filed until 1961 were thoroughly reviewed, coded and transferred to punch cards.

The experiences.of the Connecticut Tumor Registry have proved to be of great assistance in the redesigning of the operating system of the Slovene Cancer Registry. In developing the Registry's new code the Uniform Punch Card Code, used by the End Results Evalutation Section, National Cancer Insitute, Bethesda, Md., U.S.A., has been taken as a basis and adapted to the specific requirements of the cancer registration in Slovenia. The acceptance of this code as a basis has been guided by the wish to conform the registration design to the registries abroad in order to facilitate the international comparison of data.

The purposes and tasks of the Registry are, in brief, the following :

1. To compile data on all newly diagnosed cases of cancer in the population of Slovenia.
2. To compile periodical follow-up information as to the condition of the recorded patients until the end of their lives.
3. To furnish statistical surveys and reports on cancer incidence and on the survival of the patients, and on the end results of cancer therapy.

The main items of information collected by the Registry are : age, sex, area of residence, primary site of the cancer, histological type of the cancer, stage at diagnosis, when and where the diagnosis was established, when and where first treatment was given, type of treatment, findings at follow-up and survival.

The Registry can thus provide the health authorities and the medical profession with all the basic information necessary for a rational planning and evaluation of the cancer control programme, and the organisation of medical care. On the other hand the information can also serve as a sound basis for clinical and epidemiological investigations.

Compulsory notification concerns the hospitals only, as it is assumed that every patient in whom cancer diagnosis is established or suspected, is sent to a hospital. All clinically diagnosed malignant neoplastic diseases have to be reported. In this connection it should be noted that cancer cases and not cancer patients count as units in the register.

The hospitals are obliged to report every cancer patient every time when admitted or treated in the out-patient department, without regard to whether the patient had been in another hospital before, or not. The collecting of complete and accurate information about the individual patient is greatly facilitated by the fact that in average, sooner or later, about 45% of all cancer patients from Slovenia are admitted to the Institute of Oncology.

Hospitals are requested to complete their reports after discharge or death of the patient, and to submit to the Registry as complete information about the disease as possible, including histological and eventually autopsy findings.

The name and address of the physician or health institution responsible for the care and the follow-up of the patient must be given in the report.

If there are any omissions or inaccuracies in case reports submitted to the Registry, additional information and explanations are always requested from the hospitals.

Cancer patients who for one reason or another have either never been admitted to a hospital, or those whom the hospitals omitted to report, are brought to the attention of the Registry through official death certificates. Death certificates in which cancer is mentioned are passed on to the Registry by the Republic Institute of Statistics.

Death certificates of persons not reported to the Registry before are thoroughly checked and query is made for additional information by contacting the certifying physician or, if necessary, the close relatives of the deceased. If it is found that the deceased has been treated for his malignant disease in a hospital, a report is requested from the hospital concerned, and if submitted the case is not registered as obtained from the death certificate. During the last decade 11 - 19% of recorded cases have been registered annually on the basis of death certificate only. However, there have been not more than about 7% of cases in which the death certificate was the only source of data without any additional information.

In conducting the follow-up programme the Registry is responsible for obtaining information on every recorded cancer patient at least once a year. Periodical follow-up examination are more or less regularly carried out by the Institute of Oncology, and the few existing district cancer clinics (dispensaries), but unfortunately only exceptionally by hospitals.

If no information on a patient has been received for more than one year a questionnaire is sent to either the local physician or to the regional health centre. If necessary, the community, the patient's relatives, or even the patient himself, are requested for information.

In spite of considerable efforts in collecting follow-up information, still about 7% of the total number of recorded patients are lost to follow-up within the first five years following diagnosis, most of them being non-residents.

At present the responsibility for the programme, organisation and medical supervision of the Registry is entrusted to a part-time head physician, assisted by a health statistician who is in charge of routine operations. The clerical staff comprises one part-time and three full-time employees.

Bozena Ravnihar

Registry Title and Address : The Cancer Registry of Slovenia, The Institute of Oncology, Vrazov trg 4, Ljubljana, Yugoslavia. Commenced 1950. Supported financially by the University Hospitals and the Medical Faculty of Ljubljana till 1961, and by Annual Contracts from the Ministry of Health from 1961 on.

Registration. Cases are registered by doctor responsible for patient's care and clerical staff from hospital in-patients. Out-patients are registered by examining doctor and clerical staff. Radiotherapists and clerical staff register patients in conjunction with hospital staff. Cases are registered from death certificates supplied by the Republic Institute of Statistics. Doctors attending cases at home supply additional information when asked. Registration may be less than 90% completed for old people in rural areas.

Follow-up. Approximately 90% of cases are followed up at least once a year till death.

Physical Description. Slovenia is one of the six republics of the Socialist Federal Republic of Yugoslavia. It occupies the north western-most part of the territory of Yugoslavia and is bounded on the west by Italy, on the north by Austria, on the north east by Hungary, and on the east by another republic of Yugoslavia, Croatia. It lies between latitudes 45°25' and 46°53' North and longitudes 13°23' and 16°36' East. The total registration area is 20,255 square kilometres.

Demographic Description. Total population of area under survey 1,562,040. The population comprises 95.6% native Slovenes, 3.2% other Slavic nations, and 1,2% non-Slavic nationalities. The main occupational composition of the registration population is industry 31.4%, commerce 7.6%, agriculture 31.3% personal service 4.3% and others 25.4%. Of the total population 10.4% live in conurbations of more than 100,000.

Medical Services. Total number of hospital beds of all kinds 11,451 (1960). Total number of doctors in practice in registration area 1,418 (1960). Cancer caused approximately 15.8% of all deaths in 1961.

Publications. Annual reports, 1950-55 (in Slovene, 6th report for 1955 also in English). Ravnihar (1960, 1963).

TABLE 32 A

YUGOSLAVIA, SLOVENIA :

POPULATION (100,000s), MEAN 1956 - 60

AGE (in years)	MALES		FEMALES	
	No.	Per Cent	No.	Per Cent
0-	0.7619	10.26	0.7263	8.87
5-	0.7709	10.38	0.7448	9.09
10-	0.6400	8.62	0.6247	7.63
15-	0.6505	8.76	0.6374	7.78
20-	0.6671	8.98	0.6533	7.97
25-	0.6756	9.09	0.6869	8.38
30-	0.5431	7.31	0.6558	8.01
35-	0.3911	5.27	0.5130	6.26
40-	0.3358	4.52	0.4083	4.98
45-	0.4644	6.25	0.5333	6.51
50-	0.4319	5.81	0.4959	6.05
55-	0.3663	4.93	0.4426	5.40
60-	0.2620	3.53	0.3597	4.39
65-	0.1827	2.46	0.2727	3.33
70-	0.1366	1.84	0.2121	2.59
75-	0.0845	1.14	0.1311	1.60
80-	0.0450	0.61	0.0663	0.81
85- and over	0.0189	0.25	0.0279	0.34
TOTAL	7.4283	100.00	8.1921	100.00

NOTES

TO TABLES 32 A, B and C

(I)   I. L. number 193 excludes benign and unspecified tu-
      mours of the central nervous system.

(II) Carcinoma in situ excluded from I. L. number 171; a
      very few similar lesions included at some other sites.

TABLE 32 B
YUGOSLAVIA, SLOVENIA :
MALE INCIDENCE RATES, 1956 - 60.

AVERAGE ANNUAL INCIDENCE PER 100,000 — AGE IN YEARS

INTERNATIONAL LIST No.	No. of Cases — Age Unknown	No. of Cases — All Ages	Rate All Ages	85- and over	80-	75-	70-	65-	60-	55-	50-	45-	40-	35-	30-	25-	20-	15-	10-	5-	0-	INTERNATIONAL LIST No.
140	0	187	5.0	63.5	31.1	45.0	27.8	30.7	18.3	15.8	9.7	6.0	4.8	3.1	1.5	0.6	0.0	0.0	0.0	0.0	0.0	140
141	0	38	1.0	0.0	13.3	7.1	5.9	3.3	5.3	2.7	3.7	1.3	0.0	0.5	0.4	0.0	0.0	0.0	0.0	0.0	0.0	141
142	0	10	0.3	10.6	0.0	0.0	1.5	0.0	0.8	0.5	0.0	0.4	0.0	0.0	0.7	0.3	0.0	0.3	0.0	0.0	0.3	142
143-4	0	54	1.5	10.6	8.9	14.2	10.2	3.3	9.2	6.0	2.3	1.3	2.4	0.0	0.0	0.0	0.0	0.0	0.0	0.0	0.0	143-4
146	0	11	0.3	0.0	0.0	2.4	10.2	3.3	1.5	0.5	0.9	0.4	0.6	0.0	0.0	0.0	0.0	0.0	0.0	0.0	0.0	146
145,147-8	0	82	2.2	0.0	0.0	14.2	10.2	15.3	12.2	8.2	6.5	3.0	1.2	0.5	0.0	0.0	0.0	0.0	0.0	0.3	0.0	145,147-8
150	0	239	6.4	52.9	84.4	75.7	57.1	44.9	30.5	17.5	4.6	6.5	1.8	0.5	2.2	3.3	0.3	0.3	0.0	0.0	0.0	150
151	0	1739	46.8	179.9	262.2	407.1	412.9	333.9	230.5	136.0	86.6	40.9	17.3	10.7	2.2	3.3	0.6	0.6	0.0	0.0	0.0	151
152	0	12	0.3	0.0	4.4	2.4	4.4	1.1	0.8	1.6	0.5	0.4	0.0	0.0	0.0	0.0	0.0	0.0	0.3	0.0	0.0	152
153	0	176	4.7	21.2	35.6	26.0	48.3	38.3	16.8	12.0	8.3	2.6	3.0	4.6	0.4	0.6	0.0	0.0	0.3	0.0	0.3	153
154	0	235	6.3	52.9	57.8	68.6	63.0	38.3	26.0	20.2	6.9	6.0	1.8	2.6	0.4	0.3	0.3	0.0	0.0	0.0	0.3	154
155.0	0	69	1.9	0.0	22.2	11.8	13.2	14.2	11.5	5.5	2.8	1.3	0.6	0.0	0.4	0.0	0.0	0.0	0.0	0.0	0.3	155.0
155.1	0	93	2.5	10.6	22.2	33.1	14.6	23.0	12.2	7.6	3.2	1.7	0.6	0.0	0.4	0.0	0.0	0.6	0.0	0.0	0.0	155.1
156	1	128	3.4	10.6	75.6	37.9	26.4	23.0	14.5	12.6	1.9	2.2	1.2	0.0	0.4	0.0	0.0	0.0	0.0	0.8	0.0	156
157	0	134	3.6	0.0	31.1	21.3	24.9	23.0	15.3	15.3	6.5	3.9	2.4	2.0	0.4	0.0	0.0	0.0	0.0	0.3	0.3	157
160	0	32	0.9	0.0	4.4	7.1	1.5	5.5	2.3	4.9	0.0	1.3	1.2	0.5	0.4	0.3	0.0	0.0	0.0	0.3	0.3	160
161	0	158	4.3	52.9	22.2	30.8	29.3	24.1	21.4	15.8	10.2	4.7	0.6	0.5	0.4	0.0	0.0	0.0	0.0	0.0	0.0	161
162-3	0	1071	28.8	31.7	111.1	116.0	174.2	197.0	203.1	114.7	61.1	21.5	11.3	4.6	1.8	1.2	0.0	0.0	0.0	0.0	0.0	162-3
170	0	5	0.1	0.0	4.4	2.4	0.0	2.2	0.0	0.0	0.0	0.0	0.0	0.5	0.0	0.0	0.0	0.0	0.0	0.0	0.0	170
177	0	387	10.4	148.1	186.7	213.0	131.8	66.8	36.6	15.3	5.1	1.3	0.0	0.0	0.0	2.4	0.0	0.0	0.0	0.0	0.0	177
178	0	47	1.3	0.0	0.0	7.1	1.5	1.1	1.5	1.6	0.6	2.2	3.6	3.1	2.9	0.0	0.0	0.9	0.0	0.0	0.0	178
179.0	0	25	0.7	10.6	4.4	11.8	4.4	4.4	1.5	2.7	0.5	0.9	0.6	0.0	0.7	0.0	0.7	0.6	0.0	0.0	0.0	179.0
180	1	94	2.5	0.0	13.3	11.8	13.2	13.1	9.2	7.6	4.6	4.3	1.2	1.5	0.7	0.6	0.0	0.3	0.3	0.8	1.3	180
181.0	0	170	4.6	84.7	44.4	71.0	26.4	38.3	17.6	15.3	2.8	2.6	1.2	0.0	0.7	0.3	0.3	0.0	0.0	0.0	0.0	181.0
190	3	46	1.2	10.6	17.8	4.7	5.9	5.5	1.5	2.7	2.3	1.7	1.8	2.0	0.7	0.6	0.6	0.6	0.3	0.0	0.0	190
191	0	585	15.8	179.9	195.6	172.8	101.0	81.0	65.6	33.9	22.7	21.5	11.9	9.2	3.7	1.8	0.0	0.6	0.3	0.0	0.3	191
192	0	19	0.5	10.6	0.0	7.1	1.5	4.4	0.0	1.1	0.9	0.4	1.2	0.0	0.4	0.0	0.0	0.0	0.3	0.0	1.3	192
193	0	154	4.1	0.0	4.4	7.1	7.3	8.8	8.4	15.8	9.7	7.8	4.2	5.6	4.1	2.4	1.2	3.1	0.6	1.0	0.5	193
194	0	62	1.7	0.0	4.4	9.5	16.1	7.7	6.1	3.8	2.8	4.7	3.0	0.0	0.4	0.3	0.0	0.0	0.0	0.0	0.0	194
195	0	8	0.2	10.6	0.0	2.4	0.0	2.2	0.0	0.0	0.0	0.9	0.6	0.0	0.0	0.0	0.3	0.3	0.0	0.0	0.0	195
196	0	44	1.2	0.0	0.0	2.4	2.9	4.4	0.8	2.2	0.5	1.7	1.8	1.0	0.7	0.9	0.3	2.5	0.6	1.3	0.0	196
197	0	35	0.9	10.6	0.0	7.1	1.5	0.0	4.6	1.1	1.4	2.6	1.8	0.5	1.1	0.6	0.9	0.3	0.0	0.0	0.3	197
200	0	106	2.9	10.6	8.9	11.8	8.8	10.9	9.2	8.8	3.2	4.7	2.4	0.5	1.5	2.7	1.5	1.8	1.6	0.5	0.3	200
201	1	66	1.8	0.0	8.9	4.7	2.9	8.8	4.6	3.8	2.3	2.2	1.8	1.5	1.8	1.5	1.2	2.5	0.3	0.8	0.0	201
203	0	29	0.8	10.6	13.3	18.9	5.9	4.4	3.1	2.2	3.2	1.3	0.0	0.5	0.0	0.0	0.0	0.0	0.0	0.0	0.0	203
204	0	188	5.1	10.6	13.3	18.9	22.0	16.4	12.2	11.5	6.9	3.9	3.0	5.1	0.7	3.6	2.4	2.8	4.1	2.9	3.9	204
202,205	0	4	0.1	0.0	0.0	0.0	0.0	1.1	0.8	0.0	0.0	0.0	0.0	0.5	0.4	0.0	0.0	0.0	0.0	0.0	0.0	202,205
OTHER	0	208	5.6	52.9	48.9	37.9	33.7	28.5	23.7	21.3	9.7	5.2	1.8	2.0	1.5	1.2	1.2	0.0	0.0	0.5	0.8	OTHER
140-205	6	6750	181.7	1026.5	1328.9	1517.2	1311.9	1131.9	838.9	547.6	295.0	175.3	92.3	63.9	29.8	25.2	11.1	16.0	8.4	8.3	9.7	140-205
RATE PER CASE IN PERIOD	-	-	0.03	10.58	4.44	2.37	1.46	1.09	0.76	0.55	0.46	0.43	0.60	0.51	0.37	0.30	0.30	0.31	0.31	0.26	0.26	RATE PER CASE IN PERIOD

TABLE 32 C

YUGOSLAVIA, SLOVENIA :
FEMALE INCIDENCE RATES, 1956 - 60

AVERAGE ANNUAL INCIDENCE PER 100,000 — AGE IN YEARS

INTER-NATIONAL LIST No.	No. OF CASES ALL AGES	AGE UNKNOWN	0-	5-	10-	15-	20-	25-	30-	35-	40-	45-	50-	55-	60-	65-	70-	75-	80-	85- AND OVER	ALL AGES
140	27	0	0.0	0.0	0.0	0.0	0.0	0.0	0.0	0.4	0.5	1.1	1.6	0.5	1.7	1.5	2.8	4.6	9.0	21.5	0.7
141	6	0	0.0	0.0	0.0	0.0	0.0	0.0	0.0	0.0	0.5	0.0	0.4	0.9	0.0	0.7	0.0	1.5	0.0	0.0	0.1
142	24	0	0.0	0.0	0.3	0.0	0.0	0.9	1.2	0.4	0.5	0.0	0.4	0.9	2.8	1.5	1.9	0.0	3.0	7.2	0.6
143-4	15	0	0.3	0.0	0.3	0.0	0.0	0.3	0.0	0.4	0.0	0.4	0.0	1.4	1.1	1.5	0.9	4.6	6.0	0.0	0.4
146	13	0	0.0	0.3	0.0	0.0	0.3	0.3	0.0	0.0	0.0	0.4	0.4	0.5	0.6	1.5	1.9	0.0	0.0	0.0	0.3
145,147-8	20	0	0.0	0.0	0.0	0.0	0.3	0.0	0.0	0.8	0.5	0.0	1.2	1.4	2.8	3.7	2.8	3.1	0.0	0.0	0.5
150	66	2	0.0	0.0	0.0	0.0	0.0	0.0	0.0	0.8	1.0	1.5	1.2	1.8	5.6	6.6	16.0	13.7	12.1	14.3	1.6
151	1262	2	0.0	0.0	0.0	0.0	0.0	2.3	4.3	5.1	10.8	19.9	36.3	59.2	95.1	163.5	229.1	268.5	280.5	164.9	30.8
152	6	0	0.0	0.0	0.0	0.0	0.0	0.0	0.0	0.0	0.0	0.4	0.0	0.5	0.0	2.2	0.0	1.5	0.0	0.0	0.1
153	225	0	0.0	0.0	0.0	0.0	0.3	0.3	0.9	1.6	1.0	4.5	6.5	10.8	21.7	27.1	33.0	38.1	54.3	57.3	5.5
154	232	0	0.0	0.0	0.0	0.0	0.3	0.0	1.2	3.5	3.9	6.4	10.5	15.4	20.0	19.8	23.6	45.8	27.1	50.2	5.7
155.0	57	0	0.3	0.0	0.0	0.0	0.0	0.0	0.0	0.5	0.0	0.8	2.8	5.0	2.2	8.1	10.4	6.1	18.1	7.2	1.4
155.1	215	0	0.0	0.0	0.0	0.0	0.0	0.0	0.3	0.0	1.5	3.0	6.0	15.4	25.0	24.9	33.9	38.1	30.2	21.5	5.2
156	165	0	0.0	0.0	0.0	0.0	0.0	0.0	0.0	0.0	0.0	2.3	4.8	8.6	8.9	18.3	29.2	51.9	54.3	28.7	4.0
157	98	0	0.0	0.0	0.0	0.0	0.0	0.3	0.0	1.2	0.5	1.9	4.4	5.0	8.9	10.3	20.7	16.8	9.0	0.0	2.4
160	26	0	0.3	0.8	0.0	0.0	0.0	0.0	0.6	0.0	1.5	0.8	2.8	0.9	1.7	2.2	0.9	3.1	6.0	7.2	0.6
161	19	0	0.0	0.0	0.0	0.0	0.0	0.0	0.0	0.0	0.0	0.8	2.8	3.2	0.0	0.7	0.9	3.1	12.1	7.2	0.5
162-3	206	0	0.0	0.0	0.0	0.3	0.0	0.3	0.3	1.6	2.4	4.9	9.3	9.5	14.5	24.2	38.7	38.1	21.1	35.8	5.0
170	1000	0	0.0	0.0	0.0	0.3	0.6	2.0	11.0	18.7	42.1	60.4	54.0	57.8	67.3	79.2	76.4	87.0	60.3	71.7	24.4
171	1199	0	0.0	0.0	0.0	0.0	1.8	10.8	25.9	49.5	63.2	75.8	78.6	63.7	61.2	65.3	41.5	29.0	33.2	28.7	29.3
172	285	0	0.0	0.0	0.0	0.3	0.0	0.3	0.6	1.9	6.4	15.4	23.0	31.6	20.6	18.3	17.9	12.2	15.1	7.2	7.0
173	11	0	0.3	0.0	0.0	0.0	0.0	0.6	0.3	0.4	0.5	1.5	0.4	0.0	0.0	0.0	0.0	0.0	0.0	0.0	0.3
174	109	0	0.3	0.0	0.0	0.0	0.3	0.3	0.3	0.4	1.5	1.9	4.0	6.8	8.9	4.4	19.8	18.3	36.2	28.7	2.7
175	383	0	0.0	0.0	0.3	0.9	0.6	2.0	2.4	8.6	9.3	20.6	21.4	28.9	33.4	35.2	20.7	24.4	9.0	0.0	9.4
176	93	0	0.0	0.0	0.0	0.0	0.3	0.0	0.9	0.4	0.5	2.6	6.0	3.2	4.4	8.1	21.7	13.7	18.1	7.2	2.3
180	69	0	1.7	0.8	0.0	0.3	0.0	0.6	0.3	0.8	2.9	1.5	2.4	6.3	3.9	6.6	4.7	3.1	3.0	0.0	1.7
181.0	49	0	0.0	0.0	0.0	0.6	0.6	1.2	2.4	0.4	0.5	1.1	1.6	2.3	1.7	5.1	8.5	9.2	24.1	7.2	1.2
190	69	0	0.0	0.0	0.0	0.0	0.9	0.3	1.8	1.2	1.0	3.0	2.8	4.1	3.3	2.2	6.6	7.6	6.0	7.2	1.7
191	960	1	0.6	0.0	0.0	0.0	0.0	0.3	1.8	6.6	10.8	22.5	31.9	50.6	82.8	111.5	141.4	163.2	190.0	272.4	23.4
192	24	0	0.3	0.0	0.0	0.0	0.9	0.0	0.6	1.2	0.5	0.4	0.8	1.8	1.1	1.5	1.9	3.1	3.0	0.0	0.6
193	136	0	0.3	2.1	2.6	1.6	0.9	2.0	2.1	2.7	4.4	7.1	7.3	5.9	5.6	7.3	5.7	6.1	3.0	0.0	3.3
194	102	0	0.0	0.0	0.3	0.3	0.0	0.0	0.6	1.9	2.0	3.4	4.8	9.5	8.9	8.1	8.5	7.6	12.1	7.2	2.5
195	2	0	0.0	0.0	0.0	0.0	0.0	0.0	0.0	0.0	0.0	0.0	0.0	0.0	0.0	0.0	0.0	0.0	0.0	0.0	0.0
196	52	0	0.0	0.8	1.3	1.6	0.6	1.2	0.6	0.4	0.5	0.8	3.2	1.4	2.8	2.9	3.8	0.0	12.1	0.0	1.3
197	41	0	0.3	0.0	0.0	0.6	0.3	0.6	2.1	1.6	2.9	1.1	1.2	3.2	2.8	3.7	1.9	1.5	6.0	7.2	1.0
200	73	0	0.8	0.3	0.6	0.6	0.6	1.2	2.1	0.8	2.9	1.9	2.8	3.2	5.6	5.1	7.5	6.1	6.0	7.2	1.8
201	49	0	0.0	0.5	0.3	0.0	0.9	1.5	1.5	1.2	0.0	1.1	2.0	2.7	2.8	5.1	1.9	6.1	6.0	0.0	1.2
203	28	0	1.7	2.1	1.9	0.0	0.0	0.0	0.0	2.3	0.0	1.1	2.4	3.6	2.2	2.9	2.8	0.0	6.0	0.0	0.7
204	141	0	0.0	0.0	0.0	1.3	1.5	0.9	1.5	0.0	5.4	4.5	5.2	5.0	8.9	13.2	9.4	9.2	3.0	0.0	3.4
202,205	2	0	0.0	0.0	0.0	0.0	0.0	0.0	0.0	0.0	0.0	0.0	0.0	0.5	0.6	0.0	0.0	0.0	0.0	0.0	0.0
OTHER	265	0	1.1	0.3	0.6	0.0	0.6	0.6	2.7	1.9	3.4	6.4	7.7	17.2	20.0	20.5	32.1	53.4	54.3	57.3	6.5
140-205	7824	3	7.7	7.3	8.6	9.1	11.9	30.6	67.1	117.7	183.2	282.0	352.1	447.8	561.0	722.4	880.7	993.1	1043.7	924.7	191.0
RATE PER CASE IN PERIOD	-	-	0.28	0.27	0.32	0.31	0.31	0.29	0.30	0.39	0.49	0.38	0.40	0.45	0.56	0.73	0.94	1.53	3.02	7.17	0.02

NEW ZEALAND

A National Cancer Register was established in 1948 with the support of the New Zealand Branch of the British Empire Cancer Campaign Society (now the New Zealand Cancer Society). The purpose in establishing this central registry was to gain more information about the size and nature of the cancer problem in New Zealand, to compare the situation in New Zealand with that in other parts of the world and to estimate the chances of survival using different methods of treatment and to compare these with overseas figures.

The register contains particulars of patients treated at clinics and public hospitals throughout the country for all forms of malignant disease excepting skin cancers. A small number of patients treated privately are also covered by the scheme.

It is estimated that the register covers from 75 to 100 per cent of cancer patients diagnosed during their lifetime, the proportion depending on the site concerned (see paragraph headed "Registration" below).

A comprehensive report entitled "Cancer Morbity and Mortality in New Zealand" was published in 1955, covering cases registered in the years 1948 to 1953. A further special cancer report is in preparation and this will make comparisons in incidence, survival etc. in three quinquennia 1948-52; 1953-57; 1958-62.

R.J. Rose

Registry Title and Address : New Zealand National Cancer Registry, Department of Health, Medical Statistics Branch, Ford Building, P.O. Box 6314, Te Aro, Wellington C. 2, New Zealand. Commenced 1948. Supported financially by the New Zealand Cancer Society (formerly British Empire Cancer Campaign).

Registration. Cases are registered from hospital in-patients and out-patients, and radiotherapy departments by Medical Registrar and clerical staff and from death certificates. Registration is confined to public hospital cases and cancer clinics. About 85% of cases occurring are at present registered. The rates shown in Tables 33B and 33C are estimated "total rates" obtained separately for each site, by multiplying the registered rates at each age by the ratio of the total deaths in the country attributed to malignant disease in that site to the deaths from malignant disease observed among the patients on the register.

Follow-up. Follow-up, conducted by hospitals, varies from complete follow-up to none at all, but is usually from 10 to 15 years.

Physical Description. The Registry covers the whole of New Zealand, which is situated in the South Pacific, 1,100 miles south-east of Australia. It lies between latitudes 34° and 47° south and between longitudes 166° and 179° east. The total registration area is 265,149 square kilometres.

Demographic Description. Total population of area under survey 2,430,910. Ethnic groups are European 91.8%; Maori 6.9%; other races 1.3%. The main occupational groups (out of total population both sexes) are : industry 13.1%; commerce 6.8%; agriculture 5.3%; personal service 4.4%. Of the total population 60% live in conurbation of more than 100,000.

Medical Services. Total number of hospital beds of all kinds, 18,268. Total number of doctors in practice in registration area 3,200. Cancer causes approximately 16% of all deaths.

Publications. Annual reports. New Zealand Department of Health (1965).

TABLE 33 A
NEW ZEALAND :
POPULATION (100, 000s), MEAN 1960 - 62

AGE (in years)	MALES		FEMALES	
	No.	Per Cent	No.	Per Cent
0 –	1.5067	12.33	1.4431	11.94
5 –	1.3401	10.96	1.2839	10.62
10 –	1.2456	10.19	1.1905	9.85
15 –	0.9811	8.03	0.9347	7.73
20 –	0.8223	6.73	0.7911	6.55
25 –	0.7461	6.10	0.7093	5.87
30 –	0.8171	6.69	0.7566	6.26
35 –	0.8074	6.61	0.7714	6.38
40 –	0.7255	5.94	0.7349	6.08
45 –	0.7071	5.79	0.7023	5.81
50 –	0.6461	5.29	0.6245	5.17
55 –	0.5388	4.41	0.5228	4.33
60 –	0.4233	3.46	0.4501	3.72
65 –	0.3172	2.60	0.3936	3.26
70 –	0.2590	2.12	0.3269	2.70
75 –	0.1884	1.54	0.2404	1.99
80 –	0.1028	0.84	0.1392	1.15
85 – and over	0.0475	0.39	0.0717	0.59
TOTAL	12.2221	100.00	12.0870	100.00

NOTES

TO TABLES 33 A, B and C

(I)   I.L. number 191 not used; skin cancers not registered. 193 excludes benign and unspecified tumours of the central nervous system.

(II)   Carcinoma in situ excluded.

TABLE 33 B
NEW ZEALAND :
MALE INCIDENCE RATES, 1960 - 62.

INTER-NATIONAL LIST No.	0–	5–	10–	15–	20–	25–	30–	35–	40–	45–	50–	55–	60–	65–	70–	75–	80–	85– AND OVER	ALL AGES	AGE UNKNOWN	ALL AGES	INTER-NATIONAL LIST No.
					AVERAGE ANNUAL INCIDENCE PER 100,000 — AGE IN YEARS																No. OF CASES IN WHOLE PERIOD	
140	0.0	0.0	0.0	0.0	0.8	0.9	0.0	1.2	3.2	4.7	8.3	13.0	7.9	14.7	16.7	7.1	16.2	63.2	3.2	0	116	140
141	0.0	0.0	0.0	0.0	0.0	0.4	0.0	0.0	0.0	1.4	2.1	4.3	7.1	10.5	3.9	10.6	13.0	21.1	1.4	0	50	141
142	0.0	0.0	0.0	0.0	0.4	0.0	0.4	1.2	2.8	1.4	0.0	1.9	1.6	4.2	1.3	8.8	16.2	0.0	0.9	0	34	142
143–4	0.0	0.0	0.0	0.0	0.0	0.0	0.4	0.0	0.5	0.9	1.5	3.1	7.1	9.5	6.4	10.6	22.7	21.1	1.4	0	51	143–4
146	0.0	0.0	0.3	0.0	0.0	0.4	0.0	0.0	0.5	0.5	1.5	0.6	0.8	0.0	1.3	0.0	9.7	0.0	0.3	0	10	146
145,147–8	0.0	0.0	0.0	0.0	0.0	0.0	0.0	0.0	1.4	0.5	2.6	3.7	9.4	3.2	12.9	3.5	9.7	0.0	1.2	0	45	145,147–8
150	0.0	0.0	0.0	0.3	0.4	0.4	0.0	0.4	3.2	3.8	4.1	14.8	21.3	28.4	24.5	53.1	61.6	35.1	4.8	0	176	150
151	0.0	0.0	0.0	0.0	0.4	0.0	2.4	5.0	5.1	16.0	35.6	57.5	87.4	139.8	209.8	272.5	252.9	239.6	24.5	0	900	151
152	0.0	0.0	0.0	0.0	0.0	0.0	0.4	0.4	0.0	2.4	2.1	3.1	0.8	12.6	6.4	5.3	16.2	28.1	1.3	0	46	152
153	0.0	0.0	0.0	0.0	1.6	4.9	7.3	8.7	11.0	20.7	27.9	56.9	85.0	98.8	177.6	194.6	223.7	378.9	23.0	0	842	153
154	0.0	0.0	0.0	0.0	0.4	1.3	1.2	4.5	5.5	14.1	22.7	37.1	59.8	76.7	88.8	143.3	149.2	182.5	14.6	0	535	154
155.0	0.2	0.0	0.0	0.0	0.0	1.3	0.4	1.2	0.5	1.4	4.6	3.7	7.1	4.2	6.4	17.7	13.0	0.0	1.6	0	59	155.0
155.1	0.0	0.0	0.0	0.0	0.0	0.4	0.4	0.4	0.0	1.4	6.7	3.1	11.8	12.6	12.9	23.0	32.4	28.1	2.4	0	88	155.1
156	0.0	0.0	0.0	0.0	0.0	0.0	0.0	1.2	1.4	1.9	2.6	0.0	6.3	1.1	7.7	1.8	9.7	0.0	0.9	0	32	156
157	0.0	0.0	0.0	0.0	0.4	0.0	1.2	1.2	3.7	8.5	14.4	27.8	37.0	48.3	74.6	97.3	123.2	119.3	10.0	0	367	157
160	0.0	0.0	0.0	0.0	0.0	0.4	0.0	0.8	0.5	2.4	1.5	1.9	1.6	5.3	10.3	5.3	3.2	7.0	1.0	0	35	160
161	0.0	0.0	0.0	0.0	0.0	0.4	0.4	0.0	0.9	5.2	9.3	11.8	11.0	17.9	23.2	17.7	32.4	35.1	3.4	0	125	161
162–3	0.0	0.0	0.0	0.3	0.0	0.4	2.4	7.0	11.5	35.8	70.2	128.7	201.6	294.2	288.3	242.4	217.3	203.5	39.9	0	1463	162–3
170	0.0	0.0	0.0	0.0	0.0	0.0	0.4	0.0	0.0	0.0	0.5	1.9	0.0	5.3	1.3	7.1	0.0	7.0	0.4	0	16	170
177	0.0	0.0	0.0	0.0	0.0	0.0	0.0	0.0	1.4	2.4	14.4	28.5	95.3	192.3	370.7	546.7	927.4	1038.6	38.6	0	1417	177
178	0.7	0.0	0.0	1.7	8.5	8.5	10.6	6.6	3.2	5.2	0.5	4.3	0.8	1.1	1.3	1.8	0.0	0.0	3.3	0	121	178
179.0	0.0	0.2	0.0	0.0	0.0	0.0	0.8	0.0	0.0	0.0	0.0	1.4	1.4	2.1	6.4	10.6	3.2	14.0	0.8	0	28	179.0
180	1.3	0.7	0.0	0.0	0.4	0.4	1.2	2.1	2.4	7.5	12.9	13.6	35.4	38.9	30.9	37.2	25.9	28.1	6.1	0	225	180
181.0	0.0	0.0	0.3	0.0	0.4	0.0	1.6	1.7	3.2	7.5	11.4	25.4	40.2	64.1	91.4	97.3	149.2	168.4	11.0	0	404	181.0
190	0.2	0.0	1.3	0.3	2.0	3.1	2.9	7.8	6.9	7.1	7.2	14.8	14.2	5.3	19.3	15.9	42.2	7.0	4.7	0	174	190
192	1.3	0.2	0.5	0.3	0.4	2.7	0.0	0.8	0.9	1.9	3.1	2.5	1.6	4.2	1.3	5.3	3.2	0.0	1.1	0	39	192
193	5.1	4.5	2.1	0.3	2.4	1.8	2.9	5.0	3.2	10.8	15.0	16.7	14.2	12.6	18.0	12.4	0.0	0.0	5.9	0	218	193
194	0.0	0.0	0.3	0.0	0.4	0.0	0.8	0.4	0.0	1.9	2.6	3.7	1.1	1.1	7.7	5.3	6.5	0.0	0.9	0	33	194
195	1.1	0.5	0.3	0.0	0.0	1.8	0.0	0.4	0.0	1.0	0.0	0.6	2.4	1.1	0.0	5.3	0.0	0.0	0.5	0	17	195
196	0.2	1.5	2.1	2.0	1.6	0.9	0.4	2.5	1.8	0.9	2.1	5.6	3.9	1.1	0.0	1.8	0.0	28.1	1.2	0	44	196
197	0.4	0.5	0.5	1.7	1.6	3.6	3.7	0.4	4.6	3.8	0.5	8.7	5.5	6.3	11.6	35.4	6.5	56.1	1.9	0	69	197
200	0.0	1.2	0.8	0.7	0.8	3.6	3.7	3.7	3.2	3.3	7.7	8.7	22.8	28.4	21.9	35.4	25.9	0.0	5.0	0	185	200
201	0.2	0.0	0.0	2.4	1.6	4.0	3.7	3.7	3.2	4.6	4.6	5.6	5.5	2.1	5.1	5.3	9.7	0.0	2.5	0	93	201
203	0.0	0.0	0.0	0.0	0.0	0.0	0.0	0.8	0.9	0.9	2.6	5.6	8.7	13.7	15.4	19.5	19.5	14.0	2.0	0	73	203
204	5.3	2.7	2.9	5.4	4.1	1.8	1.2	3.3	3.2	6.1	8.8	10.5	19.7	28.4	57.9	84.9	51.9	112.3	8.7	0	318	204
202,205	0.4	0.2	0.0	0.0	0.0	0.0	0.0	0.0	0.5	0.5	1.0	3.1	3.1	2.1	2.6	3.5	3.2	7.0	0.7	0	24	202,205
OTHER	0.2	0.0	1.1	0.3	1.6	0.4	0.8	2.1	1.4	6.1	8.3	7.4	21.3	22.1	33.5	21.2	58.4	91.2	4.9	0	179	OTHER
140–205	16.8	12.4	12.8	16.0	29.6	40.2	49.0	70.6	88.7	190.4	320.9	533.9	861.5	1213.7	1669.2	2025.8	2545.4	2933.3	235.9	0	8651	140–205
RATE PER CASE IN PERIOD	0.22	0.25	0.27	0.34	0.41	0.45	0.41	0.41	0.46	0.47	0.52	0.62	0.79	1.05	1.29	1.77	3.24	7.02	0.03	–	–	RATE PER CASE IN PERIOD

TABLE 33 C

NEW ZEALAND :
FEMALE INCIDENCE RATES, 1960 - 62.

INTER-NATIONAL LIST No.	AVERAGE ANNUAL INCIDENCE PER 100,000 — AGE IN YEARS																		ALL AGES	No. OF CASES IN WHOLE PERIOD — AGE UNKNOWN	No. OF CASES IN WHOLE PERIOD — ALL AGES	INTER-NATIONAL LIST No.
	0-	5-	10-	15-	20-	25-	30-	35-	40-	45-	50-	55-	60-	65-	70-	75-	80-	85- AND OVER				
140	0.0	0.0	0.0	0.0	0.0	0.0	0.0	0.4	0.0	0.0	0.0	0.6	0.7	0.8	3.1	1.4	0.0	0.0	0.2	0	8	140
141	0.0	0.0	0.0	0.0	0.0	0.0	0.4	0.0	0.0	0.5	0.0	1.3	4.4	3.4	7.1	5.5	2.4	4.6	0.7	0	27	141
142	0.0	0.0	0.0	0.0	0.0	1.4	0.4	1.3	2.7	1.4	1.6	1.9	0.0	1.7	6.1	5.5	2.4	9.3	1.0	0	37	142
143-4	0.0	0.0	0.0	0.0	0.0	0.0	0.4	0.0	0.5	0.5	1.6	1.3	1.5	3.4	6.1	2.8	2.4	4.6	0.7	0	24	143-4
146	0.0	0.0	0.3	0.0	0.0	0.0	0.0	0.0	0.0	0.0	0.0	0.0	0.0	0.0	0.0	0.0	0.0	0.0	0.0	0	1	146
145,147-8	0.0	0.0	0.0	0.0	0.0	0.0	0.0	0.0	0.0	0.5	0.5	0.6	5.2	2.5	6.1	2.8	0.0	0.0	0.6	0	21	145,147-8
150	0.0	0.0	0.0	0.0	0.4	0.5	1.8	0.0	4.5	1.9	3.2	5.1	10.4	12.7	22.4	25.0	19.2	46.5	2.9	0	106	150
151	0.0	0.0	0.0	0.0	0.4	0.0	0.0	3.5	2.3	11.9	12.3	24.9	30.4	50.0	92.8	155.3	143.7	139.5	13.9	0	504	151
152	0.0	0.0	0.0	0.0	0.0	0.0	0.0	0.4	2.3	0.0	1.6	1.9	2.2	2.5	1.0	0.0	0.0	0.0	0.5	0	19	152
153	0.0	0.0	0.0	3.2	3.8	4.7	4.8	15.1	28.1	29.9	42.7	70.8	86.6	102.5	134.6	148.4	196.4	269.6	27.8	0	1007	153
154	0.0	0.3	0.0	0.0	0.0	0.9	1.8	6.0	9.1	8.1	18.1	28.1	30.4	42.3	46.9	56.8	91.0	41.8	9.9	0	360	154
155.0	0.0	0.0	0.0	0.0	0.0	0.5	0.0	0.4	0.0	0.5	0.5	1.9	0.0	5.9	5.1	1.4	7.2	0.0	0.7	0	24	155.0
155.1	0.0	0.0	0.0	0.0	0.0	0.0	0.0	0.0	1.4	1.9	4.3	5.1	13.3	19.5	24.5	43.0	47.9	23.2	4.0	0	144	155.1
156	0.0	0.0	0.0	0.0	0.0	0.0	0.0	0.4	0.0	0.5	1.1	0.0	1.5	0.0	3.1	4.2	7.2	0.0	0.4	0	15	156
157	0.0	0.0	0.0	0.0	0.4	0.0	0.4	1.3	2.7	4.3	6.9	12.8	19.3	26.3	26.5	43.0	45.5	79.0	5.6	0	203	157
160	0.0	0.0	0.0	0.4	0.0	0.0	0.0	0.0	0.5	0.5	2.1	0.0	1.5	0.0	4.1	0.0	0.0	9.3	0.4	0	15	160
161	0.0	0.3	0.0	0.0	0.0	0.0	0.0	0.0	0.0	0.0	0.0	0.0	1.5	0.8	1.0	0.0	0.0	0.0	0.1	0	4	161
162-3	0.0	0.0	0.0	0.0	1.3	7.5	15.0	3.9	3.2	10.0	12.8	15.9	26.7	35.6	28.6	33.3	19.2	9.3	6.3	0	229	162-3
170	0.0	0.0	0.0	0.0	0.4	1.9	9.7	51.4	88.0	123.4	111.0	124.3	143.7	175.3	180.5	209.4	227.5	288.2	52.8	0	1915	170
171	0.0	0.0	0.0	0.0	0.4	0.0	0.9	25.5	30.4	40.3	41.6	35.7	45.2	37.3	27.5	33.3	23.9	27.9	15.0	0	544	171
172	0.0	0.0	0.0	0.0	0.0	1.4	0.9	4.3	5.0	18.5	29.9	47.8	50.4	55.0	56.1	27.7	45.5	23.2	11.7	0	426	172
173	0.2	0.0	0.0	0.0	0.0	0.0	0.4	1.3	2.7	1.4	4.3	0.6	5.9	0.8	1.0	12.5	0.0	13.9	1.3	0	48	173
174	0.0	0.0	0.0	0.0	0.0	3.8	0.0	0.0	0.0	0.0	0.0	0.0	0.7	0.8	0.0	2.8	0.0	0.0	0.1	0	4	174
175	0.2	0.0	0.6	2.1	3.4	0.0	7.9	10.8	17.2	23.7	44.8	40.8	40.0	42.3	45.9	22.2	19.2	37.2	13.4	0	485	175
176	0.0	0.0	0.0	0.0	0.0	0.0	0.0	0.4	1.8	0.9	2.1	6.4	7.4	11.9	16.3	25.0	43.1	27.9	2.8	0	103	176
180	2.3	1.0	0.3	0.0	0.0	0.0	0.4	0.0	1.4	1.9	4.3	5.1	15.6	13.6	18.4	18.0	19.2	13.9	3.3	0	118	180
181.0	0.0	0.0	0.0	0.0	0.0	0.0	0.0	0.0	0.0	0.5	0.5	7.0	3.0	13.6	24.5	40.2	52.7	41.8	3.3	0	118	181.0
190	0.0	0.3	0.3	3.9	5.9	9.4	10.6	13.4	9.5	21.8	13.3	12.1	8.1	9.3	24.5	19.4	19.2	41.8	8.0	0	290	190
192	1.4	0.3	0.3	1.1	0.4	0.0	0.0	0.4	0.5	1.9	1.1	0.6	3.0	1.7	4.1	6.9	0.0	0.0	0.9	0	33	192
193	2.1	2.9	1.7	0.7	2.5	0.9	1.8	2.2	5.0	5.2	9.1	5.7	13.3	11.0	4.1	9.7	0.0	4.6	3.8	0	137	193
194	0.0	0.0	0.3	0.0	0.4	2.3	0.9	0.9	2.7	3.8	2.1	5.1	3.7	4.2	8.2	18.0	4.8	0.0	2.0	0	71	194
195	0.9	0.5	0.3	1.8	0.4	0.0	1.3	0.4	0.0	1.4	0.5	2.6	0.7	0.0	1.0	0.0	2.4	4.6	0.6	0	23	195
196	0.2	0.3	2.2	0.4	0.4	0.0	0.0	0.0	0.5	0.5	0.0	0.6	3.0	2.5	4.1	8.3	0.0	4.6	1.0	0	37	196
197	0.2	0.0	0.6	0.4	0.4	0.9	0.4	0.9	1.4	0.5	2.1	1.9	2.2	5.1	1.0	4.2	2.4	4.6	1.0	0	35	197
200	0.0	2.1	0.0	0.4	0.8	1.4	0.9	1.3	1.4	4.7	5.3	7.0	11.1	17.8	25.5	27.7	23.9	18.6	4.1	0	147	200
201	0.0	0.3	0.0	0.4	0.8	1.9	0.9	3.0	0.9	0.9	0.5	3.8	7.4	5.1	7.1	4.2	7.2	9.3	1.6	0	59	201
203	0.0	0.0	0.0	0.0	0.0	0.0	0.0	0.0	0.9	0.9	3.2	6.4	11.8	9.3	9.2	13.9	19.2	9.3	2.1	0	76	203
204	4.9	4.7	1.1	2.9	1.3	0.5	2.2	2.6	4.1	4.3	5.3	10.2	17.0	21.2	29.6	36.1	21.6	37.2	6.3	0	230	204
202,205	0.2	0.0	0.0	0.4	0.0	0.0	0.9	0.0	0.5	0.5	0.0	1.3	1.5	0.0	5.1	2.8	9.6	0.0	0.6	0	21	202,205
OTHER	0.2	0.0	0.6	0.0	0.8	0.9	2.2	2.6	3.6	3.8	6.4	9.6	18.5	30.5	32.6	33.3	33.5	65.1	5.7	0	206	OTHER
140-205	12.9	12.7	8.4	17.5	24.0	40.9	67.4	154.7	232.2	332.7	397.1	506.9	648.7	778.3	945.2	1103.7	1159.0	1306.4	217.1	0	7874	140-205
RATE PER CASE IN PERIOD	0.23	0.26	0.28	0.36	0.42	0.47	0.44	0.43	0.45	0.47	0.53	0.64	0.74	0.85	1.02	1.39	2.39	4.65	0.03	-	-	RATE PER CASE IN PERIOD

U.S.A., HAWAII

The Hawaii Tumor Registry is a system of individual hospital tumor registries plus a State-wide central registry participating in a program to study the prevalence of neoplastic disease and its diagnosis and treatment, to follow progress of patients and to provide data for the analysis of their management. Data on all patients admitted to hospitals with a malignant neoplasm (or with one of several selected benign neoplasms) are included.

The policy-making and administrative body of the Hawaii Tumor Registry is the six-man Cancer Commission of the Hawaii Medical Association established by the House of Delegates in 1959. Membership consists of two physicians representing the Hawaii Medical Association, two the American Cancer Society and two the State Department of Health. The Registry is financed primarily by a special grant from the United States Public Health Service.

The Hospital registry is the basic unit of the Hawaii Tumor Registry system. Following standardised definitions and procedures, and under the guidance of the Hospital's Cancer Committee (or interested members of the medical staff) the hospital registry :

Abstracts tumor information from medical records and sends copies to the central registry.

Maintains a system of following progress of the patient (via the attending physician).

Provides the hospital with a reservoir of summary information about its tumor experience.

Reports periodically to the medical staff summary data on diagnosis, treatment, survival of tumor cases and the end results of therapy.

The central registry coordinates the State-wide system of registries :

Consolidates information on tumor patients in all hospital registries.

Analyzes State-wide tumor experience and makes summary information available to physicians, hospitals, and research groups.

Gives consultation and assistance to hospitals in setting up and maintaining tumor registries and supplies forms and standardized procedures.

Provides statistical services to hospitals :

Prepares periodic reports for each hospital on its diagnosis and treatment, survival patterns and end results of therapy.

Prepares an annual diagnosis index of the hospital's cases.

Assists in special studies.

Grover H. Batten.

Registry Title and Address : Hawaii Tumor Registry, P. O. Box 3378, Honolulu, Hawaii, U.S.A. (Requests for information to Grover H. Batten, M.D., Chairman Cancer Commission of the Hawaii Medical Association, P.O. Box 3378, Honolulu). Commenced January 1st, 1960. Supported financially by Federal Funds.

Registration. Medical record librarians and others register cases from hospital in-patients and out-patients and from radiotherapy departments, and from the record rooms of hospital pathology departments. Coded lists are prepared from death certificates by the Vital Statistics Office of the State Department of Health. Doctors attending cases at home supply follow-up information only. All attending physicians are sent letters, by hospitals, requesting follow-up information. Registration is less than 90% complete for skin cancers, other than malignant melanoma and those that have spread, which are not reportable.

Follow-up. All registrations are followed up annually till death.

Physical Description. The State of Hawaii, U.S.A., comprised of the islands of Oahu, Maui, Hawaii, Molokai, Lanai, Kahoolawe, Kauai, and Niihau, lies in the North Pacific Ocean, 2,100 nautical miles from San Francisco, California. Altitudes range from 0 feet to 13,796 feet. The average temperature is 79°F in summer and 72°F in winter. Average humidity is 73% at 8. a.m., and 58% at 2 p.m. Average rainfall is 23.9 inches annually. There is 70% sunshine and the wind speed is 12 m.p.h. The State lies between latitudes 18°55' and 22°15' north and between longitudes 154°50' and 160°30' west. The total registration area is 16,638 square kilometres.

Demographic Description. Populations of area under survey are : All races 632,780; Caucasians 202,230; Japanese 203,440; Hawaiian (ethnic) 102,430. The main ethnic groups are Japanese 32%, Caucasian including Portugese 32%, Hawaiian and part-Hawaiian 14%, Filipino 11%, Chinese 6%, Others (Negro, Samoan, Korean) 5%. The only two occupational groups for whom figures are available are agiculture 6.2% and military 25.4%. Of the total population 48.5% live in conurbations of more than 100,000 (the city of Honolulu).

NOTES TO TABLES 34 to 37

(1) Population Tables 34A, 35A, 36A and 37A are grouped together on pages 208 and 209.

(2) The total population shown in Table 34A includes some ethnic groups not covered by Tables 35, 36 and 37 (e.g. Chinese).
The Hawaiian ethnic population shown in Table 37A includes Hawaiians and part Hawaiians.

(3) I.L. numbers 156 and 163 included with other tumours.
    "   numbers 170 omitted in Tables 34B, 35B, 36B, and 37B because no cases were recorded.
    "   numbers 193 includes only malignant tumours of the brain; malignant tunours of the spinal cord are classified with other tumours, and benign and unspecified tumours of the central nervous system are excluded.

(4) Carcinoma in situ included.

TABLE 35 A
HAWAII, CAUCASIAN :
POPULATION (100,000s), CENSUS 1960

AGE (in years)	MALES No.	MALES Per Cent	FEMALES No.	FEMALES Per Cent
0-	0.1307	11.58	0.1269	14.21
5-	0.1032	9.14	0.1004	11.24
10-	0.0858	7.60	0.0811	9.08
15-	0.1132	10.03	0.0579	6.48
20-	0.1822	16.14	0.0783	8.77
25-	0.0971	8.60	0.0770	8.62
30-	0.0864	7.65	0.0748	8.37
35-	0.0872	7.72	0.0765	8.56
40-	0.0735	6.51	0.0565	6.32
45-	0.0521	4.61	0.0436	4.88
50-	0.0372	3.29	0.0342	3.83
55-	0.0281	2.49	0.0254	2.84
60-	0.0192	1.70	0.0206	2.31
65-	0.0142	1.26	0.0154	1.72
70-	0.0098	0.87	0.0115	1.29
75-	0.0054	0.48	0.0072	0.81
80-	0.0024	0.21	0.0038	0.43
85- and over	0.0013	0.12	0.0022	0.25
TOTAL	1.1290	100.00	0.8933	100.00

TABLE 34 A
HAWAII, ALL GROUPS :
POPULATION (100,000s), CENSUS 1960

AGE (in years)	MALES No.	MALES Per Cent	FEMALES No.	FEMALES Per Cent
0-	0.4127	12.20	0.3970	13.48
5-	0.3717	10.99	0.3560	12.08
10-	0.3268	9.66	0.3134	10.64
15-	0.3062	9.05	0.2420	8.21
20-	0.3040	8.99	0.2020	6.86
25-	0.2241	6.63	0.2214	7.52
30-	0.2418	7.15	0.2476	8.40
35-	0.2517	7.44	0.2408	8.17
40-	0.2144	6.34	0.1891	6.42
45-	0.1957	5.79	0.1392	4.72
50-	0.1588	4.70	0.1019	3.46
55-	0.1310	3.87	0.0891	3.02
60-	0.0857	2.53	0.0720	2.44
65-	0.0553	1.64	0.0543	1.84
70-	0.0502	1.48	0.0367	1.25
75-	0.0273	0.81	0.0236	0.80
80-	0.0155	0.46	0.0130	0.44
85- and over	0.0088	0.26	0.0070	0.24
TOTAL	3.3817	100.00	2.9461	100.00

TABLE 37 A
HAWAII, HAWAIIAN ETHNIC GROUP :
POPULATION (100,000s), CENSUS 1960

AGE (in years)	MALES No.	MALES Per Cent	FEMALES No.	FEMALES Per Cent
0-	0.0922	18.01	0.0886	17.29
5-	0.0813	15.88	0.0774	15.11
10-	0.0694	13.55	0.0672	13.12
15-	0.0576	11.25	0.0552	10.77
20-	0.0328	6.41	0.0363	7.09
25-	0.0319	6.23	0.0347	6.77
30-	0.0303	5.92	0.0325	6.34
35-	0.0278	5.43	0.0286	5.58
40-	0.0237	4.63	0.0246	4.80
45-	0.0194	3.79	0.0195	3.81
50-	0.0151	2.95	0.0152	2.97
55-	0.0109	2.13	0.0117	2.28
60-	0.0084	1.64	0.0080	1.56
65-	0.0058	1.13	0.0059	1.15
70-	0.0028	0.55	0.0035	0.68
75-	0.0016	0.31	0.0021	0.41
80-	0.0006	0.12	0.0008	0.16
85- and over	0.0004	0.08	0.0005	0.10
TOTAL	0.5120	100.00	0.5123	100.00

TABLE 36 A
HAWAII, JAPANESE :
POPULATION (100,000s), CENSUS 1960

AGE (in years)	MALES No.	MALES Per Cent	FEMALES No.	FEMALES Per Cent
0-	0.1090	10.89	0.1036	10.03
5-	0.1140	11.39	0.1097	10.62
10-	0.1087	10.86	0.1047	10.13
15-	0.0839	8.38	0.0835	8.08
20-	0.0461	4.60	0.0546	5.29
25-	0.0579	5.78	0.0723	7.00
30-	0.0806	8.05	0.0993	9.61
35-	0.0906	9.05	0.1004	9.72
40-	0.0802	8.01	0.0810	7.84
45-	0.0584	5.83	0.0564	5.46
50-	0.0415	4.14	0.0355	3.44
55-	0.0364	3.64	0.0345	3.34
60-	0.0242	2.42	0.0314	3.04
65-	0.0143	1.43	0.0258	2.50
70-	0.0281	2.81	0.0180	1.74
75-	0.0144	1.44	0.0117	1.13
80-	0.0085	0.85	0.0073	0.71
85- and over	0.0045	0.45	0.0034	0.33
TOTAL	1.0013	100.00	1.0331	100.00

TABLE 34 B
HAWAII, ALL GROUPS :
MALE INCIDENCE RATES, 1960 - 63.

INTER-NATIONAL LIST No.	AVERAGE ANNUAL INCIDENCE PER 100,000 — AGE IN YEARS																		ALL AGES	No. OF CASES IN WHOLE PERIOD — AGE UNKNOWN	ALL AGES	INTER-NATIONAL LIST No.
	0-	5-	10-	15-	20-	25-	30-	35-	40-	45-	50-	55-	60-	65-	70-	75-	80-	85- AND OVER				
140	0.0	0.0	0.8	0.0	0.0	0.0	1.0	0.0	1.2	1.3	0.0	3.8	0.0	0.0	0.0	0.0	0.0	0.0	0.4	0	6	140
141	0.0	0.0	0.0	0.0	0.0	0.0	1.9	0.0	3.5	1.3	7.9	5.7	11.7	18.1	24.9	9.2	16.1	0.0	2.1	0	28	141
142	0.0	0.0	0.0	0.0	1.6	0.0	1.0	1.0	2.3	0.0	1.6	5.7	5.8	4.5	5.0	0.0	0.0	0.0	1.0	0	14	142
143-4	0.0	0.0	0.0	0.0	0.0	0.0	0.0	0.0	1.2	2.6	3.1	5.7	8.8	13.6	5.0	0.0	32.3	0.0	1.3	1	18	143-4
146	0.0	0.0	0.0	0.0	0.8	0.0	0.0	0.0	2.3	5.1	4.7	1.9	14.6	4.5	5.0	0.0	0.0	56.8	1.8	0	25	146
145,147-8	0.0	0.0	0.0	0.0	0.0	0.0	0.0	4.0	2.3	1.3	4.7	7.6	14.6	13.6	10.0	18.3	0.0	28.4	1.7	0	23	147
150	0.0	0.0	0.0	0.0	0.0	0.0	0.0	0.0	1.2	0.0	4.7	15.3	26.3	40.7	64.7	64.1	64.5	28.4	4.1	0	55	150
151	0.0	0.0	0.0	0.0	0.0	4.5	5.2	7.0	10.5	25.5	29.9	63.0	116.7	135.6	268.9	311.4	225.8	340.9	20.8	0	281	151
152	0.0	0.0	0.0	0.0	0.0	0.0	0.0	0.0	3.5	1.3	0.0	1.9	0.0	0.0	0.0	0.0	16.1	0.0	0.4	0	6	152
153	0.0	0.0	0.0	0.8	0.0	2.2	6.2	3.0	3.5	12.8	29.9	51.5	70.0	122.1	114.5	192.3	193.5	227.3	13.8	1	187	153
154	0.0	0.0	0.0	0.0	0.0	1.1	1.0	2.0	5.8	15.3	17.3	26.7	43.8	54.2	59.8	82.4	145.2	56.8	7.8	1	106	154
155.0	0.6	0.0	0.0	1.6	0.0	1.1	0.0	0.0	2.3	7.7	12.6	21.0	26.3	27.1	49.8	91.6	48.4	85.2	5.3	0	72	155.0
155.1	0.0	0.0	0.0	0.0	0.8	0.0	0.0	1.0	0.0	1.3	3.1	0.0	8.8	18.1	29.9	27.5	64.5	0.0	1.8	0	24	155.1
157	0.0	0.0	0.0	0.0	0.8	1.1	1.0	0.0	2.3	9.9	11.0	21.0	17.5	40.7	54.8	64.1	64.5	142.0	5.3	0	72	157
160	0.0	0.0	0.0	0.0	0.0	1.1	1.0	0.0	1.3	1.3	4.7	9.5	0.0	0.0	0.0	0.0	0.0	28.4	1.0	0	13	160
161	0.0	0.0	0.0	0.0	0.0	0.0	0.0	1.0	1.2	5.1	11.0	7.6	20.4	13.6	19.9	36.6	48.4	0.0	2.8	0	38	161
162	0.0	0.0	0.0	0.0	0.0	0.0	2.1	7.9	15.2	26.8	40.9	59.2	116.7	171.8	239.0	247.3	258.1	312.5	20.8	0	281	162
177	0.0	0.0	0.0	0.0	0.0	1.1	0.0	0.0	3.5	3.8	7.9	26.7	64.2	122.1	204.2	338.8	451.6	255.7	14.0	0	190	177
178	0.0	0.0	0.0	1.6	4.9	6.7	3.1	4.0	4.7	0.0	1.6	1.9	2.9	4.5	0.0	0.0	0.0	0.0	2.1	0	29	178
179	0.0	0.0	0.0	0.0	0.0	0.0	0.0	1.0	0.0	1.3	0.0	0.0	2.9	0.0	0.0	0.0	16.1	56.8	0.4	0	5	179
180	1.2	0.0	0.0	1.6	0.0	0.0	0.0	1.0	4.7	0.0	4.7	7.6	40.8	18.1	34.9	0.0	16.1	0.0	3.0	1	40	180
181	0.0	0.0	0.0	1.6	0.0	2.2	0.0	4.0	9.3	14.1	12.6	24.8	26.3	31.6	49.8	100.7	64.5	28.4	6.7	0	90	181
190	0.0	0.0	0.8	0.0	0.0	3.3	3.1	2.0	3.5	1.3	0.0	1.9	0.0	9.0	5.0	9.2	0.0	28.4	1.4	0	19	190
191	0.0	0.0	0.0	0.0	0.0	0.0	0.0	1.0	0.0	0.0	1.6	0.0	0.0	0.0	0.0	0.0	16.1	0.0	0.2	0	3	191
192	0.6	4.7	0.8	2.4	1.6	2.2	2.1	2.0	1.2	0.0	1.6	0.0	2.9	0.0	0.0	9.2	0.0	0.0	0.4	0	5	192
193	0.6	0.0	0.0	1.6	2.5	6.7	2.1	7.0	1.2	7.7	4.7	1.9	14.6	4.5	5.0	0.0	0.0	0.0	2.9	0	39	193
194	0.0	0.0	0.0	0.0	0.0	1.1	0.0	0.0	3.5	3.8	7.9	3.8	17.5	13.6	0.0	9.2	0.0	28.4	3.3	0	44	194
195	0.0	0.0	0.0	0.0	0.0	0.0	0.0	0.0	0.0	0.0	0.0	0.0	0.0	0.0	0.0	0.0	0.0	0.0	0.1	0	1	195
196	0.0	0.0	0.0	0.0	0.0	0.0	4.1	2.0	0.0	1.3	1.6	1.9	2.9	0.0	18.3	18.3	16.1	0.0	0.7	0	9	196
197	1.8	0.7	0.8	0.0	0.0	0.0	0.0	4.0	2.3	5.1	1.6	1.9	5.8	4.5	9.2	9.2	16.1	0.0	1.8	0	25	197
200	0.6	0.0	0.0	0.0	1.6	2.2	0.0	2.0	7.0	3.8	6.3	1.9	11.7	40.7	14.9	45.8	64.5	0.0	3.5	0	47	200
201	0.0	0.0	0.0	0.0	0.8	2.2	2.1	2.0	1.2	6.4	1.6	3.8	5.8	13.6	29.9	9.2	16.1	28.4	2.3	0	31	201
203	0.0	0.0	0.0	0.0	0.0	0.0	0.0	0.0	0.0	1.3	4.7	5.7	8.8	9.0	5.0	0.0	16.1	0.0	1.0	0	14	203
204	7.3	2.7	3.1	2.4	0.0	1.1	2.1	2.0	3.5	11.5	7.9	9.5	23.3	36.2	29.9	64.1	16.1	113.6	6.2	0	84	204
202,205	0.0	0.0	0.0	0.8	0.0	0.0	2.1	0.0	3.5	0.0	3.1	0.0	2.9	9.0	0.0	0.0	0.0	28.4	0.9	0	12	202,205
OTHER	0.6	0.0	0.0	1.6	0.0	0.0	0.0	1.0	1.2	7.7	4.7	11.5	17.5	45.2	24.9	73.3	112.9	113.6	4.4	0	60	OTHER
140-205	13.3	8.1	6.1	15.5	14.8	41.3	41.4	61.6	109.6	186.5	261.3	410.3	752.6	1039.8	1359.6	1822.3	1983.9	1988.5	147.6	4	1996	140-205
RATE PER CASE IN PERIOD	0.61	0.67	0.76	0.82	0.82	1.12	1.03	0.99	1.17	1.28	1.57	1.91	2.92	4.52	4.98	9.16	16.13	28.41	0.07	-	-	RATE PER CASE IN PERIOD

TABLE 34 C
HAWAII, ALL GROUPS :
FEMALE INCIDENCE RATES, 1960 - 63.

AVERAGE ANNUAL INCIDENCE PER 100,000 — AGE IN YEARS

INTER-NATIONAL LIST No.	0-	5-	10-	15-	20-	25-	30-	35-	40-	45-	50-	55-	60-	65-	70-	75-	80-	85- AND OVER	ALL AGES	No. CASES AGE UNKNOWN	No. CASES ALL AGES	INTER-NATIONAL LIST No.
140	0.0	0.0	0.0	0.0	0.0	1.1	0.0	0.0	0.0	0.0	0.0	0.0	0.0	0.0	0.0	10.6	0.0	0.0	0.2	0	2	140
141	0.0	0.0	0.0	0.0	0.0	0.0	0.0	0.0	1.3	0.0	2.5	0.0	10.4	0.0	6.8	10.6	0.0	0.0	0.6	0	7	141
142	0.0	0.0	0.0	1.0	0.0	0.0	0.0	2.1	1.3	1.8	4.9	2.8	0.0	0.0	13.6	0.0	0.0	0.0	0.8	0	10	142
143-4	0.0	0.0	0.0	0.0	0.0	0.0	0.0	0.0	2.6	1.8	0.0	5.6	3.5	4.6	0.0	0.0	38.5	0.0	0.8	0	9	143-4
146	0.0	0.0	0.0	0.0	0.0	0.0	2.0	0.0	1.3	3.6	0.0	2.8	3.5	0.0	6.8	0.0	0.0	0.0	0.6	0	7	146
145,147-8	0.0	0.0	0.0	0.0	0.0	0.0	0.0	0.0	0.0	1.8	0.0	0.0	3.5	4.6	0.0	0.0	0.0	0.0	0.3	0	3	145,147-8
150	0.0	0.0	0.0	0.0	0.0	0.0	0.0	0.0	0.0	1.8	2.5	0.0	3.5	0.0	0.0	0.0	0.0	35.7	0.3	0	3	150
151	0.0	0.0	0.0	0.0	2.5	2.3	3.0	11.4	19.8	30.5	36.8	39.3	52.1	78.3	74.9	127.1	192.3	35.7	12.3	0	145	151
152	0.0	0.0	0.0	0.0	0.0	0.0	0.0	0.0	0.0	0.0	2.5	2.8	0.0	0.0	6.8	0.0	0.0	0.0	0.3	0	3	152
153	0.0	0.0	0.0	0.0	0.0	0.0	2.0	4.2	6.6	21.6	39.3	39.3	55.6	73.7	102.2	158.9	230.8	285.7	11.5	0	135	153
154	0.0	0.0	0.0	0.0	0.0	0.0	3.0	6.2	5.3	12.6	19.6	19.5	24.3	18.4	40.9	84.7	96.2	35.7	5.6	0	66	154
155.0	0.0	0.0	0.0	0.0	0.0	0.0	1.0	0.0	2.6	0.0	2.5	5.6	13.9	9.2	6.8	10.6	0.0	35.7	1.2	0	14	155.0
155.1	0.0	0.0	0.0	0.0	0.0	0.0	0.0	0.0	1.3	0.0	4.9	8.4	13.9	23.0	47.7	21.2	38.5	35.7	2.4	0	28	155.1
157	0.0	0.0	0.8	0.0	0.0	0.0	0.0	0.0	0.0	1.8	0.0	16.8	27.8	32.2	54.5	42.4	76.9	71.4	3.5	0	41	157
160	0.0	0.0	0.0	0.0	0.0	3.0	0.0	0.0	2.6	0.0	7.4	2.9	0.0	0.0	0.0	0.0	19.2	0.0	0.3	0	4	160
161	0.0	0.0	0.0	1.0	0.0	0.0	0.0	0.0	0.0	0.0	0.0	5.6	3.5	0.0	20.4	0.0	0.0	0.0	0.8	0	9	161
162	0.0	0.0	0.0	0.0	0.0	0.0	1.0	2.1	7.9	16.2	17.2	33.7	34.7	36.8	74.9	74.2	76.9	107.1	6.8	0	80	162
170	0.0	0.0	0.0	0.0	2.5	9.0	23.2	33.2	80.6	122.1	105.5	95.4	111.1	96.7	88.6	137.7	76.9	142.9	30.4	0	358	170
171	0.0	0.0	0.0	0.0	7.4	32.7	49.5	72.7	80.6	75.4	78.5	84.2	79.9	64.5	95.4	42.4	38.5	71.4	32.2	2	380	171
172	0.0	0.0	0.0	0.0	0.0	2.3	4.0	11.4	26.4	39.5	46.6	19.6	45.1	41.4	47.7	10.5	19.2	107.1	10.1	0	119	172
173-4	0.0	0.0	0.0	0.0	0.0	0.0	0.0	0.0	0.0	0.0	2.5	0.0	0.0	0.0	0.0	0.0	0.0	0.0	0.1	0	1	173-4
175	0.0	0.0	0.0	0.0	2.5	2.3	6.1	6.2	5.3	10.8	24.5	22.4	24.3	23.0	13.6	21.2	19.2	35.7	5.3	0	62	175
176	0.0	0.0	0.0	0.0	0.0	0.0	1.0	1.0	2.6	0.0	0.0	5.6	3.5	4.6	6.8	0.0	0.0	0.0	0.7	0	8	176
180	1.9	0.0	0.0	1.0	0.0	0.0	1.0	1.0	1.3	3.6	2.5	2.8	3.5	9.2	13.6	0.0	0.0	0.0	1.4	0	16	180
181	0.0	0.0	0.0	0.0	0.0	0.0	1.0	1.0	0.0	0.0	7.4	14.0	6.9	0.0	27.2	10.6	57.7	35.7	1.8	0	21	181
190	0.0	0.0	0.0	0.0	3.7	0.0	1.0	1.0	4.0	1.8	0.0	0.0	0.0	0.0	0.0	0.0	0.0	0.0	0.8	0	9	190
191	0.0	0.0	0.0	0.0	0.0	0.0	0.0	0.0	1.3	0.0	0.0	0.0	0.0	0.0	6.8	0.0	19.2	0.0	0.2	0	2	191
192	0.0	0.0	0.0	0.0	1.2	0.0	0.0	0.0	0.0	0.0	0.0	0.0	0.0	0.0	0.0	0.0	0.0	0.0	0.1	0	1	192
193	1.3	2.8	0.8	0.0	1.2	2.3	1.0	1.0	1.3	2.6	4.9	2.8	3.5	9.2	0.0	10.6	19.2	0.0	2.0	0	23	193
194	0.0	0.0	1.6	0.0	3.7	7.9	17.2	11.4	14.5	9.0	22.1	16.8	3.5	18.4	0.0	10.6	0.0	0.0	6.6	0	78	194
195	0.6	0.0	0.0	0.0	1.2	0.0	0.0	2.1	1.3	0.0	0.0	0.0	0.0	0.0	0.0	0.0	0.0	0.0	0.4	0	5	195
196	0.0	0.0	0.8	0.0	1.2	1.1	0.0	0.0	1.3	0.0	2.5	0.0	10.4	0.0	0.0	10.6	0.0	0.0	0.3	0	4	196
197	0.0	0.7	0.0	1.0	0.0	0.0	0.0	3.1	1.3	1.8	0.0	0.0	0.0	0.0	6.8	0.0	19.2	0.0	0.9	0	11	197
200	0.0	0.0	0.8	0.0	1.2	1.1	0.0	1.0	1.3	3.6	4.9	5.6	3.5	23.0	6.8	31.8	19.2	35.7	1.8	0	21	200
201	0.0	0.0	0.0	0.0	1.2	0.0	2.0	1.0	1.3	3.6	0.0	0.0	6.9	4.6	6.8	10.6	19.2	35.7	1.2	0	14	201
203	0.0	0.0	0.0	1.0	5.0	0.0	0.0	0.0	0.0	9.0	4.9	5.6	6.9	9.2	20.4	21.2	38.5	0.0	0.6	0	7	203
204	8.8	2.1	4.8	0.0	5.0	1.1	0.0	2.1	2.6	1.8	0.0	5.6	0.0	9.2	6.8	0.0	0.0	35.7	4.6	0	54	204
202,205	0.0	0.0	0.0	0.0	0.0	0.0	0.0	1.0	1.3	1.8	0.0	5.6	0.0	0.0	6.8	0.0	0.0	0.0	0.5	0	6	202,205
OTHER	0.0	0.0	0.0	0.0	0.0	2.3	1.0	1.0	1.3	9.0	7.4	11.2	27.8	36.8	40.9	95.3	76.9	71.4	4.6	0	54	OTHER
140-205	12.6	5.6	10.4	6.2	32.2	65.5	118.1	176.5	284.2	387.9	458.8	477.0	579.9	630.8	851.5	932.2	1173.1	1214.3	154.4	2	1820	**140-205**
RATE PER CASE IN PERIOD	0.63	0.70	0.80	1.03	1.24	1.13	1.01	1.04	1.32	1.80	2.45	2.81	3.47	4.60	6.81	10.59	19.23	35.71	0.08	-	-	**RATE PER CASE IN PERIOD**

TABLE 35 B
HAWAII, CAUCASIAN :
MALE INCIDENCE RATES, 1960 - 63.

AVERAGE ANNUAL INCIDENCE PER 100,000 — AGE IN YEARS

INTER-NATIONAL LIST No.	0–	5–	10–	15–	20–	25–	30–	35–	40–	45–	50–	55–	60–	65–	70–	75–	80–	85– AND OVER	ALL AGES	No. cases AGE UNKNOWN	No. cases ALL AGES	INTER-NATIONAL LIST No.
140	0.0	0.0	2.9	0.0	0.0	0.0	2.9	0.0	3.4	4.8	0.0	17.8	0.0	0.0	0.0	0.0	0.0	0.0	1.3	0	6	140
141	0.0	0.0	0.0	0.0	0.0	0.0	0.0	0.0	3.4	4.8	20.2	8.9	13.0	35.2	51.0	0.0	0.0	0.0	2.4	0	11	141
142	0.0	0.0	0.0	0.0	2.7	0.0	0.0	0.0	0.0	0.0	0.0	0.0	13.0	0.0	25.5	0.0	0.0	0.0	0.9	0	4	142
143–4	0.0	0.0	0.0	0.0	0.0	0.0	0.0	0.0	0.0	9.6	6.7	8.9	39.1	35.2	0.0	0.0	0.0	0.0	2.0	0	9	143–4
146	0.0	0.0	0.0	0.0	0.0	0.0	0.0	2.9	0.0	0.0	6.7	0.0	26.0	17.6	0.0	0.0	0.0	0.0	0.4	0	2	146
145,147-8	0.0	0.0	0.0	0.0	0.0	0.0	0.0	0.0	3.4	0.0	6.7	17.8	39.1	52.8	0.0	0.0	0.0	0.0	1.6	0	7	145,147–8
150	0.0	0.0	0.0	0.0	0.0	0.0	0.0	0.0	3.4	0.0	20.2	26.7	52.1	35.2	25.5	46.3	0.0	192.3	2.9	0	13	150
151	0.0	0.0	0.0	0.0	0.0	0.0	0.0	0.0	10.2	4.8	20.2	44.5	52.1	35.2	229.6	46.3	0.0	0.0	6.4	0	29	151
152	0.0	0.0	0.0	0.0	0.0	0.0	0.0	0.0	0.0	0.0	0.0	0.0	0.0	0.0	0.0	0.0	0.0	0.0	0.0	0	0	152
153	0.0	0.0	0.0	0.0	0.0	2.6	5.8	0.0	6.8	14.4	33.6	62.3	78.1	88.0	127.6	138.9	416.7	192.3	10.0	0	45	153
154	0.0	0.0	0.0	2.2	0.0	0.0	2.9	0.0	3.4	9.6	33.6	8.9	26.0	52.8	76.5	46.3	104.2	0.0	4.7	1	21	154
155.0	0.0	0.0	0.0	0.0	0.0	0.0	0.0	0.0	0.0	4.8	0.0	17.8	13.0	35.2	0.0	46.3	104.2	192.3	2.0	0	9	155.0
155.1	0.0	0.0	0.0	0.0	0.0	0.0	0.0	0.0	0.0	0.0	0.0	0.0	0.0	0.0	51.0	46.3	0.0	0.0	0.7	0	3	155.1
157	0.0	0.0	0.0	0.0	1.4	0.0	0.0	5.7	0.0	9.6	13.4	53.4	26.0	17.6	51.0	46.3	0.0	192.3	4.0	0	18	157
160	0.0	0.0	0.0	0.0	0.0	0.0	0.0	5.7	0.0	4.8	6.7	8.9	0.0	0.0	51.0	0.0	0.0	0.0	0.9	0	4	160
161	0.0	0.0	0.0	0.0	0.0	0.0	0.0	2.9	17.0	14.4	20.2	35.6	26.0	17.6	25.5	92.6	0.0	0.0	3.8	0	17	161
162	0.0	0.0	0.0	0.0	0.0	0.0	0.0	14.3	17.0	43.2	87.4	106.8	195.3	211.3	408.2	185.2	0.0	384.6	20.6	0	93	162
170	0.0	0.0	0.0	0.0	0.0	0.0	0.0	0.0	0.0	0.0	0.0	0.0	0.0	0.0	0.0	0.0	0.0	0.0	0.0	0	0	170
177	0.0	0.0	0.0	0.0	0.0	2.6	0.0	0.0	6.8	9.6	26.9	80.1	117.2	246.5	433.7	787.0	729.2	576.9	18.8	0	85	177
178	0.0	0.0	0.0	4.4	8.2	7.7	5.8	2.9	6.8	0.0	0.0	0.0	13.0	0.0	0.0	0.0	0.0	0.0	3.8	0	17	178
179	0.0	0.0	0.0	0.0	0.0	0.0	0.0	0.0	0.0	4.8	0.0	0.0	0.0	0.0	0.0	0.0	0.0	0.0	0.2	0	1	179
180	1.9	0.0	0.0	0.0	0.0	0.0	0.0	0.0	6.8	0.0	6.7	0.0	78.1	0.0	51.0	0.0	0.0	0.0	2.9	1	13	180
181	0.0	0.0	0.0	0.0	0.0	5.1	0.0	5.7	10.2	28.8	26.9	53.4	52.1	70.4	102.0	185.2	0.0	0.0	9.1	0	41	181
190	0.0	0.0	0.0	0.0	0.0	5.1	5.8	5.7	10.2	4.8	0.0	0.0	0.0	17.6	25.5	0.0	0.0	0.0	2.7	0	12	190
191	0.0	0.0	0.0	0.0	0.0	0.0	0.0	2.9	0.0	0.0	6.7	8.9	0.0	0.0	0.0	0.0	0.0	0.0	0.4	0	2	191
192	0.0	0.0	0.0	0.0	0.0	0.0	0.0	2.9	0.0	0.0	6.7	0.0	0.0	0.0	0.0	0.0	0.0	0.0	0.4	0	2	192
193	1.9	2.4	2.9	2.2	2.7	10.3	2.9	8.6	3.4	24.0	13.4	0.0	0.0	17.6	46.3	46.3	0.0	0.0	3.8	0	17	193
194	0.0	0.0	0.0	4.4	2.7	2.6	0.0	0.0	0.0	4.8	0.0	8.9	0.0	35.2	0.0	0.0	0.0	192.3	4.2	0	19	194
195	0.0	0.0	0.0	0.0	0.0	0.0	5.8	0.0	0.0	0.0	0.0	0.0	0.0	0.0	0.0	0.0	0.0	0.0	0.2	0	1	195
196	0.0	0.0	0.0	0.0	0.0	0.0	0.0	2.9	0.0	0.0	0.0	0.0	0.0	0.0	0.0	0.0	104.2	0.0	0.7	0	3	196
197	0.0	0.0	0.0	0.0	0.0	2.6	5.8	0.0	0.0	9.6	6.7	0.0	0.0	17.6	0.0	46.3	0.0	0.0	1.6	0	7	197
200	0.0	2.4	0.0	0.0	1.4	2.6	0.0	0.0	6.8	0.0	13.4	8.9	26.0	70.4	0.0	46.3	0.0	0.0	2.9	0	13	200
201	0.0	0.0	0.0	0.0	1.4	5.1	2.9	5.7	3.4	0.0	0.0	0.0	13.0	17.6	51.0	0.0	0.0	0.0	2.9	0	13	201
203	0.0	0.0	0.0	0.0	0.0	0.0	0.0	0.0	0.0	0.0	6.7	0.0	13.0	0.0	0.0	0.0	0.0	0.0	0.7	0	3	203
204	5.7	4.8	5.8	2.2	0.0	0.0	0.0	2.9	0.0	4.8	13.4	17.8	0.0	70.4	25.5	92.6	0.0	192.3	4.9	0	22	204
202,205	0.0	0.0	0.0	0.0	0.0	0.0	0.0	0.0	0.0	0.0	0.0	0.0	0.0	0.0	0.0	0.0	0.0	0.0	0.0	0	0	202,205
OTHER	1.9	0.0	0.0	2.2	0.0	0.0	0.0	2.9	0.0	4.8	13.4	8.9	0.0	105.6	0.0	185.2	0.0	0.0	3.8	0	17	OTHER
140–205	11.5	9.7	11.7	22.1	20.6	46.3	40.5	65.9	105.4	225.5	403.2	596.1	859.4	1285.2	1760.2	2083.3	1458.3	2115.4	128.2	2	579	**140–205**
RATE PER CASE IN PERIOD	1.91	2.42	2.91	2.21	1.37	2.57	2.89	2.87	3.42	4.80	6.72	8.90	13.02	17.61	25.51	46.30	104.17	192.31	0.22	-	-	**RATE PER CASE IN PERIOD**

TABLE 35 C

HAWAII, CAUCASIAN :

FEMALE INCIDENCE RATES, 1960 - 63.

INTER-NATIONAL LIST No.	No. OF CASES IN WHOLE PERIOD — AGE UNKNOWN	No. OF CASES IN WHOLE PERIOD — ALL AGES	ALL AGES	85- AND OVER	80-	75-	70-	65-	60-	55-	50-	45-	40-	35-	30-	25-	20-	15-	10-	5-	0-	INTER-NATIONAL LIST No.
140	0	2	0.6	0.0	0.0	0.0	0.0	0.0	0.0	0.0	0.0	0.0	0.0	0.0	0.0	3.2	0.0	0.0	0.0	0.0	0.0	140
141	0	4	1.1	0.0	0.0	34.7	0.0	0.0	12.1	0.0	7.3	0.0	4.4	0.0	0.0	0.0	0.0	0.0	0.0	0.0	0.0	141
142	0	2	0.6	0.0	0.0	34.7	0.0	0.0	0.0	0.0	14.6	0.0	0.0	0.0	0.0	0.0	0.0	0.0	0.0	0.0	0.0	142
143-4	0	5	1.4	0.0	65.8	0.0	0.0	0.0	0.0	19.7	0.0	5.7	4.4	0.0	0.0	0.0	0.0	0.0	0.0	0.0	0.0	143-4
146	0	2	0.6	0.0	0.0	0.0	21.7	16.2	0.0	0.0	0.0	0.0	0.0	0.0	0.0	0.0	0.0	0.0	0.0	0.0	0.0	146
145,147-8	0	2	0.6	0.0	0.0	0.0	0.0	0.0	12.1	9.8	0.0	0.0	0.0	0.0	0.0	0.0	0.0	0.0	0.0	0.0	0.0	145,147-8
150	0	1	0.3	0.0	0.0	0.0	0.0	0.0	0.0	0.0	0.0	5.7	0.0	0.0	0.0	0.0	0.0	0.0	0.0	0.0	0.0	150
151	0	22	6.2	113.6	0.0	104.2	43.5	32.5	48.5	19.7	43.9	0.0	0.0	0.0	0.0	0.0	0.0	0.0	0.0	0.0	0.0	151
152	0	3	0.8	0.0	0.0	0.0	21.7	0.0	0.0	9.8	7.3	0.0	0.0	0.0	0.0	0.0	0.0	0.0	0.0	0.0	0.0	152
153	0	60	16.8	227.3	263.2	208.3	152.2	113.6	97.1	78.7	65.8	28.7	8.8	6.5	0.0	0.0	0.0	0.0	0.0	0.0	0.0	153
154	0	23	6.4	0.0	131.6	138.9	65.2	0.0	36.4	29.5	29.2	11.5	0.0	0.0	0.0	0.0	0.0	0.0	0.0	0.0	0.0	154
155.0	0	4	1.1	113.6	0.0	0.0	0.0	16.2	12.1	0.0	7.3	0.0	0.0	0.0	0.0	0.0	0.0	0.0	0.0	0.0	0.0	155.0
155.1	0	5	1.4	0.0	0.0	0.0	0.0	16.2	0.0	0.0	0.0	0.0	0.0	0.0	0.0	0.0	0.0	0.0	0.0	0.0	0.0	155.1
157	0	9	2.5	113.6	65.8	0.0	65.2	0.0	24.3	19.7	0.0	0.0	0.0	0.0	0.0	0.0	0.0	0.0	0.0	0.0	0.0	157
160	0	0	0.0	0.0	0.0	0.0	0.0	0.0	0.0	0.0	0.0	0.0	0.0	0.0	0.0	0.0	0.0	0.0	0.0	0.0	0.0	160
161	0	3	0.8	0.0	0.0	0.0	21.7	0.0	0.0	9.8	7.3	0.0	0.0	0.0	0.0	0.0	0.0	0.0	0.0	0.0	0.0	161
162	0	20	5.6	0.0	0.0	0.0	43.5	16.2	36.4	19.7	29.2	22.9	13.3	22.9	0.0	16.2	3.2	0.0	0.0	0.0	0.0	162
170	0	163	45.6	227.3	131.6	277.8	195.7	162.3	206.3	157.5	168.1	189.2	92.9	91.5	30.1	0.0	0.0	0.0	0.0	0.0	0.0	170
171	0	132	36.9	113.6	65.8	0.0	65.2	16.2	72.8	137.8	65.8	63.1	88.5	0.0	70.2	48.7	6.4	0.0	0.0	0.0	0.0	171
172	0	42	11.8	113.6	65.8	34.7	87.0	16.2	85.0	29.5	65.8	40.1	17.7	6.5	6.7	0.0	0.0	0.0	0.0	0.0	0.0	172
173-4	0	0	0.0	0.0	0.0	0.0	0.0	0.0	0.0	0.0	0.0	0.0	0.0	0.0	0.0	0.0	0.0	0.0	0.0	0.0	0.0	173-4
175	0	34	9.5	0.0	0.0	69.4	21.7	16.2	48.5	39.4	36.5	28.7	4.4	9.8	13.4	3.2	6.4	0.0	0.0	0.0	0.0	175
176	0	5	1.4	0.0	0.0	0.0	0.0	16.2	12.1	9.8	0.0	0.0	4.4	3.3	0.0	0.0	0.0	0.0	0.0	0.0	0.0	176
180	0	8	2.2	0.0	0.0	0.0	0.0	32.5	12.1	9.8	0.0	0.0	4.4	3.3	0.0	0.0	0.0	0.0	0.0	0.0	3.9	180
181	0	12	3.4	113.6	131.6	0.0	21.7	0.0	12.1	26.5	21.9	0.0	0.0	3.3	3.3	0.0	6.4	0.0	0.0	0.0	0.0	181
190	0	8	2.2	113.6	0.0	0.0	0.0	0.0	0.0	0.0	0.0	5.7	13.3	3.3	0.0	0.0	6.4	0.0	0.0	0.0	0.0	190
191	0	1	0.3	0.0	65.8	0.0	0.0	0.0	0.0	0.0	0.0	0.0	4.4	0.0	3.3	0.0	0.0	0.0	0.0	0.0	0.0	191
192	0	1	0.3	0.0	0.0	0.0	0.0	0.0	12.1	9.8	0.0	0.0	4.4	0.0	0.0	6.5	0.0	0.0	0.0	0.0	0.0	192
193	0	10	2.8	0.0	0.0	0.0	0.0	0.0	0.0	0.0	14.6	0.0	13.3	6.5	13.4	3.2	3.2	4.3	6.2	7.5	2.0	193
194	0	17	4.8	0.0	0.0	0.0	0.0	0.0	0.0	0.0	14.6	5.7	0.0	6.5	0.0	0.0	0.0	0.0	0.0	0.0	0.0	194
195	0	3	0.8	0.0	0.0	0.0	0.0	0.0	0.0	0.0	0.0	0.0	0.0	0.0	0.0	0.0	0.0	0.0	0.0	0.0	2.0	195
196	0	1	0.3	0.0	0.0	0.0	0.0	0.0	12.1	0.0	0.0	0.0	0.0	6.5	0.0	0.0	0.0	0.0	0.0	0.0	0.0	196
197	0	2	0.6	0.0	0.0	0.0	0.0	0.0	0.0	0.0	7.3	0.0	0.0	0.0	0.0	0.0	3.2	0.0	0.0	0.0	0.0	197
200	0	9	2.5	0.0	65.8	0.0	0.0	48.7	12.1	0.0	14.6	5.7	0.0	0.0	0.0	3.2	0.0	0.0	0.0	0.0	0.0	200
201	0	4	1.1	0.0	0.0	0.0	21.7	0.0	0.0	0.0	0.0	5.7	0.0	0.0	3.3	0.0	3.2	0.0	0.0	0.0	0.0	201
203	0	3	0.8	0.0	65.8	69.4	21.7	16.2	0.0	0.0	0.0	0.0	0.0	0.0	0.0	0.0	0.0	0.0	0.0	0.0	0.0	203
204	0	18	5.0	0.0	131.6	0.0	21.7	16.2	0.0	9.8	14.6	0.0	0.0	0.0	0.0	0.0	6.4	0.0	3.1	2.5	9.9	204
202,205	0	0	0.0	0.0	0.0	0.0	0.0	0.0	0.0	0.0	0.0	0.0	0.0	0.0	0.0	0.0	0.0	0.0	0.0	0.0	0.0	202,205
OTHER	0	22	6.2	0.0	131.6	69.4	87.0	64.9	48.5	19.7	14.6	5.7	0.0	0.0	0.0	3.2	0.0	0.0	0.0	0.0	0.0	OTHER
140-205	0	662	185.3	1136.4	1447.4	1041.7	1065.2	616.9	813.1	669.3	636.0	424.3	278.8	179.7	143.8	87.7	38.3	4.3	9.2	10.0	17.7	**140-205**
RATE PER CASE IN PERIOD	-	-	0.28	113.64	65.79	34.72	21.74	16.23	12.14	9.84	7.31	5.73	4.42	3.27	3.34	3.25	3.19	4.32	3.08	2.49	1.97	**RATE PER CASE IN PERIOD**

AVERAGE ANNUAL INCIDENCE PER 100,000 — AGE IN YEARS

TABLE 36 B
HAWAII, JAPANESE :
MALE INCIDENCE RATES, 1960 - 63.

AVERAGE ANNUAL INCIDENCE PER 100,000 — AGE IN YEARS

INTER-NATIONAL LIST No.	No. of cases — ALL AGES	No. of cases — AGE UNKNOWN	ALL AGES	85– and over	80–	75–	70–	65–	60–	55–	50–	45–	40–	35–	30–	25–	20–	15–	10–	5–	0–
140	0	0	0.0	0.0	0.0	0.0	0.0	0.0	0.0	0.0	0.0	0.0	0.0	0.0	0.0	0.0	0.0	0.0	0.0	0.0	0.0
141	9	0	2.2	0.0	29.4	17.4	17.8	35.0	10.3	0.0	6.0	0.0	0.0	0.0	3.1	0.0	0.0	0.0	0.0	0.0	0.0
142	2	0	0.5	0.0	0.0	0.0	0.0	17.5	0.0	0.0	0.0	0.0	0.0	0.0	3.1	0.0	0.0	0.0	0.0	0.0	0.0
143–4	2	0	0.5	0.0	0.0	0.0	8.9	0.0	0.0	0.0	0.0	0.0	3.1	0.0	0.0	0.0	0.0	0.0	0.0	0.0	0.0
146	2	0	0.5	55.6	0.0	0.0	0.0	0.0	0.0	0.0	0.0	0.0	0.0	0.0	0.0	0.0	0.0	0.0	0.0	0.0	0.0
145,147–8	6	0	1.5	0.0	0.0	17.4	17.8	17.5	0.0	6.9	6.0	0.0	0.0	0.0	0.0	0.0	0.0	0.0	0.0	0.0	0.0
150	26	0	6.5	0.0	117.6	104.2	71.2	52.4	31.0	13.7	0.0	0.0	0.0	0.0	0.0	17.3	0.0	0.0	0.0	0.0	0.0
151	169	0	42.2	388.9	352.9	520.8	302.5	314.7	155.0	103.0	54.2	59.9	15.6	11.0	6.2	17.3	0.0	0.0	0.0	0.0	0.0
152	3	0	0.7	0.0	29.4	0.0	0.0	0.0	0.0	6.9	0.0	4.3	0.0	0.0	0.0	0.0	0.0	0.0	0.0	0.0	0.0
153	73	0	18.2	277.8	205.9	208.3	115.7	104.9	82.6	34.3	42.2	25.7	3.1	2.8	6.2	0.0	0.0	0.0	0.0	0.0	0.0
154	45	0	11.2	111.1	176.5	86.8	62.3	52.4	31.0	41.2	24.1	21.4	6.2	2.8	0.0	4.3	0.0	3.0	0.0	0.0	0.0
155.0	29	0	7.2	111.1	58.8	86.8	62.3	17.5	41.3	13.7	18.1	4.3	0.0	0.0	0.0	4.3	0.0	0.0	0.0	0.0	0.0
155.1	16	0	4.0	0.0	117.6	34.7	26.7	17.5	20.7	0.0	12.0	4.3	0.0	2.8	0.0	0.0	0.0	0.0	0.0	0.0	0.0
157	26	0	6.5	166.7	117.6	52.1	53.4	52.4	10.3	13.7	6.0	8.6	0.0	0.0	6.2	4.3	0.0	0.0	0.0	0.0	0.0
160	4	0	1.0	55.6	0.0	0.0	0.0	0.0	0.0	6.9	6.0	0.0	3.1	0.0	0.0	0.0	0.0	0.0	0.0	0.0	0.0
161	10	0	2.5	0.0	58.8	17.4	17.8	35.0	20.7	0.0	6.0	0.0	0.0	0.0	0.0	0.0	0.0	0.0	0.0	0.0	0.0
162	84	0	21.0	277.8	323.5	260.4	169.0	192.3	72.3	34.3	12.0	12.8	9.4	5.5	3.1	0.0	0.0	0.0	0.0	0.0	0.0
170	0	0	0.0	0.0	0.0	0.0	0.0	0.0	0.0	0.0	0.0	0.0	0.0	0.0	0.0	0.0	0.0	0.0	0.0	0.0	0.0
177	54	0	13.5	166.7	352.9	225.7	106.8	69.9	62.0	13.7	0.0	4.3	3.1	0.0	0.0	0.0	0.0	0.0	0.0	0.0	0.0
178	5	0	1.2	0.0	0.0	0.0	0.0	17.5	0.0	0.0	0.0	0.0	3.1	2.8	3.1	4.3	0.0	0.0	0.0	0.0	0.0
179	2	0	0.5	0.0	29.4	0.0	0.0	0.0	10.3	0.0	0.0	0.0	0.0	0.0	0.0	0.0	0.0	0.0	0.0	0.0	0.0
180	11	0	2.7	0.0	58.8	86.8	35.6	35.0	10.3	6.9	0.0	0.0	6.2	0.0	0.0	0.0	0.0	0.0	0.0	0.0	2.3
181	27	0	6.7	55.6	58.8	86.8	44.5	17.5	0.0	20.6	0.0	17.1	15.6	2.8	0.0	4.3	0.0	0.0	0.0	0.0	0.0
190	3	0	0.7	55.6	0.0	17.4	0.0	0.0	0.0	0.0	0.0	0.0	0.0	0.0	3.1	4.3	0.0	0.0	0.0	0.0	0.0
191	0	0	0.0	0.0	0.0	0.0	0.0	0.0	0.0	0.0	0.0	0.0	0.0	0.0	0.0	0.0	0.0	0.0	0.0	0.0	0.0
192	0	0	0.0	0.0	0.0	0.0	0.0	0.0	0.0	0.0	0.0	0.0	0.0	0.0	0.0	0.0	0.0	0.0	0.0	0.0	0.0
193	7	0	1.7	0.0	0.0	0.0	0.0	0.0	10.3	6.9	0.0	4.3	3.1	2.8	0.0	8.6	0.0	0.0	0.0	2.2	0.0
194	5	0	1.2	0.0	0.0	0.0	0.0	0.0	20.7	0.0	6.0	0.0	3.1	0.0	0.0	0.0	0.0	0.0	0.0	0.0	0.0
195	0	0	0.0	0.0	0.0	0.0	0.0	0.0	0.0	0.0	0.0	0.0	0.0	0.0	0.0	0.0	0.0	0.0	0.0	0.0	0.0
196	1	0	0.2	0.0	0.0	0.0	0.0	0.0	0.0	0.0	0.0	0.0	0.0	2.8	0.0	0.0	0.0	0.0	0.0	0.0	0.0
197	8	0	2.0	0.0	29.4	34.7	26.7	17.5	0.0	0.0	12.0	8.6	3.1	2.8	3.1	0.0	0.0	0.0	0.0	2.2	2.3
200	15	0	3.7	0.0	88.2	34.7	26.7	17.5	0.0	0.0	12.0	0.0	9.4	2.8	0.0	0.0	0.0	0.0	0.0	0.0	0.0
201	7	0	1.7	55.6	0.0	0.0	17.8	17.5	10.3	6.9	0.0	8.6	0.0	0.0	0.0	0.0	0.0	0.0	0.0	0.0	0.0
203	2	0	0.5	0.0	0.0	17.4	26.7	0.0	10.3	0.0	6.0	0.0	3.1	0.0	0.0	0.0	0.0	3.0	0.0	0.0	0.0
204	19	0	4.7	111.1	29.4	17.4	26.7	0.0	20.7	0.0	6.0	12.8	0.0	0.0	3.1	4.3	0.0	3.0	4.6	2.2	0.0
202,205	5	0	1.2	55.6	0.0	0.0	0.0	17.5	10.3	0.0	0.0	0.0	0.0	0.0	3.1	0.0	0.0	0.0	0.0	0.0	0.0
OTHER	28	0	7.0	111.1	176.5	52.1	44.5	35.0	10.3	27.5	0.0	17.1	3.1	0.0	0.0	0.0	0.0	0.0	0.0	0.0	0.0
140–205	**705**	**0**	**176.0**	2055.6	2352.9	1840.3	1227.8	1136.4	640.5	357.1	228.9	214.0	93.5	41.4	31.0	51.8	0.0	8.9	4.6	6.6	4.6
RATE PER CASE IN PERIOD	–	–	**0.25**	55.56	29.41	17.36	8.90	17.48	10.33	6.87	6.02	4.28	3.12	2.76	3.10	4.32	5.42	2.98	2.30	2.19	2.29

TABLE 36 C

HAWAII, JAPANESE :

FEMALE INCIDENCE RATES, 1960 - 63.

INTER-NATIONAL LIST No.	AVERAGE ANNUAL INCIDENCE PER 100,000 — AGE IN YEARS																		ALL AGES	No. OF CASES IN WHOLE PERIOD		INTER-NATIONAL LIST No.
	0-	5-	10-	15-	20-	25-	30-	35-	40-	45-	50-	55-	60-	65-	70-	75-	80-	85- AND OVER		AGE UNKNOWN	ALL AGES	
140	0.0	0.0	0.0	0.0	0.0	0.0	0.0	0.0	0.0	0.0	0.0	0.0	0.0	0.0	0.0	0.0	0.0	0.0	0.0	0	0	140
141	0.0	0.0	0.0	0.0	0.0	0.0	0.0	0.0	0.0	4.4	0.0	0.0	0.0	0.0	0.0	0.0	0.0	0.0	0.2	0	1	141
142	0.0	0.0	0.0	0.0	0.0	0.0	0.0	2.5	3.1	4.4	0.0	0.0	0.0	0.0	27.8	0.0	0.0	0.0	1.2	0	5	142
143-4	0.0	0.0	0.0	0.0	0.0	0.0	0.0	0.0	0.0	0.0	0.0	0.0	8.0	9.7	0.0	0.0	34.2	0.0	0.7	0	3	143-4
146	0.0	0.0	0.0	0.0	0.0	0.0	0.0	0.0	0.0	0.0	0.0	0.0	0.0	0.0	0.0	0.0	0.0	0.0	0.0	0	0	146
145,147-8	0.0	0.0	0.0	0.0	0.0	0.0	0.0	0.0	0.0	0.0	0.0	0.0	0.0	0.0	13.9	0.0	0.0	0.0	0.2	0	1	145,147-8
150	0.0	0.0	0.0	0.0	0.0	0.0	0.0	0.0	0.0	0.0	7.0	0.0	0.0	0.0	0.0	0.0	0.0	73.5	0.5	0	2	150
151	0.0	0.0	0.0	0.0	9.2	6.9	7.6	14.9	34.0	48.8	35.2	43.5	71.7	87.2	111.1	149.6	342.5	0.0	21.5	0	89	151
152	0.0	0.0	0.0	0.0	0.0	0.0	0.0	0.0	0.0	0.0	0.0	0.0	0.0	0.0	0.0	0.0	0.0	0.0	0.0	0	0	152
153	0.0	0.0	0.0	0.0	0.0	0.0	5.0	2.5	9.3	17.7	49.3	7.2	15.9	67.8	69.4	106.8	239.7	147.1	11.1	0	46	153
154	0.0	0.0	0.0	0.0	0.0	0.0	5.0	5.0	6.2	22.2	14.1	14.5	23.9	29.1	27.8	64.1	68.5	73.5	7.0	0	29	154
155.0	0.0	0.0	0.0	0.0	0.0	0.0	0.0	0.0	0.0	0.0	0.0	0.0	15.9	0.0	0.0	0.0	0.0	0.0	0.5	0	2	155.0
155.1	0.0	0.0	0.0	0.0	0.0	0.0	2.5	0.0	3.1	0.0	7.0	14.5	8.0	38.8	27.8	21.4	34.2	73.5	3.6	0	15	155.1
157	0.0	0.0	0.0	0.0	0.0	0.0	0.0	0.0	0.0	0.0	0.0	14.5	8.0	19.4	41.7	64.1	102.7	73.5	3.6	0	15	157
160	0.0	0.0	0.0	0.0	0.0	0.0	0.0	0.0	3.1	0.0	0.0	0.0	0.0	0.0	0.0	0.0	34.2	0.0	0.7	0	3	160
161	0.0	0.0	0.0	0.0	0.0	0.0	0.0	0.0	0.0	0.0	0.0	0.0	8.0	0.0	27.8	0.0	0.0	0.0	0.7	0	3	161
162	0.0	0.0	0.0	0.0	0.0	0.0	0.0	0.0	3.1	13.3	14.1	7.2	8.0	19.4	55.6	128.2	137.0	147.1	6.3	0	26	162
170	0.0	0.0	0.0	0.0	0.0	6.9	22.7	34.9	77.2	62.1	28.2	58.0	39.8	29.1	13.9	21.4	68.5	147.1	21.8	0	90	170
171	0.0	0.0	0.0	0.0	0.0	13.8	35.2	52.3	58.6	66.5	63.4	43.5	63.7	67.8	97.2	42.7	34.2	73.5	28.1	2	116	171
172	0.0	0.0	0.0	0.0	0.0	0.0	0.0	12.5	21.6	44.3	35.2	14.5	15.9	38.8	27.8	0.0	0.0	73.5	9.2	0	38	172
173-4	0.0	0.0	0.0	3.0	0.0	0.0	0.0	0.0	0.0	0.0	0.0	0.0	0.0	0.0	0.0	0.0	0.0	0.0	0.2	0	1	173-4
175	0.0	0.0	0.0	0.0	0.0	3.5	2.5	10.0	12.3	35.5	28.2	21.7	8.0	19.4	0.0	0.0	34.2	0.0	7.3	0	30	175
176	0.0	0.0	0.0	3.0	0.0	0.0	0.0	0.0	0.0	0.0	0.0	0.0	0.0	0.0	0.0	0.0	0.0	0.0	0.2	0	1	176
180	0.0	0.0	0.0	3.0	0.0	0.0	0.0	0.0	0.0	4.4	0.0	0.0	0.0	0.0	13.9	0.0	0.0	0.0	0.7	0	3	180
181	0.0	0.0	0.0	0.0	0.0	0.0	0.0	0.0	0.0	4.4	0.0	0.0	0.0	0.0	27.8	21.4	0.0	0.0	1.0	0	4	181
190	0.0	0.0	0.0	0.0	0.0	0.0	0.0	0.0	0.0	0.0	0.0	0.0	0.0	0.0	0.0	0.0	0.0	0.0	0.0	0	0	190
191	0.0	0.0	0.0	0.0	0.0	0.0	0.0	0.0	0.0	0.0	0.0	0.0	0.0	0.0	13.9	0.0	0.0	0.0	0.2	0	1	191
192	0.0	0.0	0.0	0.0	0.0	0.0	0.0	0.0	0.0	0.0	0.0	0.0	0.0	0.0	0.0	0.0	0.0	0.0	0.0	0	0	192
193	0.0	0.0	0.0	0.0	0.0	0.0	12.6	5.0	3.1	8.9	0.0	0.0	0.0	9.7	0.0	0.0	0.0	0.0	1.0	0	4	193
194	0.0	0.0	0.0	0.0	4.6	13.8	12.6	0.0	12.3	4.4	21.1	7.2	0.0	38.8	0.0	21.4	0.0	0.0	6.3	0	26	194
195	0.0	0.0	0.0	0.0	0.0	0.0	0.0	0.0	3.1	0.0	0.0	0.0	0.0	0.0	0.0	0.0	0.0	0.0	0.2	0	1	195
196	0.0	2.3	0.0	0.0	0.0	0.0	0.0	5.0	0.0	0.0	0.0	0.0	0.0	0.0	0.0	0.0	0.0	0.0	0.2	0	1	196
197	0.0	0.0	2.4	0.0	0.0	0.0	0.0	0.0	0.0	0.0	0.0	7.2	0.0	9.7	0.0	0.0	0.0	0.0	0.7	0	3	197
200	0.0	0.0	2.4	0.0	0.0	0.0	0.0	2.5	3.1	0.0	0.0	0.0	0.0	9.7	0.0	64.1	34.2	0.0	1.9	0	8	200
201	0.0	0.0	2.4	0.0	0.0	0.0	0.0	0.0	3.1	0.0	0.0	0.0	0.0	0.0	0.0	21.4	0.0	0.0	1.0	0	4	201
203	0.0	0.0	0.0	0.0	0.0	0.0	0.0	0.0	0.0	13.3	0.0	0.0	0.0	2.7	13.9	0.0	0.0	0.0	0.5	0	2	203
204	2.4	0.0	4.8	0.0	4.6	0.0	0.0	5.0	6.2	13.3	0.0	7.2	15.9	9.7	13.9	0.0	0.0	73.5	4.1	0	17	204
202,205	0.0	0.0	0.0	0.0	0.0	0.0	0.0	0.0	0.0	0.0	0.0	0.0	0.0	0.0	13.9	0.0	0.0	0.0	0.7	0	3	202,205
OTHER	0.0	0.0	0.0	0.0	0.0	0.0	2.5	2.5	3.1	13.3	0.0	7.2	0.0	29.1	13.9	64.1	34.2	73.5	3.9	0	16	OTHER
140-205	2.4	2.3	9.6	6.0	18.3	45.0	95.7	156.9	268.5	363.5	316.9	297.1	310.5	532.9	638.9	790.6	1198.6	1029.4	147.4	2	609	140-205
RATE PER CASE IN PERIOD	2.41	2.28	2.39	2.99	4.58	3.46	2.52	2.49	3.09	4.43	7.04	7.25	7.96	9.69	13.89	21.37	34.25	73.53	0.24	-	-	RATE PER CASE IN PERIOD

TABLE 37 B
HAWAII, HAWAIIAN ETHNIC GROUP
MALE INCIDENCE RATES, 1960 - 63.

AVERAGE ANNUAL INCIDENCE PER 100,000 — AGE IN YEARS

INTER-NATIONAL LIST No.	0-	5-	10-	15-	20-	25-	30-	35-	40-	45-	50-	55-	60-	65-	70-	75-	80-	85- AND OVER	ALL AGES	No. OF CASES AGE UNKNOWN	No. OF CASES ALL AGES	INTER-NATIONAL LIST No.
140	0.0	0.0	0.0	0.0	0.0	0.0	0.0	0.0	0.0	0.0	0.0	0.0	0.0	0.0	0.0	0.0	0.0	0.0	0.0	0	0	140
141	0.0	0.0	0.0	0.0	0.0	0.0	0.0	0.0	10.5	0.0	0.0	7.0	29.8	0.0	0.0	0.0	0.0	0.0	1.0	0	2	141
142	0.0	0.0	0.0	0.0	0.0	0.0	0.0	0.0	10.5	0.0	0.0	45.9	0.0	0.0	0.0	0.0	0.0	0.0	1.5	0	3	142
143-4	0.0	0.0	0.0	0.0	0.0	0.0	0.0	0.0	0.0	0.0	0.0	0.0	0.0	0.0	0.0	0.0	0.0	0.0	0.5	1	1	143-4
146	0.0	0.0	0.0	0.0	7.6	0.0	0.0	0.0	0.0	12.9	0.0	0.0	59.5	0.0	89.3	0.0	0.0	625.0	2.9	0	6	146
145,147-8	0.0	0.0	0.0	0.0	0.0	0.0	0.0	0.0	10.5	0.0	16.6	0.0	0.0	0.0	0.0	156.3	0.0	0.0	1.5	0	3	145,147-8
150	0.0	0.0	0.0	0.0	0.0	0.0	0.0	0.0	0.0	0.0	16.6	0.0	59.5	86.2	267.9	0.0	0.0	0.0	3.9	0	8	150
151	0.0	0.0	0.0	0.0	0.0	0.0	16.5	27.0	0.0	51.5	33.1	160.6	386.9	129.3	714.3	156.3	0.0	0.0	21.5	0	44	151
152	0.0	0.0	0.0	0.0	0.0	0.0	0.0	0.0	0.0	12.9	0.0	0.0	0.0	0.0	0.0	0.0	416.7	0.0	1.5	0	3	152
153	0.0	0.0	0.0	0.0	0.0	0.0	8.3	0.0	0.0	12.9	49.7	68.8	59.5	43.1	178.6	312.5	0.0	0.0	7.3	0	15	153
154	0.0	0.0	0.0	0.0	0.0	0.0	0.0	9.0	0.0	12.9	49.7	0.0	29.8	43.1	0.0	0.0	0.0	0.0	2.4	0	5	154
155.0	0.0	0.0	0.0	0.0	0.0	0.0	0.0	0.0	10.5	12.9	16.6	68.8	29.8	0.0	178.6	0.0	0.0	0.0	4.4	0	9	155.0
155.1	0.0	0.0	0.0	0.0	0.0	0.0	0.0	0.0	0.0	0.0	0.0	0.0	0.0	0.0	0.0	0.0	0.0	0.0	0.0	0	0	155.1
157	0.0	0.0	0.0	0.0	0.0	0.0	8.3	0.0	10.5	0.0	33.1	22.9	29.8	86.2	178.6	156.3	0.0	0.0	5.4	0	11	157
160	0.0	0.0	0.0	0.0	0.0	0.0	0.0	0.0	0.0	0.0	0.0	0.0	0.0	0.0	0.0	0.0	0.0	0.0	0.0	0	0	160
161	0.0	0.0	0.0	0.0	0.0	0.0	0.0	0.0	0.0	0.0	49.7	0.0	29.8	0.0	0.0	0.0	0.0	0.0	2.0	0	4	161
162	0.0	0.0	0.0	0.0	0.0	0.0	8.3	0.0	42.2	64.4	82.8	206.4	297.6	301.7	267.9	312.5	416.7	0.0	22.9	0	47	162
177	0.0	0.0	0.0	0.0	0.0	0.0	0.0	0.0	0.0	0.0	0.0	22.9	89.3	215.5	357.1	0.0	416.7	0.0	6.8	0	14	177
178	0.0	0.0	0.0	8.7	0.0	15.7	0.0	9.0	10.5	0.0	16.6	0.0	0.0	0.0	0.0	0.0	0.0	0.0	2.4	0	5	178
179	0.0	0.0	0.0	0.0	0.0	0.0	0.0	0.0	0.0	0.0	0.0	0.0	0.0	0.0	0.0	0.0	0.0	0.0	0.0	0	0	179
180	0.0	0.0	0.0	0.0	0.0	0.0	0.0	0.0	0.0	0.0	16.6	22.9	29.8	0.0	0.0	0.0	0.0	0.0	1.5	0	3	180
181	0.0	0.0	0.0	0.0	0.0	0.0	0.0	9.0	0.0	0.0	33.1	0.0	89.3	0.0	0.0	156.3	0.0	0.0	3.4	0	7	181
190	0.0	0.0	3.6	0.0	0.0	0.0	0.0	0.0	0.0	0.0	0.0	0.0	0.0	0.0	0.0	0.0	0.0	0.0	0.5	0	1	190
191	0.0	0.0	0.0	0.0	0.0	0.0	0.0	0.0	0.0	0.0	0.0	0.0	0.0	0.0	0.0	0.0	0.0	0.0	0.0	0	0	191
192	0.0	0.0	0.0	0.0	0.0	0.0	0.0	0.0	0.0	0.0	0.0	0.0	0.0	0.0	0.0	0.0	0.0	0.0	0.0	0	0	192
193	0.0	3.1	0.0	0.0	0.0	0.0	0.0	0.0	0.0	0.0	0.0	22.9	29.8	0.0	0.0	0.0	0.0	0.0	2.0	0	4	193
194	0.0	0.0	0.0	0.0	7.6	7.8	0.0	0.0	0.0	0.0	33.1	22.9	59.5	0.0	0.0	0.0	0.0	0.0	3.4	0	7	194
195	0.0	0.0	0.0	0.0	0.0	0.0	0.0	0.0	0.0	0.0	0.0	0.0	0.0	0.0	0.0	0.0	0.0	0.0	0.0	0	0	195
196	0.0	0.0	0.0	0.0	0.0	7.8	0.0	0.0	0.0	0.0	0.0	0.0	29.8	0.0	0.0	0.0	0.0	0.0	1.0	0	2	196
197	5.4	0.0	0.0	0.0	7.6	0.0	8.3	9.0	10.5	0.0	0.0	22.9	0.0	0.0	0.0	0.0	0.0	0.0	2.9	0	6	197
200	0.0	0.0	3.6	0.0	0.0	0.0	0.0	0.0	0.0	12.9	16.6	0.0	0.0	43.1	0.0	312.5	0.0	0.0	3.4	0	7	200
201	0.0	0.0	0.0	4.3	0.0	0.0	8.3	0.0	0.0	12.9	16.6	22.9	0.0	43.1	0.0	0.0	0.0	0.0	2.4	0	5	201
203	0.0	0.0	0.0	0.0	0.0	0.0	0.0	0.0	0.0	0.0	0.0	0.0	0.0	43.1	0.0	0.0	0.0	0.0	1.5	0	3	203
204	16.3	0.0	0.0	0.0	0.0	0.0	16.5	0.0	0.0	25.8	33.1	22.9	59.5	43.1	0.0	312.5	0.0	0.0	7.8	0	16	204
202,205	0.0	0.0	0.0	0.0	0.0	0.0	8.3	0.0	0.0	0.0	0.0	0.0	59.5	86.2	0.0	0.0	0.0	0.0	1.5	0	3	202,205
OTHER	0.0	0.0	0.0	4.3	0.0	0.0	0.0	0.0	0.0	0.0	0.0	0.0	0.0	0.0	0.0	0.0	0.0	0.0	2.4	0	5	OTHER
140-205	21.7	3.1	7.2	17.4	22.9	31.3	82.5	71.9	158.2	219.1	463.3	711.0	1458.3	1163.8	2232.1	1875.0	1250.0	625.0	121.6	1	249	**140-205**
RATE PER CASE IN PERIOD	2.71	3.08	3.60	4.34	7.62	7.84	8.25	8.99	10.55	12.89	16.56	22.94	29.76	43.10	89.29	156.25	416.67	625.00	0.49	-	-	**RATE PER CASE IN PERIOD**

TABLE 3/C

HAWAII, HAWAIIAN ETHNIC GROUP :

FEMALE INCIDENCE RATES, 1960 - 63.

INTER-NATIONAL LIST No.	AVERAGE ANNUAL INCIDENCE PER 100,000 — AGE IN YEARS																		ALL AGES	No. OF CASES IN WHOLE PERIOD		INTER-NATIONAL LIST No.
	0-	5-	10-	15-	20-	25-	30-	35-	40-	45-	50-	55-	60-	65-	70-	75-	80-	85- AND OVER		AGE UNKNOWN	ALL AGES	
140	0.0	0.0	0.0	0.0	0.0	0.0	0.0	0.0	0.0	0.0	0.0	0.0	0.0	0.0	0.0	0.0	0.0	0.0	0.0	0	0	140
141	0.0	0.0	0.0	0.0	0.0	0.0	0.0	0.0	0.0	0.0	0.0	0.0	62.5	0.0	0.0	0.0	0.0	0.0	1.0	0	2	141
142	0.0	0.0	0.0	4.5	0.0	0.0	0.0	0.0	0.0	0.0	0.0	0.0	0.0	0.0	0.0	0.0	0.0	0.0	0.5	0	1	142
143-4	0.0	0.0	0.0	0.0	0.0	0.0	0.0	0.0	0.0	0.0	0.0	0.0	0.0	0.0	0.0	0.0	0.0	0.0	0.0	0	0	143-4
146	0.0	0.0	0.0	0.0	0.0	0.0	0.0	0.0	0.0	0.0	0.0	0.0	0.0	0.0	0.0	0.0	0.0	0.0	0.0	0	0	146
145,147-8	0.0	0.0	0.0	0.0	0.0	0.0	0.0	0.0	0.0	0.0	0.0	0.0	0.0	0.0	0.0	0.0	0.0	0.0	0.0	0	0	145,147-8
150	0.0	0.0	0.0	0.0	0.0	0.0	0.0	0.0	0.0	0.0	0.0	0.0	0.0	0.0	0.0	0.0	0.0	0.0	0.0	0	0	150
151	0.0	0.0	0.0	0.0	0.0	0.0	0.0	17.5	20.3	51.3	49.3	106.8	31.3	84.7	71.4	119.0	0.0	0.0	10.2	0	21	151
152	0.0	0.0	0.0	0.0	0.0	0.0	0.0	0.0	0.0	0.0	0.0	0.0	0.0	0.0	0.0	0.0	0.0	0.0	0.0	0	0	152
153	0.0	0.0	0.0	0.0	0.0	0.0	0.0	8.7	0.0	0.0	16.4	42.7	31.3	42.4	142.9	119.0	0.0	500.0	4.9	0	10	153
154	0.0	0.0	0.0	0.0	0.0	0.0	0.0	0.0	0.0	0.0	16.4	0.0	31.3	0.0	0.0	119.0	312.5	0.0	1.5	0	3	154
155.0	0.0	0.0	0.0	0.0	0.0	0.0	0.0	0.0	0.0	0.0	16.4	42.7	31.3	0.0	0.0	119.0	0.0	0.0	2.4	0	5	155.0
155.1	0.0	0.0	0.0	0.0	0.0	0.0	0.0	0.0	10.2	0.0	16.4	0.0	31.3	0.0	0.0	119.0	312.5	0.0	2.0	0	4	155.1
157	0.0	0.0	0.0	0.0	0.0	0.0	0.0	0.0	0.0	0.0	0.0	21.4	93.8	84.7	71.4	0.0	0.0	0.0	3.9	0	8	157
160	0.0	0.0	0.0	0.0	0.0	0.0	0.0	0.0	0.0	0.0	0.0	0.0	0.0	0.0	0.0	0.0	0.0	0.0	0.0	0	0	160
161	0.0	0.0	0.0	0.0	0.0	0.0	0.0	0.0	0.0	0.0	16.4	21.4	0.0	0.0	0.0	0.0	0.0	0.0	1.0	0	2	161
162	0.0	0.0	0.0	0.0	0.0	0.0	0.0	8.7	10.2	25.6	16.4	64.1	62.5	84.7	285.7	0.0	0.0	0.0	7.8	0	16	162
170	0.0	0.0	0.0	0.0	6.9	0.0	23.1	35.0	61.0	141.0	115.1	128.2	218.8	254.2	71.4	0.0	0.0	0.0	26.4	0	54	170
171	0.0	0.0	0.0	0.0	6.9	43.2	69.2	113.6	111.8	89.7	131.6	106.8	156.3	127.1	142.9	0.0	0.0	0.0	34.2	0	70	171
172	0.0	0.0	0.0	0.0	0.0	14.4	15.4	8.7	20.3	12.8	65.8	0.0	93.8	169.5	71.4	238.1	0.0	0.0	9.8	0	20	172
173-4	0.0	0.0	0.0	0.0	0.0	0.0	0.0	0.0	0.0	0.0	0.0	0.0	0.0	0.0	0.0	0.0	0.0	0.0	0.0	0	0	173-4
175	0.0	0.0	0.0	0.0	0.0	7.2	0.0	17.5	20.3	12.8	49.3	21.4	93.8	127.1	71.4	0.0	0.0	0.0	8.3	0	17	175
176	0.0	0.0	0.0	0.0	0.0	0.0	0.0	0.0	0.0	0.0	0.0	0.0	0.0	0.0	0.0	0.0	0.0	0.0	0.0	0	0	176
180	2.8	0.0	0.0	0.0	0.0	0.0	0.0	0.0	0.0	12.8	16.4	0.0	0.0	0.0	0.0	0.0	0.0	0.0	1.5	0	3	180
181	0.0	0.0	0.0	4.5	0.0	0.0	0.0	0.0	0.0	0.0	0.0	21.4	0.0	0.0	71.4	0.0	0.0	0.0	1.5	0	3	181
190	0.0	0.0	0.0	0.0	0.0	0.0	0.0	0.0	0.0	0.0	0.0	0.0	0.0	0.0	0.0	0.0	0.0	0.0	0.0	0	0	190
191	0.0	0.0	0.0	0.0	0.0	0.0	0.0	0.0	0.0	0.0	0.0	0.0	0.0	0.0	0.0	0.0	0.0	0.0	0.0	0	0	191
192	0.0	0.0	0.0	0.0	0.0	0.0	0.0	0.0	0.0	0.0	0.0	0.0	0.0	0.0	0.0	0.0	0.0	0.0	0.0	0	0	192
193	2.8	0.0	3.7	0.0	6.9	0.0	30.8	0.0	0.0	0.0	0.0	0.0	31.3	0.0	0.0	0.0	0.0	0.0	2.4	0	5	193
194	0.0	0.0	0.0	0.0	6.9	0.0	0.0	17.5	10.2	12.8	65.8	21.4	31.3	0.0	0.0	0.0	0.0	0.0	6.8	0	14	194
195	0.0	0.0	0.0	0.0	0.0	0.0	0.0	0.0	0.0	0.0	16.4	0.0	0.0	0.0	0.0	0.0	0.0	0.0	0.5	0	1	195
196	0.0	0.0	3.7	0.0	0.0	7.2	0.0	0.0	0.0	0.0	0.0	0.0	0.0	0.0	0.0	0.0	0.0	0.0	1.0	0	2	196
197	0.0	0.0	0.0	0.0	0.0	0.0	0.0	8.7	10.2	0.0	0.0	0.0	31.3	0.0	71.4	0.0	0.0	0.0	1.5	0	3	197
200	0.0	0.0	0.0	0.0	0.0	0.0	0.0	0.0	0.0	0.0	0.0	21.4	31.3	0.0	0.0	0.0	0.0	0.0	1.0	0	2	200
201	0.0	0.0	0.0	0.0	0.0	0.0	0.0	0.0	0.0	0.0	16.4	0.0	31.3	0.0	0.0	0.0	0.0	0.0	0.5	0	1	201
203	0.0	0.0	0.0	0.0	0.0	0.0	0.0	0.0	0.0	0.0	0.0	0.0	0.0	0.0	71.4	0.0	0.0	500.0	1.0	0	2	203
204	14.1	3.2	7.4	4.5	0.0	0.0	0.0	0.0	10.2	12.8	0.0	0.0	0.0	0.0	71.4	0.0	0.0	0.0	5.4	0	11	204
202,205	0.0	0.0	0.0	0.0	0.0	0.0	0.0	0.0	10.2	12.8	0.0	21.4	0.0	0.0	0.0	0.0	0.0	0.0	1.5	0	3	202,205
OTHER	0.0	0.0	0.0	0.0	0.0	7.2	0.0	0.0	0.0	0.0	15.4	21.4	93.6	0.0	0.0	119.0	0.0	500.0	3.9	0	8	OTHER
140-205	19.8	3.2	14.9	13.6	27.5	79.3	****	236.0	294.7	397.4	608.6	662.4	1125.0	974.6	1142.9	952.4	625.0	1500.0	142.0	0	291	140-205
RATE PER CASE IN PERIOD	2.82	3.23	3.72	4.53	6.89	7.20	7.69	8.74	10.16	12.82	16.45	21.37	31.25	42.37	71.43	119.05	312.50	500.0	0.49	-		RATE PER CASE IN PERIOD

Chapter V
COMPARISON BETWEEN REGISTRIES

SYSTEMATIC BIASSES

Comparison of statistical data is often difficult and particularly when the data have been collected in different countries under different conditions. On superficial examination the data may seem to represent the same things; yet, in fact, they may have very different characters, and conclusions drawn from comparisons between them may be grossly misleading. The reasons which may invalidate comparisons between cancer incidence rates are well known, and many of them have been referred to in previous chapters. They are brought together here, partly for ease of reference and partly to re-emphasize the need for caution in drawing conclusions from the gross differences between some of the recorded rates.

Differences in reporting

The most important bias, and the one least amenable to quantitative assessment, is that due to differences in the standard of reporting. The rates may be artificially low if some known cases fail to be registered, if diagnostic standards are inadequate, if the provision of medical services is incomplete, and if some people fail to make use of the available service. Alternatively, they may, on occasions, be artificially high if the diagnosis is not commonly supported by good histological evidence. In many countries, the automatic reporting of deaths attributed to cancer serves to ensure that there is no serious under-reporting of diagnosed cases of those types of cancer that are commonly fatal. The proportions of these cancers that are recorded directly as a result of death certification may, therefore, be taken as a first indication of the efficiency of the recording system and of the extent to which people make use of the medical services before the terminal stage of their disease. If the proportion of cases diagnosed histologically is also high it is usually safe to assume that the figures provide a close estimate of the true incidence. Unfortunately, it was not possible to obtain such evidence for all registries, but those data that were obtained are illuminating and have been brought together in the Appendix.

The factor that is most difficult to measure is the extent to which people make use of the services. This is always important in the oldest age groups (say, age 75 years and over), but it can probably be ignored at younger ages in most of the countries in which cancer registries have been established on a continuing basis. The situation is different in the developing countries and failure to seek medical attention - or, having sought it, to be adequately investigated - must be regarded as an important potential source of error. Moreover, this source of error is likely to affect different age groups to different extents and it will be particularly important among the older sections of the community where cancer would normally be expected to be most common (Maclean, 1965). Not only are older people less likely to turn to new services for help, but economic pressures, which encourage the wage earner to seek treatment, are more likely to keep them away. How far this provides an explanation for some of the very low rates recorded in Africa is a matter for conjecture, and can be decided only on the basis of an intimate knowledge of the individual communities.

Differences in prophylactic services

It is the hope of many of those concerned with preventive medicine that cancer can be prevented by the treatment of precancerous conditions. If this is indeed so, the adequacy of the preventive services might have a major effect on the cancer incidence rate, and a low rate might indicate a high standard of prophylaxis rather than a relative lack of exposure to carcinogenic factors. Whether prophylaxis of this sort can have an important effect on cancer incidence remains to be proved. At present the question is largely theoretical as few prophylactic programmes are sufficiently developed to have to be taken seriously into account. The most important exceptions are the cytological screening programmes for the detection of pre-invasive lesions of the cervix uteri, and the routine medical treatment of papilloma of the bladder. These have been discussed previously in chapter III.

Differences in classification

Differences in classification, due to difficulty in deciding whether a particular growth is malignant or benign and in determining its histological type and its site of origin, have been discussed in chapter III. They do not generally provide such large sources of bias as those derived from differences in reporting; but they vary from one type of cancer to another and may occasionally have substantial effects. The rates recorded in the present volume that are most likely to have been affected by this factor are those for cancers of the colon (I.L. no. 153), rectum (I.L. no. 154), cervix uteri (I.L. no. 171), bladder (I.L. no. 181.0) and central nervous system (I.L. no. 193).

Differences in age distribution

Comparison of the incidence of cancer in different populations is complicated by the fact that cancer incidence varies with age. With some cancers (for example, cancer of the prostate, stomach, rectum, bronchus and bladder) the incidence may increase 500 times or more over a span of 50 years, and differences in the proportion of the population living at different ages can produce differences in the crude incidence as big as those produced by differences in the prevalence of carcinogenic factors. Clearly, therefore, comparisons of total incidence rates uncorrected for age are of little value in the study of aetiology.

The most suitable comparisons are those made directly between the individual age-specific rates. Not only may differences be noted between the rates, but the trends in incidence with age can be compared and differences in these trends may be equally important. Such comparisons are, however, not easy. The mental effort required to master so many separate figures and the interrelationship between them is considerable; moreover, the numbers of cases in any one sex and age group may be extremely small. The size of the individual age-specific rates may, therefore, be affected materially by chance and some degree of condensation is essential.

STANDARDIZED INCIDENCE RATES

The traditional way of overcoming the difficulty introduced by differences in the age distribution of the populations is by the use of rates standardized for age; that is, of rates which, it is claculated, would have been observed, if the age-specific rates recorded by each registry had occurred in a standard population with a specified age distribution. The difficulty is, however, not wholly resolved by this means. It would be, if the incidence of each cancer varied with age in the same way in different populations, at different places, and at different times; but it does not. In Denmark, for example, the male incidence rate for cancer of the stomach is 66 times greater at 70-74 years of age than at 35-39 years; in England and Wales and the U.S.A. it is about 50 times greater; in Cali, Colombia and Japan it is about 30 times greater; in Chile about 20 times greater; in the Johannesburg, South African Bantu about 10 times greater; while in the Kampala Registry, Uganda there was no case of cancer of the stomach in men of 70 years of age or over at all. Accurate incidence data have not been recorded for sufficiently long to demonstrate whether similar differences may also occur with the passage of time. Notable differences have, however, been found in mortality rates (Case, 1956) and it seems only reasonable to presume that they do. A comparison of incidence rates standardized for age may, therefore, give different results depending on the age distribution of the population that is taken as the standard. If the standard population has a high proportion of persons at old ages, standardized rates will be relatively high when the incidence of cancer rises rapidly and progressively with age, and relatively low when it levels off or falls in the oldest age groups. If the standard population has a low proportion of persons at old ages, the reverse will be true. In the study of aetiology, therefore, standardized rates are little better than crude rates. They reduce the effect of differences in age distribution; but they do not eliminate it, and if their limitations are forgotten they may be grossly misleading.

There is, in fact, no way of compressing the age-specific incidence rates without losing some - and often vital - information. Many solutions have been suggested; but none have achieved international acceptance. Stocks (1959) recommended a simple form of standardization using six age groups, and suggested that the rates in these groups could also be shown conveniently as percentages of the standardized rate. Doll (1966) thought that any form of standardization that included age groups over 65 years of age would be misleading when African populations were included and recommended limiting comparisons to standardized rates within the limits of 45 and 64 years of age. In the present report we have confined ourselves to traditional methods and have calculated standardized rates, including all ages. We have, however, used three standard populations differing widely in the proportion of persons at different ages (Table 38), and we give in this chapter the three rates which result for each type of cancer for each registry (Tables 39A to 39F and 40A to 40F). The population with the lowest proportion of old people that we have used is the standard "African" population suggested by Knowelden and Oettlé (1962). As an intermediate "world" population, we have rounded off the figures that Segi (1960) derived from data for 46 countries, and we have used Scandinavian figures to provide an old "European" population. For each, we have used five-year age groups up to ages 80-84 years and, if necessary, have interpolated in the published figures to be able to do so. We would stress, however, that the standardized rates are included only as a guide and that the figures of greatest value are the age-specific rates given in chapter IV.

TABLE 38

Standard populations (100,000s)

Age (in years)	African	World	European
0-	1.00	1.20	0.80
5-	1.00	1.00	0.70
10-	1.00	0.90	0.70
15-	1.00	0.90	0.70
20-	1.00	0.80	0.70
25-	1.00	0.80	0.70
30-	1.00	0.60	0.70
35-	1.00	0.60	0.70
40-	0.50	0.60	0.70
45-	0.50	0.60	0.70
50-	0.30	0.50	0.70
55-	0.20	0.40	0.60
60-	0.20	0.40	0.50
65-	0.10	0.30	0.40
70-	0.10	0.20	0.30
75-	0.05	0.10	0.20
80-	0.03	0.05	0.10
85 and over	0.02	0.05	0.10
Total	10.00	10.00	10.00

Incidence of different types of cancer recorded by each Registry standardized for age : male rates

INCIDENCE RATE PER 100,000 PER YEAR IN:

INTER-NATIONAL LIST No.	STANDARD POPU-LATION	Mozambique Lourenço Marques	Nigeria Ibadan	S. Africa Johannesburg (Bantu)	Uganda Kyadondo	CANADA 5 provinces	Alberta	Manitoba	New Brunswick	Newfoundland	Saskatchewan	Chile	Colombia Cali	Jamaica Kingston	Puerto Rico	U.S.A. Connecticut	N.Y. State	Israel	Japan Miyagi	Singapore (Chinese)
140	African	0.0	0.2	0.2	0.0	10.8	9.7	7.2	11.1	14.7	14.2	0.1	1.3	0.3	1.4	1.8	1.6	3.6	0.3	0.1
	World	0.0	0.5	0.2	0.0	17.7	15.8	11.8	19.1	22.1	23.1	1.1	2.7	0.5	2.2	3.1	2.9	4.6	0.5	0.1
	European	0.0	0.6	0.3	0.0	24.9	22.1	16.6	28.1	31.4	32.2	1.6	3.9	0.7	3.0	4.7	4.3	6.0	0.9	0.2
141	African	0.0	0.2	1.2	0.0	0.5	0.6	0.3	0.4	0.7	0.4	0.4	2.2	1.6	4.3	2.1	1.1	0.3	0.5	1.0
	World	0.0	0.3	2.1	0.0	0.8	1.0	0.6	0.8	1.4	0.7	0.6	4.1	3.4	7.1	3.6	2.1	0.5	0.9	1.6
	European	0.0	0.5	2.9	0.0	1.2	1.5	0.8	1.2	2.2	0.9	0.9	6.6	5.1	10.0	5.1	3.0	0.7	1.5	2.2
142	African	0.0	1.2	0.4	0.3	1.2	0.5	1.6	1.2	1.1	2.1	0.4	2.1	1.1	0.2	0.9	0.7	0.7	0.3	0.1
	World	0.0	1.8	0.3	0.2	1.5	0.8	2.0	1.4	1.5	2.2	0.5	2.1	1.4	0.4	1.2	1.0	0.9	0.3	0.2
	European	0.0	2.2	0.3	0.2	1.9	1.0	2.6	1.7	1.9	2.8	0.8	3.2	1.8	0.6	1.6	1.3	1.1	0.3	0.2
143-4	African	2.2	0.8	1.5	0.0	0.9	0.9	0.9		0.7	0.6	0.3	0.8	1.5	3.9	2.0	1.4	0.8	0.3	1.3
	World	3.9	1.1	3.2	0.0	1.7	1.5	1.6		1.6	1.3	0.5	1.6	2.3	7.1	3.7	2.6	1.2	0.6	1.9
	European	5.4	1.4	4.6	0.0	2.7	2.2	2.5		2.3	2.0	0.7	2.3	2.9	10.1	5.5	3.9	1.5	0.7	2.5
146	African	1.6	0.4	0.8	0.0	0.3	0.3	0.2		0.8	0.3	0.0	0.0	0.8	0.2	0.4	0.3	1.1	0.5	14.2
	World	2.2	0.8	0.9	0.0	0.5	0.5	0.4		1.3	0.4	0.1	0.0	1.7	0.4	0.7	0.5	1.5	0.7	16.1
	European	3.1	1.0	1.0	0.0	0.7	0.7	0.6		1.7	0.6	0.1	0.0	2.3	0.6	0.9	0.6	1.9	0.9	19.7
145,147-8	African		0.0	0.1	0.3	0.4	0.4	0.6	0.0	0.2	0.5	0.3	1.9	1.2	4.2	2.1	1.2	0.6	0.2	1.4
	World		0.0	0.1	0.4	0.7	0.7	0.9	0.1	0.4	0.9	0.5	3.3	2.0	7.2	3.9	2.3	0.8	0.3	2.5
	European		0.0	0.1	0.5	1.0	1.0	1.2	0.1	0.6	1.3	0.7	4.5	3.0	10.0	5.6	3.4	1.1	0.4	3.5
150	African	3.4	0.9	7.7	1.1	1.2	0.8	1.1	1.1	1.5	1.4	5.8	2.7	10.0	9.6	3.1	2.1	2.1	6.7	7.3
	World	4.4	1.2	12.9	1.8	2.3	1.6	2.4	2.1	2.9	2.8	10.7	5.4	17.2	18.0	6.0	4.2	3.9	13.4	11.9
	European	6.0	1.5	20.2	2.4	3.5	2.5	4.0	2.9	4.4	4.2	15.5	7.9	23.8	26.1	8.7	6.3	6.3	19.4	16.2
151	African	1.4	6.3	5.9	1.9	11.5	8.3	13.1	12.1	21.7	9.8	25.9	31.8	15.8	15.2	9.2	7.1	14.9	53.1	8.0
	World	3.0	10.6	10.2	2.3	21.5	16.6	24.1	21.4	40.1	18.9	45.9	55.3	27.2	29.0	17.9	13.7	28.3	95.5	12.9
	European	4.3	14.1	14.4	2.8	32.1	24.4	36.1	31.8	60.1	28.4	65.4	76.3	38.0	42.6	27.6	20.8	42.5	135.5	17.5
152	African	0.0	0.0	0.1	0.4	0.4	0.3	0.5	0.7	0.3	0.2	0.1	1.0	0.1	0.2	0.6	0.4	0.4	0.1	0.0
	World	0.0	0.0	0.2	0.3	0.6	0.4	1.0	1.2	0.5	0.3	0.2	1.6	0.1	0.4	1.1	0.6	0.6	0.1	0.1
	European	0.0	0.0	0.2	0.3	0.9	0.6	1.4	1.8	0.7	0.4	0.2	2.5	0.1	0.7	1.6	0.9	0.8	0.2	0.1
153	African	1.8	0.8	0.9	0.2	9.5	8.4	11.5	9.3	14.1	7.1	2.0	3.4	4.4	2.4	13.4	11.1	6.5	2.2	1.6
	World	1.9	1.0	1.8	0.3	16.9	15.2	20.7	16.7	21.8	13.3	3.5	5.4	8.5	4.4	25.4	21.2	11.2	3.9	2.6
	European	2.4	1.3	2.4	0.5	24.9	22.5	31.0	24.1	31.3	20.0	5.2	7.3	12.4	6.4	38.8	32.1	16.0	5.7	3.6
154	African	0.0	1.2	1.1	0.6	5.6	4.9	6.0	6.3	2.8	6.5	1.9	1.2	2.4	2.2	7.7	7.0	4.6	2.8	3.1
	World	0.0	1.3	2.0	1.1	10.4	9.0	11.1	11.6	4.7	12.8	3.3	2.2	4.3	3.5	15.1	13.4	7.8	4.9	5.0
	European	0.0	1.6	3.1	1.5	15.6	13.5	16.9	17.2	6.9	19.0	4.8	3.1	6.3	4.9	22.7	20.3	11.1	7.0	7.1
155.0	African	113.4	8.6	13.5		0.5	0.2	1.2	0.4	0.3	0.3		2.3	2.3	1.6	1.3	0.8	1.3		6.3
	World	103.8	9.8	19.2		1.0	0.4	2.2	0.7	0.4	0.6		4.0	3.3	2.8	2.4	1.5	2.3		8.6
	European	112.9	11.7	25.5		1.4	0.6	3.1	0.9	0.5	1.4		5.6	4.1	4.1	3.4	2.3	3.0		11.2
155.1	African	0.0	0.0	0.0		0.8	0.8	1.0	0.9	0.5	0.7		1.7	1.2	0.7	1.2	0.9	1.7		0.3
	World	0.0	0.0	0.0		1.6	1.5	1.8	1.7	1.0	1.5		3.4	2.3	1.5	2.3	1.7	3.2		0.6
	European	0.0	0.0	0.0		2.4	2.1	2.8	2.6	1.6	2.4		4.7	3.4	2.2	3.5	2.6	4.8		0.9
155	African				6.2							2.4							3.1	
	World				6.2							4.0							6.0	
	European				7.7							5.5							8.4	
156	African			0.2	1.1	0.4	0.6		0.5	0.8	0.4	2.1		0.6	1.6	0.7	1.1	1.5	5.1	1.0
	World			0.6	1.3	0.7	1.0		1.0	1.3	0.8	3.4		0.8	2.8	1.4	2.0	2.8	9.6	1.3
	European			0.8	1.6	1.0	1.2		1.4	2.0	1.2	4.7		0.9	3.9	2.2	3.0	4.0	14.2	1.7

TABLE 39B

Incidence of different types of cancer recorded by each Registry standardized for age : male rates

INCIDENCE RATE PER 100,000 PER YEAR IN:

INTER-NATIONAL LIST No.	STANDARD POPULATION	Denmark	ENGLAND and WALES 4 regions	Birmingham region	Liverpool region	South. Met. region	S. Western region	Finland	Germany F.R. Hamburg	Iceland	Netherlands 3 provinces	Norway	Sweden	Yugoslavia Slovenia	N. Zealand	HAWAII All groups*	Caucasian	Japanese	Hawaiian ethnic
140	African	2.9	1.2	1.0	1.5	0.7	1.8	5.6	0.9	3.2	1.6	1.9	1.5	3.1	1.9	0.4	1.3	0.0	0.0
	World	4.8	2.0	1.8	2.8	1.2	3.2	9.3	1.4	6.3	2.8	3.5	2.7	5.2	3.2	0.4	1.6	0.0	0.0
	European	6.8	2.9	2.7	4.1	1.7	4.8	13.4	1.9	9.6	4.1	5.3	4.0	7.6	4.5	0.5	2.0	0.0	0.0
141	African	0.4	0.8	1.1	0.8	0.7	0.6	0.4	0.4	0.6	0.6	0.4	0.3	0.6	0.7	1.5	2.3	1.4	1.1
	World	0.7	1.5	1.9	1.5	1.3	1.2	0.7	0.8	0.6	1.0	0.8	0.5	1.0	1.3	2.7	4.5	2.6	1.8
	European	1.1	2.2	2.9	2.5	1.9	1.8	1.0	1.1	1.0	1.4	1.2	0.8	1.4	2.0	3.7	6.1	3.7	2.2
142	African	0.8	0.9	1.0	0.8	0.8	0.9	1.1	2.5*	0.3	0.7	0.3	0.4	0.2	0.6	0.9	0.8	0.5	1.4
	World	1.0	1.1	1.2	1.0	1.0	1.1	1.5	3.7*	0.4	1.0	0.4	0.6	0.3	0.8	1.2	1.3	0.7	2.5
	European	1.2	1.4	1.6	1.4	1.3	1.4	1.9	5.1*	0.5	1.3	0.6	0.8	0.4	1.2	1.5	1.6	0.9	3.5
143-4	African	0.4	0.9	0.9	1.1	0.9	0.6	0.5		0.2	0.5	0.7	0.6	0.8	0.7	1.1	2.0	0.2	2.0
	World	0.7	1.7	1.7	2.0	1.6	1.1	0.8		0.4	0.9	1.3	1.1	1.5	1.3	1.9	3.9	0.4	2.0
	European	1.1	2.5	2.5	3.1	2.5	1.8	1.3		0.7	1.4	2.0	1.6	2.2	2.0	2.6	5.0	0.5	2.0
146	African		0.3	0.3	0.3	0.3	0.3	0.3		0.7	0.2	0.2	0.5	0.2	0.2	1.6	0.5	0.3	4.7
	World		0.5	0.5	0.4	0.5	0.4	0.3		1.1	0.2	0.3	0.7	0.3	0.3	2.2	0.5	0.6	8.7
	European		0.6	0.7	0.5	0.6	0.6	0.4		1.7	0.3	0.4	0.9	0.4	0.3	3.0	0.7	1.0	13.3
145,147-8	African	0.4	1.1	1.1	1.1	1.0	1.0	0.8		0.2	0.8	0.5	0.5	1.2	0.6	1.2	1.4	0.8	1.8
	World	0.7	2.1	2.1	2.3	2.0	2.0	1.3		0.4	1.4	1.0	1.0	2.2	1.2	2.3	2.8	1.6	3.0
	European	1.1	3.2	3.3	3.5	3.1	3.0	1.9		0.5	2.1	1.5	1.5	3.1	1.7	3.3	3.8	2.4	5.0
150	African	1.8	2.3	2.3	2.5	2.2	1.9	3.5	2.4	4.8	1.3	1.6	1.2	3.4	2.3	2.7	2.7	3.0	5.2
	World	3.6	4.5	4.6	5.0	4.4	3.8	7.1	4.8	8.5	2.5	3.3	2.5	6.7	4.5	5.6	5.7	6.4	11.2
	European	5.6	6.9	7.1	7.9	6.9	5.8	10.7	7.4	13.1	4.0	5.1	3.8	10.0	6.7	8.4	8.1	9.9	15.6
151	African	16.2	13.4	15.2	18.0	11.0	10.1	27.6	18.7	37.1	10.9	16.7	13.7	25.2	11.9	14.9	6.6	24.6	29.3
	World	31.8	24.8	28.1	34.6	20.9	20.1	53.2	36.9	70.8	20.4	33.0	26.5	48.2	22.9	27.3	12.8	44.9	51.1
	European	48.8	36.4	41.2	51.8	30.8	29.5	79.4	56.6	104.0	30.6	50.4	40.2	69.3	34.6	40.8	18.9	64.9	71.8
152	African	0.3	0.4	0.4	0.3	0.4	0.2	0.5	0.2	0.8	0.2	0.2	0.5	0.2	0.7	0.3	0.0	0.4	1.6
	World	0.6	0.6	0.6	0.5	0.6	0.3	0.7	0.4	1.1	0.3	0.4	0.8	0.3	1.2	0.4	0.0	0.7	1.9
	European	0.8	0.8	0.9	0.6	0.8	0.4	1.0	0.6	1.3	0.4	0.5	1.1	0.5	1.8	0.6	0.0	1.0	2.2
153	African	7.7	7.7	8.1	10.2	6.8	6.4	3.5	6.3	7.0	5.1	5.7	7.4	2.9	12.7	10.0	10.4	10.4	9.3
	World	14.3	13.9	14.9	18.8	12.3	12.3	6.1	11.9	11.1	9.3	10.5	13.4	5.0	22.0	18.4	18.0	19.0	16.9
	European	21.9	21.0	22.8	28.3	18.6	18.5	9.0	17.9	16.2	13.3	16.0	20.1	7.0	32.6	27.4	28.4	28.5	25.4
154	African	8.5	7.0	8.0	6.3	6.3	6.5	3.3	5.3	2.3	4.1	3.3	5.5	3.5	7.5	5.8	5.4	6.6	3.1
	World	16.3	13.1	15.6	11.7	12.1	12.2	6.3	10.4	4.3	8.0	6.5	10.3	6.5	13.8	10.2	9.0	11.4	4.4
	European	24.6	19.5	23.4	17.7	18.0	18.4	9.4	16.3	6.6	12.4	10.0	15.5	9.7	20.6	14.7	12.6	16.7	5.5
155.0	African	1.4		0.5	0.8	0.5		0.8			0.4	0.5	0.9	1.0	1.0		2.1	4.2	5.4
	World	2.7		0.8	1.5	0.8		1.4			0.7	0.9	1.8	1.9	1.5		4.5	7.5	9.7
	European	4.1		1.1	2.1	1.1		2.1			1.0	1.4	2.6	2.7	2.1		7.4	11.0	13.8
155.1	African	0.7		0.8	0.8	0.6		0.4	4.0		1.2	0.5	0.8	1.2	1.2	1.2	0.7	2.2	0.0
	World	1.4		1.5	1.6	1.1		0.7	8.1		2.3	1.0	1.7	2.6	2.3	2.4	1.5	3.8	0.0
	European	2.2		2.2	2.3	1.7		1.1	12.4		3.6	1.5	2.5	3.8	3.4	3.6	2.5	5.7	0.0
155	African		1.2	0.9			1.0	0.8		1.4				1.9		3.7			
	World		2.2	1.8			1.9	1.6		2.6				3.6		6.8			
	European		3.2	2.7			2.8	2.5		3.6				5.3		10.1			
156	African	0.6	0.6	0.9	0.6	0.5	0.4	0.8	0.8	0.9	0.0	0.4	0.3	1.9	0.5				
	World	1.2	1.2	1.8	1.1	1.0	0.7	1.6	1.5	2.0	0.1	0.9	0.7	3.6	0.9				
	European	1.8	1.8	2.7	1.7	1.5	1.0	2.5	2.3	3.3	0.2	1.3	1.0	5.3	1.2				

* See notes to Tables 27 and 34.

INCIDENCE RATE PER 100,000 PER YEAR IN:

INTERNATIONAL LIST No.	STANDARD POPULATION	Mozambique Lourenço Marques	Nigeria Ibadan	S.Africa Johannesburg (Bantu)	Uganda Kyadondo	CANADA 5 provinces	Alberta	Manitoba	New Brunswick	Newfoundland	Saskatchewan	Chile	Colombia Cali	Jamaica Kingston	Puerto Rico	U.S.A. Connecticut	U.S.A. N.Y. State	Israel	Japan Miyagi	Singapore (Chinese)
157	African	0.9	1.6	1.5	1.0	3.7	2.4	5.5	3.7	3.4	3.6	1.8	1.1	2.0	2.2	4.6	4.1	4.6	3.1	0.4
	World	1.5	1.5	2.4	1.3	7.0	4.8	10.3	7.3	5.8	6.7	3.5	2.9	3.2	4.4	9.1	8.0	8.7	6.1	0.7
	European	2.0	1.8	3.6	1.7	10.4	7.1	15.5	11.0	8.2	10.0	5.1	4.1	4.6	6.5	13.7	11.9	12.6	9.1	0.9
160	African	0.0	1.5	1.1	0.6	0.4	0.3	0.4	0.4	0.9	0.2	0.2	0.2	0.4	0.4	0.3	0.5	0.4	1.6	1.4
	World	0.0	1.9	1.9	0.8	0.7	0.5	0.7	0.7	1.8	0.4	0.3	0.3	0.8	0.6	0.6	0.7	0.6	2.7	2.1
	European	0.0	1.9	2.7	1.1	1.0	0.7	1.0	1.1	2.4	0.6	0.4	0.4	1.2	0.8	0.8	1.0	0.7	3.8	2.8
161	African	0.8	0.8	1.2	0.5	1.2	1.0	1.8	1.6	1.7	0.3	1.1	4.9	2.2	3.4	3.9	2.5	4.4	1.4	2.2
	World	1.2	1.4	2.3	0.9	2.1	1.8	3.3	3.3	2.9	0.7	2.0	8.6	4.4	6.1	7.1	4.8	8.0	2.8	3.8
	European	1.7	1.8	3.1	1.2	3.1	2.7	4.7	4.6	4.0	0.9	2.7	12.4	6.6	8.9	10.1	6.8	11.5	4.5	5.2
162-3	African	2.5	1.2	4.6	0.8	13.6	11.1	20.0	11.1	13.6	11.8	7.5	8.4	7.2	6.4	23.0	19.4	13.2	7.3	8.0
	World	4.1	1.2	7.4	0.9	25.8	21.9	38.7	20.3	22.0	21.9	13.2	15.9	14.0	12.5	43.2	37.4	25.4	14.1	12.9
	European	5.6	1.5	10.4	1.0	36.5	30.9	55.7	28.0	30.2	30.9	18.5	22.1	19.2	18.2	61.4	53.3	37.2	19.9	17.2
170	African	0.0	0.0	0.5	0.2	0.2	0.2	0.2	0.0	0.1	0.1	0.3	0.2	0.4	0.5	0.4	0.3	0.9	0.2	0.1
	World	0.0	0.0	0.8	0.3	0.3	0.4	0.5	0.1	0.3	0.3	0.4	0.3	0.8	0.7	0.8	0.5	1.5	0.3	0.1
	European	0.0	0.0	1.1	0.4	0.5	0.6	0.6	0.2	0.5	0.4	0.6	0.4	1.5	0.9	1.2	0.7	2.1	0.5	0.2
177	African	4.9	4.9	4.3	2.4	12.4	9.9	14.6	11.2	6.5	15.7	5.5	13.7	6.4	8.0	16.0	11.1	7.0	1.8	0.5
	World	9.2	10.2	9.4	4.4	26.2	21.3	30.6	23.1	12.9	33.4	11.3	27.7	14.1	16.6	33.9	23.5	14.1	3.8	0.9
	European	13.4	15.2	14.1	6.4	42.9	34.8	50.5	37.0	20.7	54.6	17.9	42.5	21.4	26.7	55.2	39.1	22.4	5.7	1.5
178	African	0.4	0.7	0.4	0.1	2.9	3.4	3.3	1.8	2.4	2.5	2.2	2.1	0.5	0.4	2.9	2.4	1.7	0.5	0.5
	World	0.6	0.6	0.6	0.1	2.5	3.0	3.0	1.6	1.5	2.2	2.2	2.6	0.8	0.3	2.4	2.1	1.6	0.6	0.5
	European	0.6	0.6	0.6	0.1	2.7	3.2	3.3	1.9	1.6	2.4	2.8	2.6	1.0	0.4	2.6	2.3	1.9	0.8	0.5
179.0	African	2.1	0.2	0.9		0.5	0.6	0.4	0.8	1.4	0.4		3.1		4.4	0.4	0.4	0.0		1.0
	World	2.7	0.3	1.5		0.9	0.8	0.7	1.5	1.7	0.7		5.5		6.7	0.8	0.7	0.1		1.6
	European	3.5	0.5	2.0		1.3	1.0	0.9	2.2	2.2	1.1		8.5		9.5	1.1	1.0	0.1		2.2
179	African			0.9	4.7							0.9		5.8					0.4	
	World			1.5	6.8							1.6		8.7					0.7	
	European			2.0	9.4							2.4		12.0					1.0	
180	African	1.1	0.5	0.6	0.1	3.5	3.2	4.2	4.0	1.4	3.7	0.9	1.9	1.8	0.8	3.6	2.8	3.4	0.5	0.9
	World	2.4	0.6	1.1	0.1	5.7	5.1	6.9	6.2	2.2	6.1	1.5	3.3	2.7	1.2	6.3	5.0	6.4	0.9	1.3
	European	3.5	0.7	1.5	0.1	7.9	6.9	9.8	8.3	2.6	8.8	2.0	4.3	3.1	1.6	8.8	6.8	9.0	1.1	1.7
181.0	African	11.1	2.5		3.9	6.5	4.9	6.9	6.9	8.7	6.9		7.3		4.2	9.0	6.9	6.9		1.2
	World	17.5	4.7		7.0	12.1	9.5	12.8	13.2	13.8	13.3		14.2		7.9	16.9	13.4	12.4		2.1
	European	24.1	6.5		9.5	18.2	14.3	19.1	20.1	19.6	20.1		20.6		12.0	25.3	20.3	18.0		3.0
181	African			2.1										3.2					2.1	
	World			3.6										6.7					4.1	
	European			4.7										9.7					6.4	
190	African		0.6	0.8	0.9	1.4	1.5	1.0	1.3	1.2	1.8	0.6	3.2	0.7	0.7	2.9	2.0	2.2	0.2	0.4
	World		0.8	1.2	1.4	2.1	2.2	1.5	1.8	1.8	2.3	1.0	4.7	1.2	0.9	3.0	2.3	2.4	0.3	0.6
	European		1.1	1.5	2.1	2.7	3.0	2.0	2.4	2.5	3.1	1.5	6.7	2.0	1.2	3.8	2.9	2.9	0.4	0.8
191	African	6.7	1.8	1.0	5.5	30.9	25.3	28.2	42.8	24.9	35.1	1.6	23.1	9.2	19.1	31.8	22.1	31.2	1.0	3.1
	World	7.9	2.0	1.4	6.6	54.0	43.9	44.7	78.2	40.3	65.4	2.7	39.5	15.6	32.0	47.0	36.1	44.9	1.5	5.4
	European	10.5	2.1	1.9	8.5	79.8	64.6	63.7	116.3	57.8	99.1	3.9	54.3	21.3	45.2	63.7	51.9	59.4	2.2	7.9
192	African	1.8	0.3	0.5	1.0	1.0	0.3	0.9	0.8	0.2	2.3	0.2	1.1	0.5	0.9	0.5	0.3	1.0	0.4	0.3
	World	1.4	0.4	0.7	1.0	1.3	0.4	1.4	1.0	0.4	2.8	0.3	1.4	0.5	1.1	0.6	0.4	1.4	0.5	0.4
	European	1.3	0.3	0.7	1.1	1.6	0.5	1.8	1.5	0.6	3.4	0.3	1.9	0.4	1.4	0.7	0.6	1.7	0.4	0.4

Incidence of different types of cancer recorded by each Registry
standardized for age : male rates

INCIDENCE RATE PER 100,000 PER YEAR IN:

INTER-NATIONAL LIST No.	STANDARD POPU-LATION	Denmark	England and Wales 4 regions	Birmingham region	Liverpool region	Sorth. Met. region	S. Western region	Finland	Germany F.R. Hamburg	Iceland	Netherlands 3 provinces	Norway	Sweden	Yugoslavia Slovenia	N. Zealand	Hawaii All groups*	Hawaii Caucasian	Hawaii Japanese	Hawaii Hawaiian ethnic
157	African	3.1	3.4	3.5	3.7	3.4	2.8	4.2	4.0	2.8	2.2	3.1	3.5	2.0	4.9	3.7	3.9	3.5	6.8
	World	6.0	6.6	6.7	7.4	6.4	5.6	8.1	7.3	5.5	4.2	5.9	6.8	3.6	9.4	7.0	7.5	6.7	12.6
	European	8.9	9.7	10.0	11.1	9.6	8.3	11.7	10.8	8.7	6.1	8.7	10.1	5.1	14.1	10.5	11.3	10.2	18.4
160	African	0.7	0.8	0.8	0.6	0.5	0.2	0.8	0.3	0.8	0.6	0.4	0.5	0.6	0.6	0.7	0.9	0.6	0.0
	World	1.1	1.0	0.8	0.9	0.7	0.5	1.4	0.6	1.2	0.9	0.8	0.9	0.9	0.9	1.1	1.2	1.0	0.0
	European	1.6	1.1	1.2	1.3	1.0	0.7	2.0	0.8	1.9	1.3	1.2	1.3	1.2	1.3	1.5	1.5	1.6	0.0
161	African	0.9	1.9	1.8	2.0	2.0	1.6	4.3	2.4	0.8	2.2	0.9	1.0	2.3	1.7	2.0	3.7	1.4	2.1
	World	1.5	3.6	3.5	3.8	3.7	3.0	6.9	4.4	1.6	3.9	1.6	1.8	4.4	3.3	3.5	6.5	3.0	3.7
	European	2.1	5.1	5.1	5.5	5.2	4.2	9.4	6.2	2.4	5.5	2.2	2.6	6.4	4.8	5.1	9.4	4.3	5.0
162-3	African	13.1	37.7	37.8	40.5	37.0	26.3	33.4	29.5	8.3	21.8	7.3	8.3	15.5	20.2	14.6*	21.0*	10.9*	27.2*
	World	24.4	70.3	71.7	77.6	73.7	50.2	64.7	58.7	13.6	41.7	13.6	16.1	29.5	39.3	27.5*	39.2*	21.5*	50.6*
	European	34.4	98.1	100.7	109.7	93.6	70.0	91.6	83.3	18.6	57.7	18.8	22.6	41.0	56.2	40.6*	55.7*	32.7*	71.6*
170	African	0.2	0.3	0.2	0.3	0.3	0.2	0.2	0.3	0.0	0.4	0.1	0.2	0.1	0.2		0.0	0.0	
	World	0.4	0.5	0.4	0.5	0.5	0.4	0.4	0.6	0.1	0.6	0.3	0.4	0.1	0.4		0.0	0.0	
	European	0.6	0.7	0.7	0.7	0.8	0.6	0.5	0.9	0.2	0.9	0.4	0.6	0.2	0.6		0.0	0.0	
177	African	8.4	8.4	8.3	8.2	7.3	7.8	8.3	7.8	9.7	7.7	12.0	12.5	5.2	16.3	9.4	19.9	6.2	9.2
	World	17.7	16.7	17.4	16.8	15.0	16.4	17.6	16.5	17.7	16.3	25.2	26.5	10.9	34.4	19.2	40.5	12.6	20.2
	European	29.0	27.2	28.8	28.7	24.8	27.2	28.5	27.5	28.1	27.0	41.6	42.9	17.4	57.2	30.8	65.5	20.2	29.3
178	African	4.4	2.7	2.4	2.4	2.9	2.4	1.1	3.0	3.2	3.0	4.0	2.8	1.4	4.3	2.5	3.5	1.3	3.5
	World	3.8	3.7	2.1	2.3	2.4	2.1	1.3	2.6	3.3	2.8	3.3	2.4	1.3	3.5	2.2	3.1	1.3	3.3
	European	4.2	2.5	2.2	2.3	2.6	2.3	1.4	2.8	3.2	3.1	3.7	2.7	1.5	3.6	2.3	3.2	1.6	3.6
179.0	African	0.7		0.5	0.6	0.5		0.6		0.4	0.4	0.4	0.6	0.4	0.4				
	World	1.1		0.9	1.0	0.8		0.9		1.0	0.7	0.7	0.9	0.7	0.7				
	European	1.5		1.4	1.4	1.2		1.3		1.6	1.1	1.1	1.4	1.1	1.1				
179	African		0.5				0.6		0.3							0.3	0.0	0.3	0.0
	World		0.9				1.0		0.6							0.6	0.3	0.6	0.0
	European		1.3				1.4		0.9							1.0	0.3	0.8	
180	African	3.1	2.3	2.0	2.1	2.2	2.3	2.3	9.0	5.2	2.6	3.0	4.2	1.8	3.5	2.4	3.7	1.6	1.6
	World	5.3	3.7	3.4	3.5	3.6	3.5	4.0	16.7	8.9	3.9	5.4	7.5	2.7	6.1	4.2	6.0	3.1	2.9
	European	7.4	4.9	4.7	4.9	4.9	4.5	5.4	24.6	12.5	5.1	7.5	10.6	3.4	8.4	5.4	7.4	4.0	4.0
181.0	African	5.8	6.5	5.3	5.8	6.8	6.2	3.3		3.2	3.9	2.5	4.5	2.8	5.4				
	World	10.8	12.1	10.2	11.4	12.9	11.7	6.7		5.9	7.7	4.9	8.4	4.8	10.4				
	European	15.8	17.9	15.4	17.4	19.1	17.3	10.2		8.8	11.8	7.4	12.3	7.4	15.8				
181	African															4.9	9.0	3.7	4.5
	World															8.1	15.1	5.8	7.3
	European															11.6	21.1	8.6	10.5
190	African	1.2	0.8	0.8	0.6	0.9	0.9	1.4	6.1	0.3	1.2	2.4	2.0	1.0	3.7	1.4	2.8	0.6	0.4
	World	1.6	1.0	0.9	0.7	1.1	1.2	1.9	9.0	0.7	1.4	2.7	2.4	1.3	4.5	1.6	3.0	0.8	0.3
	European	2.1	1.3	1.2	0.9	1.5	1.5	2.5	12.6	1.2	1.8	3.5	3.1	1.7	5.9	2.1	3.7	1.2	0.3
191	African	11.6	19.0	13.8	15.7	16.3	15.3	12.8		9.4	12.5		2.6	10.0		0.2	0.5	0.0	0.0
	World	21.1	29.9	23.5	28.2	27.1	26.7	21.6		14.4	21.6		4.9	16.6		0.2	0.5	0.0	0.0
	European	31.8	42.2	34.5	42.4	39.2	39.9	31.4		20.5	32.5		7.9	24.2		0.3	0.7	0.0	0.0
192	African	0.6	0.7	0.5	0.3	0.6	0.4	0.8	0.5	0.5	0.3	0.6	0.7	0.4	0.7	0.3	0.5	0.0	0.0
	World	0.9	0.7	0.5	0.4	0.7	0.5	1.1	0.5	0.8	0.3	0.9	1.0	0.6	1.0	0.4	0.5	0.0	0.0
	European	1.1	0.8	0.6	0.5	0.8	0.6	1.3	0.6	1.0	0.4	1.1	1.2	0.7	1.2	0.5	0.7	0.0	0.0

* See notes to Tables 34, 35, 36 and 37.

Incidence of different types of cancer recorded by each Registry standardized for age : male rates

INCIDENCE RATE PER 100,000 PER YEAR IN:

INTER-NATIONAL LIST No.	STANDARD POPU-LATION	Mozambique Lourenço Marques	Nigeria Ibadan	S. Africa Johannesburg (Bantu)	Uganda Kyadondo	CANADA 5 provinces	Alberta	Manitoba	New Brunswick	Newfoundland	Saskatchewan	Chile	Colombia Cali	Jamaica Kingston	Puerto Rico	U.S.A. Connecticut	N.Y. State	Israel	Japan Miyagi	Singapore (Chinese)
193	African	1.7	0.6	1.8	0.2	4.4	3.9	6.4	3.4	5.5	3.3	0.8	2.5	1.8	1.7	4.5	4.4	9.1	0.3	1.3
	World	1.4	1.0	1.4	0.2	5.4	4.6	8.0	4.0	6.1	4.0	0.9	2.9	2.0	2.0	5.5	5.5	10.7	0.4	1.4
	European	1.2	1.1	1.3	0.1	6.2	5.4	9.3	4.3	6.8	4.8	1.0	3.0	2.0	2.3	6.5	6.4	12.2	0.3	1.6
194	African	0.9	0.9	0.1	0.1	0.7	0.5	0.5	0.6	1.2	0.8	0.6	3.0	0.7	0.5	0.9	0.8	1.5	0.6	0.4
	World	1.8	0.8	0.1	0.1	0.9	0.6	0.8	0.9	1.4	1.2	0.9	4.5	0.9	0.7	1.2	1.1	2.1	1.1	0.5
	European	2.6	0.9	0.1	0.1	1.2	0.8	1.2	1.0	1.5	1.6	1.3	5.8	1.2	1.0	1.5	1.3	2.8	1.6	0.7
195	African	0.0	0.0	0.4	0.4	0.3	0.2	0.8	0.3	0.0	0.1	0.1	0.0	0.2	0.1	0.6	0.4	0.4	0.1	0.1
	World	0.0	0.0	0.4	0.4	0.4	0.3	0.9	0.3	0.0	0.1	0.1	0.0	0.2	0.2	0.7	0.5	0.5	0.1	0.1
	European	0.0	0.0	0.3	0.4	0.4	0.3	0.9	0.3	0.0	0.2	0.1	0.0	0.2	0.2	0.8	0.6	0.6	0.1	0.1
196	African	2.0	1.2	0.3	0.5	1.0	0.9	1.7	1.1	1.1	0.5	1.9	2.6	1.2	1.0	1.1	0.9	1.1	1.8	0.7
	World	3.0	1.1	0.4	0.5	1.2	1.1	1.9	1.1	1.3	0.5	2.7	3.4	0.9	1.2	1.2	1.1	1.3	2.4	0.7
	European	3.9	1.1	0.5	0.4	1.3	1.2	2.0	1.3	1.6	0.6	3.6	3.7	0.9	1.3	1.3	1.5	1.4	3.0	0.7
197	African	3.7	1.4	2.2	1.1	1.8	1.9	1.6	1.9	1.2	2.1	0.3	4.4	1.5	1.2	2.1	1.0	2.2	0.1	0.5
	World	3.8	1.4	2.9	1.6	2.3	2.4	1.7	3.0	1.8	2.5	0.5	5.5	1.6	1.4	2.8	1.8	2.9	0.1	0.7
	European	4.2	1.3	3.8	1.9	2.8	3.1	2.0	3.7	2.3	3.0	0.6	7.3	2.0	1.7	3.5	1.9	3.6	0.0	1.0
200	African	6.3	8.3	0.8	3.7	3.0	2.7	3.7	1.6	1.8	3.9	0.8	3.7	2.5	2.4	2.1	3.7	7.6	1.8	1.2
	World	5.1	8.9	0.9	3.9	4.2	3.2	5.1	2.3	2.5	5.9	1.0	4.6	3.1	3.1	3.1	5.3	9.6	2.9	1.4
	European	4.4	9.1	0.9	3.9	5.4	4.2	6.8	2.8	3.1	7.9	1.3	5.6	4.1	3.9	4.1	7.0	11.8	3.8	1.5
201	African		2.1	1.3	1.7	2.6	2.2	3.9	2.2	2.6	2.4	1.9	2.5	2.7	2.9	3.4	3.1	2.7	0.6	0.7
	World		2.6	1.1	1.7	2.8	2.3	4.0	2.7	2.7	2.5	2.1	3.4	3.0	3.4	3.4	3.2	2.9	0.9	0.8
	European		2.9	1.0	1.8	3.3	2.6	4.6	3.4	2.9	2.9	2.4	4.2	3.8	3.9	3.9	3.7	3.3	1.4	0.8
203	African		0.3	0.7	0.3	1.2	1.0	1.7	0.9	0.7	1.2	0.6	0.4	0.8	0.7	1.1	1.0	1.2	0.1	0.1
	World		0.2	0.9	0.5	2.1	1.7	3.1	1.8	1.2	2.3	0.9	0.4	1.6	1.4	2.2	1.8	2.1	0.3	0.1
	European		0.2	1.1	0.7	3.1	2.4	4.6	2.7	1.6	3.2	1.2	0.4	2.3	2.0	3.3	2.6	2.9	0.4	0.2
204	African	2.9	4.6	2.3	2.3	4.8	3.6	6.4	3.8	3.7	5.4	3.4	3.6	3.2	4.2	6.8	5.8	6.7	3.3	0.9
	World	3.8	4.8	2.7	2.4	7.0	5.1	9.4	5.3	4.3	8.6	3.7	4.1	4.3	5.1	9.9	8.6	9.4	3.8	0.9
	European	4.8	5.4	2.8	2.5	9.2	6.7	12.6	6.3	4.9	11.7	4.1	4.9	5.2	6.0	12.8	11.2	12.0	4.3	0.9
202,205	African			0.6		0.5	0.4	0.8	0.0	0.5	0.8	0.2	1.6	0.2*	0.1	1.8	0.6	0.3	0.0	
	World			0.5		0.7	0.6	1.1	0.0	1.0	0.9	0.2	1.9	0.3**	0.2	2.5	0.8	0.4	0.1	
	European			0.5		1.0	0.9	1.4	0.0	1.6	1.3	0.3	2.2	0.3**	0.3	3.2	1.0	0.4	0.1	
OTHER	African	0.4	5.0	2.5	1.5	2.6	2.0	4.9	2.8	2.2	1.2	6.7	13.2	5.0	4.5	6.9	5.2	6.9	3.3	9.3
	World	0.7	7.6	4.3	2.1	4.4	3.2	8.8	4.4	4.4	2.0	10.7	22.8	8.7	8.0	12.4	8.9	10.8	4.8	12.5
	European	1.1	9.3	5.9	3.0	6.3	4.4	12.9	5.8	6.9	2.6	15.0	31.1	12.3	11.7	18.2	12.9	15.2	6.9	16.1
140-205	African	173.7	61.8	65.9	45.7	145.1	119.9	165.2	151.6	147.0	150.7	83.3	159.2	103.3	118.2	177.1	138.5	156.8	107.7	81.3
	World	186.7	82.7	103.9	58.9	250.1	206.9	280.5	265.6	235.0	266.9	139.6	271.1	175.4	204.3	304.3	242.9	249.5	192.1	117.2
	European	221.9	102.0	142.7	74.8	363.1	298.4	406.7	385.7	333.6	392.0	197.1	377.0	242.9	292.6	439.5	353.5	346.6	273.0	154.3

TABLE 39F

Incidence of different types of cancer recorded by each Registry standardized for age : male rates

INCIDENCE RATE PER 100,000 PER YEAR IN:

INTER-NATIONAL LIST No.	STANDARD POPU-LATION	Denmark	ENGLAND and WALES					Finland	Germany F.R. Hamburg	Iceland	Netherlands 3 provinces	Norway	Sweden	Yugoslavia Slovenia	N. Zealand	HAWAII			
			4 regions	Birmingham region	Liverpool region	South. Met. region	S. Western region									All groups*	Caucasian	Japanese	Hawaiian ethnic
193	African	5.4	4.8	4.9	4.7	4.5	4.6	4.6	3.2	6.5	4.0	6.2	6.0	3.4	4.6	2.7	3.8	1.8	1.8
	World	6.6	5.9	5.8	5.4	5.5	5.8	5.4	4.0	7.7	5.0	7.4	7.3	4.0	5.8	3.1	4.6	1.9	2.3
	European	7.9	6.9	6.6	6.3	6.5	6.9	6.3	4.8	9.6	5.9	8.6	8.9	4.9	6.8	3.5	5.5	2.2	2.3
194	African	0.3	0.3	0.3	0.4	0.3	0.3	0.6	0.5	1.0	0.5	0.6	0.9	1.0	0.7	3.3	4.5	1.0	4.2
	World	0.5	0.5	0.5	0.6	0.5	0.5	0.8	0.8	1.8	0.7	1.0	1.2	1.7	0.9	3.8	5.2	1.5	6.2
	European	0.7	0.7	0.7	0.9	0.7	0.7	1.1	1.1	2.6	0.9	1.4	1.6	2.3	1.2	4.5	6.7	1.9	7.8
195	African	0.2	0.6	0.5	0.4	0.7	0.5	0.6	0.4	0.4	0.4	0.2	1.1	0.2	0.3	0.1	0.3	0.0	0.0
	World	0.3	0.7	0.6	0.5	0.8	0.5	0.6	0.4	0.7	0.5	0.3	1.4	0.3	0.4	0.1	0.2	0.0	0.0
	European	0.4	0.8	0.8	0.5	0.9	0.6	0.7	0.5	0.8	0.5	0.2	1.7	0.3	0.5	0.1	0.2	0.0	0.0
196	African	0.9	0.9	0.7	1.0	0.9	0.9	1.8	2.1	1.2	1.0	0.6	1.1	1.1	1.2	0.6	0.8	0.3	1.4
	World	0.9	1.0	0.8	1.2	1.0	1.1	2.4	2.5	1.6	1.0	0.7	1.1	1.2	1.2	0.7	1.0	0.2	1.8
	European	1.0	1.1	1.0	1.5	1.1	1.3	3.0	2.9	2.1	1.1	0.7	1.2	1.4	1.2	1.1	1.6	0.2	2.0
197	African	0.9	1.2	1.3	1.4	1.2	1.0	1.2	0.5	3.1	0.9	0.7	1.5	0.8	1.5	1.8	1.7	1.7	3.3
	World	1.2	1.5	1.5	1.8	1.4	1.2	1.5	0.5	3.6	1.1	1.0	2.0	0.9	1.9	1.9	2.3	1.9	3.2
	European	1.6	1.8	1.9	2.2	1.9	1.4	1.8	0.6	4.2	1.4	1.3	2.5	1.1	2.4	2.3	3.2	1.9	3.8
200	African	1.4	2.1	2.0	1.6	2.1	2.4	1.6	2.5	2.3	1.0	2.1	2.3	2.1	3.2	2.7	2.6	2.0	4.7
	World	2.0	2.8	2.7	2.3	2.7	3.3	2.3	3.1	2.9	1.2	2.9	3.5	2.8	5.0	4.4	5.0	3.2	6.7
	European	2.7	3.6	3.5	3.0	3.4	4.2	3.0	3.9	3.9	1.5	3.6	4.8	3.5	6.9	6.0	6.7	4.8	10.3
201	African	2.6	2.4	2.6	2.6	2.3	1.9	2.2	2.3	1.4	2.5	2.5	2.7	1.6	2.5	2.0	3.1	1.0	2.8
	World	2.9	2.5	2.6	2.7	2.7	2.0	2.6	2.7	1.5	2.4	2.7	2.9	1.9	2.5	2.8	3.9	1.9	3.8
	European	2.9	2.8	2.9	3.1	2.8	2.4	3.1	3.3	1.6	2.6	3.2	3.5	2.1	3.0	3.8	4.9	2.8	4.7
203	African	1.0	0.7	0.6	0.5	0.8	0.8	0.7		1.5	0.7	1.4	1.4	0.4	1.0	0.7	0.6	0.4	1.4
	World	1.9	1.3	1.0	0.9	1.4	1.3	1.2		2.0	1.3	2.9	2.5	0.8	1.9	1.3	1.4	0.7	3.0
	European	2.7	1.7	1.4	1.3	1.9	1.9	1.7		2.4	1.9	4.3	3.7	1.1	2.8	1.9	1.8	0.9	4.3
204	African	5.8	4.6	4.0	4.4	7.6	4.1	5.0	4.9	6.2	2.2	5.3	6.1	4.1	5.7	5.0	5.0	3.5	8.2
	World	8.3	6.0	5.1	6.2	12.2	5.6	6.9	6.1	8.3	3.2	7.5	8.9	5.1	8.3	7.6	8.3	4.7	12.2
	European	10.3	7.5	6.3	7.9	15.2	6.8	8.5	7.6	9.7	4.4	9.4	11.6	6.0	11.0	9.8	11.3	6.1	16.6
202,205	African	0.2	0.6	0.8	0.5	0.6	0.6	0.1	1.3*	0.2	0.7*	1.1	0.3	0.1	0.4	0.8	0.0	1.1	1.8
	World	0.3	0.8	1.0	0.6	0.8	0.7	0.2	2.2*	0.2	0.8*	1.4	0.3	0.1	0.6	1.1	0.0	1.7	2.2
	European	0.4	1.0	1.2	0.8	1.0	0.9	0.3	3.0*	0.3	1.1*	1.7	0.4	0.1	0.9	1.5	0.0	2.2	2.9
OTHER	African	3.5	2.9	3.2	2.6	2.6	2.7	6.9	4.5	1.5	5.2	4.5	3.7	3.3	2.9	3.1	3.5	3.6	2.5
	World	6.1	5.0	5.7	4.4	4.5	4.8	12.2	7.7	2.5	8.5	8.1	6.4	5.7	4.8	5.9	6.9	6.6	5.4
	European	8.9	7.0	8.3	6.4	6.4	6.7	18.2	11.3	3.7	12.1	12.1	9.1	8.1	6.9	9.0	10.2	10.2	6.7
140-205	African	117.5	143.6	139.7	142.7	136.9	118.5	147.7	126.7	129.5	105.1	94.9*	104.7	106.1	128.7*	110.3	131.8	101.1	152.2
	World	204.9	246.0	246.7	265.5	239.7	210.1	263.8	227.1	216.3	182.6	165.0	182.0	186.9	224.7	190.0	229.6	179.8	261.0
	European	299.3	350.4	356.1	388.1	342.7	302.2	380.0	331.6	312.2	263.8	241.1	264.5	265.7	328.5	275.3	329.6	264.7	364.4

Incidence of different types of cancer recorded by each Registry standardized for age : female rates

INCIDENCE RATE PER 100,000 PER YEAR IN:

International List No.	Standard Population	Mozambique Lourenço Marques	Nigeria Ibadan	S. Africa Johannesburg (Bantu)	Uganda Kyadondo	CANADA 5 provinces	Alberta	Manitoba	New Brunswick	Newfoundland	Saskatchewan	Chile	Colombia Cali	Jamaica Kingston	Puerto Rico	U.S.A. Connecticut	U.S.A. N.Y. State	Israel	Japan Miyagi	Singapore (Chinese)
140	African	0.0	0.0	0.0	0.0	0.6	1.0	0.3	0.3	0.2	0.6	0.1	0.8	0.2	0.4	0.1	0.1	0.8	0.0	0.0
	World	0.0	0.0	0.0	0.0	1.0	1.7	0.6	0.5	0.4	1.0	0.2	1.8	0.5	0.7	0.2	0.2	1.2	0.0	0.0
	European	0.0	0.0	0.0	0.0	1.4	2.6	1.0	0.7	0.6	1.4	0.3	2.2	0.7	1.0	0.3	0.3	1.8	0.0	0.1
141	African	0.0	0.0	0.4	0.2	0.4	0.2	0.3	0.6	0.5	0.4	0.2	1.0	0.7	1.1	0.4	0.4	0.3	0.4	0.3
	World	0.0	0.0	0.9	0.4	0.6	0.4	0.5	0.9	1.0	0.6	0.3	1.8	1.0	2.3	0.6	0.7	0.5	0.5	0.3
	European	0.0	0.0	1.2	0.6	0.9	0.5	0.7	1.3	1.3	0.9	0.5	2.8	1.3	3.0	0.9	1.0	0.8	0.7	0.4
142	African	2.4	0.5	0.3	1.0	1.3	0.9	2.3	1.0	0.7	1.5	0.3	1.3	0.7	0.2	0.5	0.6	0.9	0.3	0.3
	World	3.8	0.6	0.8	1.9	1.6	1.2	3.2	1.1	0.7	1.8	0.4	2.0	1.2	0.4	0.7	0.8	1.1	0.5	0.3
	European	5.2	0.7	1.0	1.0	2.0	1.5	4.0	1.5	0.7	2.3	0.5	2.2	1.7	0.5	1.0	1.1	1.3	0.6	0.4
143-4	African	2.5	0.0	0.1	0.5	0.4	0.3	0.5	0.3	0.3	0.6	0.2	1.1	0.9	1.5	0.7	0.4	0.6	0.2	0.3
	World	3.1	0.0	0.2	0.6	0.7	0.4	0.8	0.5	0.6	0.8	0.2	2.2	1.6	2.6	1.1	0.7	0.9	0.3	0.5
	European	3.6	0.0	0.2	0.7	1.0	0.7	1.2	0.9	1.1	1.3	0.3	3.6	2.2	3.8	1.6	1.0	1.3	0.3	0.7
146	African	0.0	0.0	0.6	0.0	0.2	0.1	0.1	0.1	0.8	0.3	0.0	0.0	0.3	0.2	0.3	0.1	0.6	0.0	0.3
	World	0.0	0.0	1.2	0.0	0.3	0.2	0.2	0.2	1.1	0.6	0.0	0.0	0.5	0.3	0.3	0.2	0.8	0.1	0.5
	European	0.0	0.0	1.6	0.0	0.4	0.2	0.3	0.2	1.5	0.8	0.0	0.0	0.7	0.3	0.4	0.2	0.9	0.1	0.7
145, 147-8	African															1.2				0.1	
	World															2.3				0.2	
	European															3.2				0.3	
150	African	0.0	0.2	0.6	0.2	0.3	0.2	0.5	0.1	0.3	0.1	0.1	0.9	0.2	4.1	0.4	0.3	0.2	3.4	0.3
	World	0.0	0.2	1.2	0.5	0.4	0.3	0.7	0.1	0.4	0.3	0.2	1.6	0.3	7.7	0.7	0.4	0.4	6.3	0.4
	European	0.0	0.2	1.6	0.7	0.6	0.5	0.9	0.1	0.5	0.4	0.2	2.6	0.3	11.2	1.0	0.6	0.6	9.4	0.5
151	African	1.1	3.3	3.8	0.8	5.7	3.8	7.2	5.7	12.2	3.9	2.8	14.6	3.5	7.4	4.9	3.5	1.5	28.4	1.1
	World	2.4	4.9	6.2	0.9	10.4	7.2	12.8	10.7	23.1	7.2	5.0	23.9	5.5	13.9	8.9	6.6	2.6	47.7	2.2
	European	3.5	6.1	8.9	1.3	15.5	10.2	19.2	15.7	33.4	10.7	7.0	31.9	7.9	21.0	13.6	10.2	3.8	67.4	2.7
152	African	0.0	0.0	0.1	0.0	0.4	0.2	0.5	0.6	0.6	0.5	0.1	0.3	0.0	0.5	0.4	0.3	0.4	0.3	0.3
	World	0.0	0.0	0.1	0.0	0.7	0.3	0.8	0.9	0.8	0.9	0.1	0.7	0.0	0.6	0.7	0.5	0.6	0.4	0.3
	European	0.0	0.0	0.1	0.0	1.0	0.4	1.2	1.4	1.1	1.2	0.2	1.0	0.0	0.9	1.1	0.7	0.8	0.5	0.3
153	African	0.9	1.2	2.3	0.6	11.0	8.8	13.7	12.9	11.4	9.9	2.2	1.9	5.4	2.7	13.9	11.2	8.0	2.4	1.4
	World	1.9	2.1	4.1	0.6	19.3	16.1	23.0	24.1	19.6	16.3	3.7	3.0	9.4	4.8	25.4	20.7	12.7	4.1	2.2
	European	2.9	3.1	5.5	0.8	28.1	23.4	33.3	35.1	28.7	23.5	5.3	4.1	13.3	7.1	38.2	30.9	18.2	6.2	2.9
154	African	0.0	0.8	1.2	1.8	4.5	3.2	5.7	5.9	2.7	5.0	3.4	3.3	3.2	1.9	5.6	4.7	4.7	2.6	1.7
	World	0.0	0.9	2.2	2.5	7.9	5.7	9.5	9.9	4.7	8.9	3.4	5.3	5.0	3.3	10.1	8.6	7.9	4.4	2.6
	European	0.0	1.0	2.9	3.3	11.4	8.3	13.5	14.4	6.4	13.1	4.7	7.1	7.1	4.8	14.8	12.7	11.1	6.2	3.5
155.0	African	28.8	1.7	5.4		0.3	0.1	0.7	0.2	0.4	0.4			0.9	0.6	0.5	0.5	0.7		1.0
	World	30.8	2.3	9.9		0.5	0.1	1.2	0.4	0.6	0.4			0.9	1.1	1.0	0.9	1.0		1.2
	European	35.9	3.1	14.1		0.8	0.2	2.0	0.4	0.7	0.6			1.1	1.6	1.5	1.3	1.4		1.4
155.1	African	0.0	0.2	0.7		1.6	1.6	1.7	1.5	1.0	1.9		1.5	1.4	1.5	1.5	1.3	4.4		0.2
	World	0.0	0.4	1.5		3.3	3.3	3.6	2.8	2.2	3.6		1.9	2.6	2.9	3.0	2.5	8.3		0.4
	European	0.0	0.6	1.9		5.0	4.8	5.7	4.0	3.3	5.8		2.4	3.8	4.3	4.7	3.8	12.2		0.6
155	African				2.2							4.3	5.4		1.1				2.7	
	World				2.3							7.8	8.9		1.9				4.7	
	European				2.6							10.9	12.4		2.7				6.6	
156	African		1.1	0.0	1.0	0.4	0.4		0.6	0.7	0.5	2.3		0.2		0.5	0.7	1.5	3.5	0.3
	World		1.6	0.0	1.6	0.7	0.8		1.3	1.4	0.8	3.7		0.2		1.0	1.4	2.8	6.7	0.4
	European		2.0	0.0	2.1	1.0	1.1		1.8	2.2	1.2	5.1		0.2		1.5	2.1	4.4	10.1	0.6

TABLE 40B

Incidence of different types of cancer recorded by each Registry standardized for age : female rates

INCIDENCE RATE PER 100,000 PER YEAR IN:

INTER-NATIONAL LIST No.	STANDARD POPU-LATION	Denmark	ENGLAND and WALES — 4 regions	Birmingham region	Liverpool region	South. Met. region	S. Western region	Finland	Germany F.R. Hamburg	Iceland	Netherlands 3 provinces	Norway	Sweden	Yugoslavia Slovenia	N. Zealand	HAWAII — All groups*	Caucasian	Japanese	Hawaiian ethnic
140	African	0.2	0.2	0.3	0.1	0.1	0.1	0.4	0.1	0.1	0.0	0.1	0.1	0.3	0.1	0.2	0.5	0.0	0.0
	World	0.4	0.3	0.5	0.2	0.1	0.1	0.6	0.1	0.1	0.1	0.1	0.2	0.6	0.2	0.2	0.6	0.0	0.0
	European	0.6	0.4	0.7	0.2	0.2	0.2	1.0	0.2	0.2	0.1	0.2	0.3	0.9	0.3	0.3	0.9	0.0	0.0
141	African	0.2	0.3	0.3	0.3	0.3	0.3	0.4	0.2	2.4	0.3	0.3	0.3	0.1	0.3	0.5	0.9	0.2	1.3
	World	0.4	0.6	0.5	0.5	0.5	0.6	0.6	0.4	2.6	0.6	0.5	0.6	0.2	0.6	0.9	1.5	0.3	2.5
	European	0.6	0.8	0.7	0.7	0.8	0.8	0.8	0.5	2.8	0.9	0.7	0.8	0.2	0.9	1.2	2.1	0.3	3.1
142	African	1.0	1.1	1.2	1.2	1.0	1.0	1.3	2.0*	1.7	0.8	0.2	0.4	0.4	0.7	0.8	0.4	0.9	0.5
	World	1.1	1.2	1.4	1.3	1.1	1.1	1.5	2.5*	2.0	1.1	0.3	0.6	0.5	0.9	1.0	0.7	1.2	0.4
	European	1.5	1.5	1.7	1.6	1.3	1.4	1.9	3.2*	2.3	1.3	0.4	0.8	0.7	1.2	1.4	1.0	1.5	0.3
143-4	African	0.1	0.4	0.3	0.4	0.4	0.3	0.4		0.1	0.1	0.3	0.3	0.2	0.3	0.6	1.1	0.4	0.0
	World	0.3	0.6	0.5	0.8	0.6	0.6	0.6		0.2	0.3	0.6	0.6	0.3	0.6	1.0	1.7	0.8	0.0
	European	0.5	0.9	0.8	1.1	0.9	0.8	0.9		0.3	0.4	0.9	0.9	0.4	0.8	1.4	2.6	1.1	0.0
146	African		0.1	0.2	0.2	0.1	0.0	0.1		0.9	0.1	0.1	0.2	0.2	0.0	0.6	0.4	0.0	0.0
	World		0.2	0.3	0.3	0.1	0.1	0.2		1.3	0.1	0.1	0.4	0.3	0.0	0.7	0.8	0.0	0.0
	European		0.2	0.3	0.3	0.2	0.1	0.3		1.7	0.2	0.1	0.6	0.3	0.0	0.9	1.2	0.0	0.0
145.147-8	African	0.2	0.7	0.6	1.1	0.5	0.6	0.5	0.4	0.3	0.2	0.2	0.3	0.2	0.3	0.2	0.4	0.1	0.0
	World	0.4	1.1	1.1	1.8	0.9	1.1	0.7	0.8	0.4	0.4	0.5	0.7	0.4	0.5	0.4	1.0	0.3	0.0
	European	0.5	1.6	1.5	2.5	1.3	1.6	1.1	1.4	0.4	0.5	0.7	0.9	0.6	0.7	0.6	1.3	0.4	0.0
150	African	0.8	1.3	1.3	1.6	1.2	1.3	2.9	0.4	3.6	0.5	0.4	0.6	0.7	1.2	0.2	0.3	0.4	0.0
	World	1.6	2.4	2.4	3.1	2.2	2.5	5.8	0.8	6.2	0.8	0.8	1.2	1.3	2.3	0.4	0.3	0.7	0.0
	European	2.7	3.6	3.5	4.7	3.3	3.9	9.1	1.4	9.7	1.3	1.2	1.9	2.0	3.5	0.7	0.4	1.2	0.0
151	African	10.4	7.1	8.2	8.6	5.1	4.3	15.7	10.3	16.3	4.9	9.9	7.2	13.6	5.8	10.2	4.8	15.1	11.7
	World	20.1	12.4	15.0	16.8	9.5	8.0	29.5	19.4	30.1	8.8	18.8	13.4	25.3	10.5	16.0	8.8	22.0	18.5
	European	32.4	18.4	22.4	26.1	14.5	12.1	45.2	30.1	46.0	13.5	29.4	20.2	37.3	16.2	22.6	13.0	30.4	25.6
152	African	0.3	0.3	0.3	0.3	0.3	0.1	0.3	0.3	0.5	0.3	0.2	0.4	0.1	0.3	0.2	0.6	0.0	0.0
	World	0.5	0.4	0.4	0.5	0.4	0.2	0.6	0.5	0.6	0.4	0.3	0.6	0.1	0.6	0.4	1.1	0.0	0.0
	European	0.7	0.6	0.6	0.6	0.6	0.3	0.8	0.7	0.8	0.5	0.4	0.9	0.2	0.7	0.5	1.8	0.0	0.0
153	African	8.9	8.6	8.5	9.9	7.7	6.9	3.9	6.5	10.4	6.6	5.6	7.4	2.5	14.7	8.9	13.0	7.0	6.7
	World	15.9	14.5	15.2	17.8	12.8	12.3	7.2	12.2	15.0	11.2	10.2	13.0	4.6	23.7	16.2	24.0	11.9	12.9
	European	24.4	21.0	22.8	26.7	18.5	18.1	10.9	18.4	21.3	16.2	15.3	19.0	6.7	33.6	24.6	35.4	17.9	21.2
154	African	5.7	4.5	4.9	3.8	4.2	3.8	2.7	4.0	2.1	2.9	2.2	3.5	2.9	5.0	4.7	5.2	4.8	1.6
	World	10.2	7.8	8.7	7.0	7.4	6.7	5.1	7.2	3.5	5.4	4.2	6.2	4.8	8.3	7.2	8.5	7.3	2.7
	European	15.0	11.3	13.0	10.5	10.8	9.8	7.4	10.6	5.3	8.0	6.3	9.0	6.9	11.9	10.6	12.9	10.4	3.4
155.0	African	1.5		0.1	0.2	0.3		0.4			0.1	0.5	0.5	1.1	0.5		0.9	0.3	
	World	2.7		0.3	0.3	0.4		0.8			0.2	0.5	0.8	1.1	0.6		1.9	0.6	
	European	4.4		0.4	0.5	0.6		1.1			0.3	0.6	1.2	1.7	0.8		2.9	0.8	
155.1	African	1.5		1.0	0.9	0.7		0.8		1.4	1.9	0.8	1.5	2.3	1.5	1.8	1.0	2.1	2.7
	World	3.1		2.0	1.8	1.4		1.5		2.8	3.6	1.6	3.0	4.3	3.0	3.5	2.2	4.1	4.8
	European	4.6		3.1	2.8	2.1		2.2		4.2	5.5	2.4	4.6	6.2	4.6	5.2	3.3	6.0	8.2
155	African		1.1				1.1		4.5					1.6		0.9			
	World		2.0				2.1		9.0					3.1		1.8			
	European		3.0				3.1		13.9					4.9		2.5			
156	African		0.6	0.8	0.4	0.5	0.3	0.6	0.6	1.2	0.0	0.4	0.4		0.2				2.6
	World		1.0	1.4	0.8	0.8	0.5	1.2	1.0	1.8	0.0	0.8	0.6		0.3				4.8
	European		1.4	2.1	1.3	1.2	0.8	1.9	1.4	2.8	0.1	1.3	0.9		0.5				7.2

* See notes to Tables 27 and 34.

Incidence of different types of cancer recorded by each Registry standardized for age : female rates

INCIDENCE RATE PER 100,000 PER YEAR IN:

INTER-NATIONAL LIST No.	STANDARD POPU-LATION	Mozambique Lourenço Marques	Nigeria Ibadan	S. Africa Johannesburg (Bantu)	Uganda Kyadondo	CANADA 5 provinces	Alberta	Manitoba	New Brunswick	Newfoundland	Saskatchewan	Chile	Colombia Cali	Jamaica Kingston	Puerto Rico	U.S.A. Connecticut	U.S.A. N.Y. State	Israel	Japan Miyagi	Singapore (Chinese)
157	African	0.9	1.1	0.9	1.0	2.4	2.0	3.6	2.0	2.3	1.9	1.4	2.6	0.8	1.3	3.0	2.5	3.0	1.7	0.4
	World	1.9	1.5	1.7	1.0	4.7	3.8	7.0	4.0	4.6	3.7	2.5	4.0	1.3	2.7	5.7	4.9	5.7	3.2	0.5
	European	2.9	1.9	2.9	1.3	7.2	5.5	11.1	6.4	6.9	5.5	3.5	5.5	2.1	4.1	8.7	7.5	8.4	4.6	0.5
160	African	0.0	0.0	0.0	0.9	0.4	0.2	0.4	0.5	0.3	0.4	0.2	0.4	1.1	0.3	0.3	0.3	0.4	1.5	0.7
	World	0.0	0.0	0.0	1.0	0.5	0.3	0.4	0.8	0.7	0.7	0.3	0.8	1.3	0.5	0.5	0.5	0.5	2.1	0.9
	European	0.0	0.0	0.0	1.2	0.8	0.5	0.6	0.9	0.9	1.1	0.5	1.3	1.6	0.8	0.6	0.7	0.6	2.8	1.2
161	African	1.3	0.0	0.3	0.0	0.2	0.1	0.1	0.5	0.5	0.0	0.3	0.7	0.1	0.7	0.4	0.3	0.5	0.4	0.1
	World	1.6	0.0	0.3	0.0	0.3	0.1	0.2	0.9	0.8	0.0	0.4	1.1	0.2	1.3	0.6	0.5	0.8	0.7	0.2
	European	1.8	0.0	0.3	0.0	0.5	0.2	0.4	1.4	1.3	0.0	0.5	1.5	0.4	1.9	0.8	0.6	1.1	1.0	0.3
162-3	African	1.2	1.2	1.7	0.0	2.5	2.6	3.5	1.9	2.1	1.7	2.3	2.1	2.3	2.7	4.0	2.8	4.1	3.2	2.1
	World	1.4	1.4	3.1	0.0	4.4	4.6	6.3	3.3	3.8	2.9	4.0	3.6	3.4	4.7	6.7	4.8	7.7	5.5	3.2
	European	2.2	1.7	4.5	0.0	6.3	6.5	9.2	4.6	5.5	4.1	5.5	4.9	4.0	6.8	9.5	6.9	11.4	7.7	4.2
170	African	1.9	11.9	9.5	7.9	36.8	35.4	40.3	34.7	25.7	40.7	14.0	21.8	22.2	11.1	40.3	32.4	37.2	11.1	6.3
	World	3.2	16.8	15.3	9.7	53.3	51.2	58.5	51.5	37.4	57.4	19.9	31.6	31.1	16.1	59.3	49.1	51.2	13.3	8.0
	European	4.4	21.8	20.9	12.5	72.2	69.3	79.4	70.6	50.6	77.0	26.5	43.0	41.5	21.9	81.9	67.9	67.4	16.8	10.2
171	African	22.5	14.1	35.6	18.1	24.0	18.6	37.6	32.7	18.5	14.8	37.7	77.0	37.6	37.9	10.7	11.6	4.4	15.4	18.0
	World	30.0	21.9	52.0	22.2	25.3	21.1	36.4	33.6	21.8	16.3	44.9	100.6	51.4	47.1	13.6	14.6	5.9	22.1	21.4
	European	39.4	29.8	69.9	27.9	31.6	26.9	44.6	41.8	27.4	20.5	57.3	129.9	67.4	61.2	17.7	19.2	7.7	29.2	26.9
172	African	2.4	0.0	0.1	1.9	7.8	7.5	9.1	8.0	0.4	9.8	2.0	5.3	2.6	1.8	7.8	6.8	6.4	1.2	2.9
	World	2.3	0.0	0.2	3.2	12.6	12.5	14.3	12.7	0.6	15.4	3.3	8.1	4.3	3.0	12.8	12.0	10.1	2.0	4.2
	European	3.0	0.0	0.2	4.2	17.0	16.9	19.5	17.0	0.8	20.8	4.4	10.9	5.6	4.2	17.7	16.7	13.4	2.6	5.5
173	African		2.5	1.5	0.7	0.5	0.1	0.1	0.7	3.3	0.3	0.7	1.0	1.6	0.1	0.0	0.0	0.3	2.1	1.6
	World		2.0	2.0	0.6	0.6	0.1	0.1	0.6	5.3	0.2	0.7	0.8	1.8	0.1	0.0	0.2	0.3	1.8	1.2
	European		2.1	2.4	0.7	0.8	0.1	0.1	0.5	6.6	0.2	0.7	1.0	2.3	0.1	0.0	0.2	0.3	2.0	1.3
174	African		0.0	1.1		0.4	0.0		0.0	2.7	0.0	4.1	0.0	0.0	0.9	2.5	0.9	0.8	4.2	2.6
	World		0.0	2.2		0.4	0.0		0.0	4.6	0.0	5.5	0.0	0.0	1.4	3.9	1.5	1.4	6.9	3.2
	European		0.0	3.6		0.6	0.0		0.0	6.5	0.0	7.3	0.0	0.0	2.0	5.4	2.2	2.1	9.5	4.0
175	African	1.6	5.9	3.2	6.0	7.4	6.1	10.4	6.9	6.1	6.9	1.4	9.7	5.4	3.4	9.2	6.7	8.3	1.7	2.6
	World	2.9	8.5	3.8	7.7	11.0	9.3	15.4	9.6	9.0	10.0	2.0	12.8	7.4	4.9	13.2	10.2	11.9	2.3	3.2
	European	3.8	11.1	4.5	9.8	14.7	12.4	20.9	13.0	11.6	13.4	2.5	16.3	9.5	6.3	17.4	13.8	15.6	2.6	4.0
176	African		0.5		1.8	1.3	1.3	1.1	1.5	1.5	1.2	1.9	3.9	2.0	2.0	1.2	1.2	0.9	0.3	0.8
	World		0.8		2.1	2.1	2.1	2.1	2.5	2.5	1.7	2.8	6.2	2.8	3.4	2.0	2.0	1.7	0.5	1.1
	European		1.1		2.8	3.1	3.0	3.1	3.7	3.5	2.7	3.8	8.3	3.7	5.1	3.0	2.9	2.4	0.8	1.4
180	African	0.6	0.3	0.4	0.1	2.0	2.0	2.2	1.6	1.7	2.0	0.7	1.0	0.9	0.7	1.9	1.7	2.6	0.7	0.6
	World	0.6	0.2	0.5	0.1	3.2	3.4	3.6	2.7	2.2	3.3	1.0	1.3	1.0	1.1	3.3	2.7	4.1	1.0	0.8
	European	0.5	0.2	0.4	0.1	4.4	4.7	4.7	3.5	2.9	4.7	1.3	1.3	1.0	1.2	4.5	3.7	5.4	1.1	0.9
181.0	African	10.0	1.1			1.8	1.3	1.5	2.6	2.2	1.2		2.8		2.0	2.9	1.9	1.8		0.3
	World	14.2	1.6			2.9	2.5	2.4	5.1	3.4	2.4		4.7		3.7	5.1	3.6	2.9		0.5
	European	18.9	2.2			4.5	3.9	3.8	7.5	5.1	3.9		6.6		5.5	7.7	5.6	4.2		0.7
181	African			0.6	1.2							0.5		2.6					1.0	
	World			1.0	1.5							0.8		4.1					1.8	
	European			1.5	1.9							1.2		5.4					2.5	

TABLE 40D

Incidence of different types of cancer recorded by each Registry standardized for age : female rates

INCIDENCE RATE PER 100,000 PER YEAR IN:

INTER-NATIONAL LIST No.	STANDARD POPULATION	Denmark	ENGLAND and WALES 4 regions	Birmingham region	Liverpool region	South. Met. region	S. Western region	Finland	Germany F.R. Hamburg	Iceland	Netherlands 3 provinces	Norway	Sweden	Yugoslavia Slovenia	N. Zealand	HAWAII All groups*	Caucasian	Japanese	Hawaiian ethnic
157	African	2.1	2.0	2.1	2.3	2.0	1.6	2.4	2.2	2.9	1.2	2.0	2.3	1.1	2.5	2.5	2.0	1.8	4.5
	World	4.0	3.9	4.1	4.5	3.9	3.0	4.6	4.4	4.6	2.3	3.8	4.4	1.9	4.6	5.2	4.0	3.8	9.8
	European	5.9	5.9	6.3	6.8	5.9	4.5	7.0	6.7	6.5	3.5	5.6	6.5	2.8	6.8	7.8	6.1	6.3	13.9
160	African	0.2	0.3	0.3	0.3	0.3	0.2	0.4	0.4	0.3	0.2	0.3	0.4	0.4	0.2	0.2	0.0	0.6	0.0
	World	0.3	0.5	0.5	0.5	0.5	0.3	0.7	0.5	0.7	0.2	0.4	0.6	0.6	0.4	0.4	0.0	0.9	0.0
	European	0.4	0.6	0.7	0.7	0.6	0.3	0.9	0.7	1.0	0.3	0.6	0.9	0.8	0.5	0.5	0.0	1.0	0.0
161	African	0.1	0.2	0.2	0.3	0.2	0.1	0.3	0.3	0.1	0.3	0.0	0.1	0.2	0.0	0.6	0.6	0.4	0.9
	World	0.2	0.4	0.3	0.6	0.4	0.2	0.4	0.5	0.2	0.4	0.0	0.2	0.4	0.1	1.1	1.2	0.9	1.7
	European	0.3	0.5	0.5	0.8	0.6	0.3	0.6	0.7	0.3	0.5	0.1	0.3	0.6	0.1	1.6	1.8	1.2	2.4
162–3	African	2.5	5.2	4.4	5.6	5.6	3.7	2.3	4.2	4.0	1.6	1.8	2.2	2.3	3.3	5.3*	4.7*	3.6*	9.4*
	World	4.4	8.9	7.5	9.6	9.9	6.7	4.0	7.6	5.8	2.6	2.8	3.9	4.2	5.6	9.5*	7.4*	6.7*	16.8*
	European	6.4	12.5	10.5	13.5	13.9	9.3	5.9	10.9	8.1	3.6	4.0	5.6	6.1	7.7	13.9*	9.8*	10.8*	23.2*
170	African	28.6	32.8	31.9	27.7	32.4	30.5	17.8	25.8	27.8	29.4	26.0	29.1	14.8	32.6	27.3	39.5	17.2	31.4
	World	43.8	46.9	46.8	40.4	46.7	44.0	26.3	37.8	39.4	45.1	39.0	45.2	21.3	47.2	37.2	58.0	20.1	47.2
	European	60.6	63.2	64.2	55.3	63.2	59.4	35.5	51.5	53.7	62.0	53.5	62.4	28.6	64.2	49.1	77.9	25.9	62.4
171	African	25.7	10.0	9.8	10.6	8.9	10.1	13.0	31.7	12.6	16.6	13.5	15.6	22.0	11.1	32.4	36.7	24.5	45.3
	World	28.3	12.5	12.6	13.8	11.2	12.4	16.0	36.5	16.2	18.9	15.3	17.2	26.2	14.1	35.9	37.6	28.2	50.8
	European	35.6	16.2	16.6	18.1	14.5	16.0	20.8	45.6	20.6	24.2	19.5	21.6	33.3	18.4	44.9	46.7	35.6	63.2
172	African	6.2	5.4	4.6	4.9	5.4	5.4	5.6	8.1*	4.7	5.5	4.5	6.2	3.6	6.0	9.0	10.1	7.0	11.8
	World	10.7	9.1	8.1	8.4	9.0	9.5	9.2	12.7*	7.7	9.8	7.7	11.1	5.9	10.6	12.9	15.6	9.8	18.1
	European	14.7	12.5	11.1	11.6	12.5	13.2	12.4	17.3*	10.4	13.6	10.6	15.6	8.0	14.6	17.1	21.3	12.7	23.2
173	African	0.1	0.5	0.5	0.3	0.2	0.5	0.2		0.2	0.0	0.3	0.3	0.3	0.9	0.1	0.0	0.2	0.0
	World	0.1	0.7	0.7	0.4	0.2	0.5	0.2		0.3	0.0	0.2	0.2	0.3	1.2	0.1	0.0	0.4	0.0
	European	0.1	0.9	0.9	0.5	0.2	0.5	0.2		0.4	0.0	0.2	0.2	0.3	1.6	0.2	0.0	0.5	0.0
174	African	1.1		0.4	0.0	0.4	0.4	1.4		1.0	0.2	0.6	1.5	1.3	0.0				
	World	1.7		0.6	0.0	0.7	0.7	2.2		1.6	0.4	1.0	2.2	2.2	0.1				
	European	2.5		0.8	0.0	1.0	1.0	3.0		2.5	0.5	1.4	2.9	3.3	0.1				
175	African	8.6	7.2	6.9	6.3	7.2	7.1	6.1	11.6	9.1	5.2	7.9	8.7	5.6	9.0	4.8	8.7	6.0	9.9
	World	13.1	10.5	10.1	9.7	10.6	10.1	9.0	17.6	13.1	7.4	11.5	13.1	8.1	12.6	6.6	11.4	7.5	15.9
	European	17.7	13.9	13.5	13.0	14.1	13.5	11.9	23.6	17.1	9.9	15.3	17.5	10.6	16.5	8.9	15.3	9.5	20.7
176	African	1.6	1.2	1.4	1.2	1.2	1.1	1.3		1.3	0.9	1.5	1.2	1.1	1.1	0.5	1.1	0.1	0.0
	World	2.5	2.1	2.4	2.1	1.9	1.9	2.4		1.9	1.6	2.4	2.1	1.8	2.1	0.9	1.8	0.3	0.0
	European	3.6	3.0	3.5	3.1	2.7	2.9	3.4		2.6	2.4	3.5	3.1	2.7	3.3	1.2	2.4	0.4	0.0
180	African	2.1	1.1	1.2	1.2	1.2	0.9	2.0	2.7	3.5	1.2	1.8	2.6	1.6	1.6	1.2	1.7	0.7	1.4
	World	3.8	1.8	1.8	2.0	1.9	1.4	3.0	4.9	6.4	1.8	3.4	4.6	1.6	2.8	1.7	2.8	0.8	1.9
	European	5.3	2.3	2.4	2.6	2.4	1.9	4.0	7.0	9.4	2.4	4.8	6.4	1.9	3.7	2.0	3.3	0.9	2.3
181.0	African	1.8	1.7	1.2	1.7	1.7	1.8	0.8		1.7	1.1	1.0	1.5	0.5	1.1				
	World	3.4	3.0	2.3	3.2	5.1	3.2	1.4		3.2	2.3	2.0	2.9	1.0	2.3				
	European	5.1	4.5	3.6	4.8	2.6	4.8	2.1		4.9	3.5	3.1	4.3	1.4	3.7				
181	African															1.4	2.7	0.5	1.6
	World															2.5	4.6	1.1	2.7
	European															3.8	7.2	1.7	3.7

* See notes to Tables 27, 34, 35, 36 and 37.

TABLE 40E

Incidence of different types of cancer recorded by each Registry standardized for age : female rates

INCIDENCE RATE PER 100,000 PER YEAR IN:

INTER-NATIONAL LIST No.	STANDARD POPU-LATION	Mozambique Lourenço Marques	Nigeria Ibadan	S. Africa Johannesburg (Bantu)	Uganda Kyadondo	CANADA 5 provinces	CANADA Alber.	CANADA Manitoba	CANADA New Brunswick	CANADA Newfoundland	CANADA Saskatchewan	Chile	Colombia Cali	Jamaica Kingston	Puerto Rico	U.S.A. Connecticut	U.S.A. N.Y. State	Israel	Japan Miyagi	Singapore (Chinese)
190	African		0.8	1.3	0.0	1.9	2.5	1.9	1.5	1.4	1.8	0.6	2.3	1.2	0.5	3.2	2.0	2.9	0.1	0.5
	World		1.6	2.0	0.0	2.2	2.7	2.3	1.5	2.5	1.9	0.9	3.4	1.9	0.7	3.6	2.3	3.3	0.2	0.6
	European		2.1	2.7	0.0	2.8	3.4	2.8	1.9	3.4	2.4	1.3	4.1	1.9	0.9	4.3	2.8	4.0	0.3	0.8
191	African	4.5	0.7	1.7	2.4	21.5	18.6	20.4	28.2	18.1	22.9	1.7	18.9	8.9	20.2	20.9	15.2	29.0	0.5	2.0
	World	7.7	1.0	2.8	3.0	35.6	31.7	32.5	47.9	25.1	39.7	2.5	32.0	13.5	34.2	29.7	23.4	40.2	0.8	3.0
	European	10.8	1.2	3.6	3.9	52.2	46.5	47.0	70.4	34.1	59.4	3.5	44.4	18.3	49.9	40.0	33.2	52.5	1.0	4.1
192	African	2.7	0.1	0.3	1.4	0.5	0.3	0.6	0.6	0.0	0.6	0.2	0.5	0.6	0.5	0.3	0.1	0.8	0.2	0.2
	World	2.9	0.1	0.3	1.6	0.6	0.6	0.7	0.9	0.0	0.8	0.3	0.5	0.7	0.7	0.5	0.2	1.2	0.2	0.3
	European	3.2	0.1	0.2	1.9	0.8	0.8	0.8	1.1	0.0	0.8	0.4	0.5	0.7	0.9	0.6	0.3	1.4	0.1	0.3
193	African	1.6	0.2	2.2	0.2	3.4	2.8	5.5	2.4	4.3	2.1	0.6	1.3	0.8	1.6	3.2	3.4	8.1	0.4	1.4
	World	1.4	0.2	3.5	0.3	4.0	3.2	7.2	2.8	5.1	2.2	0.6	1.6	0.9	2.0	3.9	4.2	10.0	0.5	1.4
	European	1.1	0.1	4.4	0.3	4.7	3.6	8.5	3.1	5.9	2.5	0.7	1.6	1.1	2.3	4.5	4.7	11.7	0.5	1.4
194	African	1.4	2.6	1.1	2.2	2.3	2.2	3.1	2.7	2.2	1.4	1.4	5.6	1.5	2.1	2.9	2.6	3.9	1.9	0.9
	World	2.3	3.5	1.7	2.6	2.6	2.2	3.6	3.2	2.5	1.6	2.0	6.6	1.8	2.3	3.1	2.6	4.6	2.6	1.0
	European	3.2	4.3	2.4	3.2	3.2	2.6	4.3	4.1	2.9	2.1	2.7	8.5	2.2	3.1	3.8	3.2	5.6	3.5	1.2
195	African	0.0	0.0	0.3	1.1	0.2	0.2	0.5	0.0	0.0	0.3	0.1	0.2	0.1	0.1	0.5	0.3	0.4	0.0	0.1
	World	0.0	0.0	0.3	1.1	0.3	0.3	0.6	0.0	0.0	0.3	0.1	0.2	0.2	0.1	0.6	0.3	0.4	0.1	0.1
	European	0.0	0.0	0.3	1.2	0.3	0.4	0.7	0.0	0.0	0.2	0.1	0.2	0.2	0.2	0.7	0.4	0.5	0.1	0.1
196	African	1.5	0.4	0.3	0.5	0.9	1.2	0.9	0.4	0.9	1.0	1.3	0.9	0.7	0.4	0.7	0.5	0.8	0.9	0.4
	World	1.7	0.4	0.3	0.5	1.0	1.1	0.9	0.5	1.2	1.0	1.9	1.0	0.7	0.4	0.9	0.7	0.8	1.2	0.4
	European	1.9	0.3	0.4	0.6	0.9	1.1	0.8	0.5	1.4	1.0	2.4	1.0	0.7	0.5	1.0	0.8	0.8	1.5	0.5
197	African	1.7	1.2	1.5	1.4	1.5	1.7	1.0	2.7	0.0	1.8	0.2	1.3	1.6	0.8	1.9	1.0	2.4	0.2	0.3
	World	1.1	1.8	2.1	1.3	1.9	2.2	1.1	3.4	0.0	2.1	0.3	1.8	2.2	0.8	2.3	1.2	2.7	0.3	0.4
	European	1.2	2.2	2.7	1.3	2.3	2.8	1.2	4.5	0.0	2.4	0.3	2.2	2.8	0.9	2.7	1.6	3.1	0.3	0.4
200	African	2.8	7.3	1.0	2.0	1.7	1.2	2.1	1.4	0.8	2.3	0.5	2.3	2.3	1.1	1.3	2.2	4.7	0.6	1.0
	World	2.7	8.5	1.6	2.9	2.5	1.8	3.2	1.9	1.3	3.7	0.7	4.1	2.8	1.8	2.1	3.3	6.3	0.7	1.2
	European	2.9	9.4	2.5	3.3	3.5	2.5	4.4	2.8	1.6	5.0	0.9	5.3	3.5	2.3	2.9	4.5	8.0	0.9	1.4
201	African		0.4	0.9	0.8	1.8	1.5	2.2	2.0	1.1	1.9	1.0	1.3	0.2	1.4	1.8	1.9	2.4	0.1	0.2
	World		0.7	1.4	0.7	1.8	1.5	2.4	2.3	1.1	1.7	1.1	1.6	0.3	2.0	1.9	1.9	2.3	0.1	0.2
	European		0.9	1.8	0.7	2.0	1.7	2.7	2.8	1.5	1.6	1.2	1.9	0.5	2.7	2.1	2.2	2.6	0.2	0.2
203	African		0.0	1.0	0.0	0.6	0.7	0.9	0.5	0.3	0.5	0.4	0.3	0.6	0.4	0.9	0.7	1.2	0.1	0.1
	World		0.0	2.4	0.0	1.1	1.1	2.0	0.8	0.6	1.0	0.4	0.6	1.0	0.7	1.8	1.3	2.2	0.1	0.1
	European		0.0	3.5	0.0	1.8	1.6	2.9	1.2	0.8	1.4	0.5	0.8	1.3	0.9	2.6	1.8	3.1	0.1	0.1
204	African	2.2	3.1	3.0	2.6	3.4	2.6	4.5	3.7	3.8	3.5	2.8	1.3	2.3	2.7	3.1	4.0	5.3	2.8	0.4
	World	2.3	4.5	3.8	3.2	4.5	3.3	6.1	4.9	4.8	4.1	2.8	2.0	3.0	3.3	4.6	5.5	7.1	3.3	0.5
	European	2.9	5.4	4.5	4.0	5.6	4.0	8.0	5.8	6.4	4.8	3.1	2.4	3.4	3.9	5.9	6.9	9.0	2.7	0.5
202,205	African	0.6		0.3		0.5	0.4	0.6	0.1	0.5	0.5	0.2	0.6	0.2*	0.1	2.5	0.5	0.4	0.1	
	World	0.8		0.3		0.7	0.5	1.1	0.1	1.0	0.6	0.2	0.7	0.2*	0.2	3.5	0.6	0.6	0.1	
	European	0.9		0.2		0.9	0.6	1.5	0.2	1.3	0.8	0.2	1.0	0.2*	0.2	4.3	0.8	0.7	0.1	
OTHER	African		4.2	2.8	1.2	2.8	2.4	5.3	2.1	2.5	1.1	7.0	11.5	5.6	3.6	5.4	3.7	7.7	2.4	5.1
	World		5.9	4.6	2.0	4.6	4.2	8.4	3.5	4.3	1.8	10.6	19.0	8.5	6.5	8.9	6.6	13.1	3.4	6.9
	European		7.5	6.3	2.7	6.6	6.1	12.1	5.0	6.6	2.6	14.7	25.3	11.6	9.3	13.0	9.6	18.9	4.5	9.0
140-205	African	97.0	68.6	88.3	64.3	157.8	136.7	193.8	172.2	135.3	148.5	110.6	210.5	129.3	124.8	163.3	131.8	174.6	99.2	64.2
	World	123.3	95.7	137.5	79.5	233.5	206.0	276.7	255.9	204.1	220.1	155.9	304.7	186.5	190.4	248.6	205.9	256.4	151.5	81.5
	European	155.9	122.5	185.6	99.8	322.0	283.5	379.5	353.5	280.8	304.3	207.9	403.5	248.0	264.7	345.3	288.0	345.6	207.4	103.1

TABLE 40F

Incidence of different types of cancer recorded by each Registry standardized for age : female rates

INCIDENCE RATE PER 100,000 PER YEAR IN:

INTER-NATIONAL LIST No.	STANDARD POPULATION	Denmark	ENGLAND and WALES 4 regions	Birmingham region	Liverpool region	South. Met. region	S. Western region	Finland	Germany F.R. Hamburg	Iceland	Netherlands 3 provinces	Norway	Sweden	Yugoslavia Slovenia	N. Zealand	HAWAII All groups*	Caucasion	Japanese	Hawaiian ethnic
190	African	2.0	1.8	1.5	1.4	1.9	1.9	1.7	4.8*	1.5	1.7	2.2	2.4	1.2	7.3	0.9	2.3	0.0	0.0
	World	2.2	2.0	1.6	1.5	2.1	2.3	2.1	6.3	1.8	2.1	2.6	2.8	1.4	7.7	0.8	2.0	0.0	0.0
	European	2.8	2.5	1.9	2.0	2.6	2.9	2.7	8.2	2.2	2.6	3.3	3.5	1.9	9.4	0.8	2.2	0.0	0.0
191	African	7.3	11.5	9.7	9.4	9.0	9.3	10.7		7.2	7.0		1.5	10.8		0.1	0.2	0.1	0.0
	World	13.0	17.2	15.6	16.1	14.5	15.3	18.2		10.2	12.5		2.6	19.8		0.2	0.3	0.3	0.0
	European	19.7	23.9	22.4	24.1	20.5	22.4	26.5		13.7	19.0		4.1	29.1		0.4	0.7	0.4	0.0
192	African	0.5	0.4	0.5	0.4	0.4	0.2	0.6	0.2	0.5	0.3	0.5	0.7	0.4	0.6	0.1	0.2	0.0	0.0
	World	0.7	0.5	0.6	0.5	0.5	0.3	0.8	0.2	0.7	0.5	0.7	0.9	0.5	0.8	0.1	0.3	0.0	0.0
	European	0.9	0.6	0.6	0.5	0.6	0.4	1.0	0.3	0.9	0.4	0.9	1.1	0.7	1.0	0.1	0.3	0.0	0.0
193	African	4.8	3.7	3.6	3.3	3.7	4.2	4.1	1.9	5.9	3.2	5.3	5.5	2.6	2.9	1.8	2.7	0.7	2.4
	World	5.7	4.5	4.3	3.9	4.5	5.0	4.5	2.4	7.5	3.9	6.3	6.9	3.1	3.7	2.2	2.6	1.0	3.5
	European	6.7	5.1	4.8	4.6	5.1	5.7	5.1	2.9	8.9	4.4	7.4	8.3	3.6	4.2	2.4	2.5	1.2	4.1
194	African	1.0	0.9	0.9	1.0	0.9	0.8	1.8	0.7	4.6	1.5	1.5	2.5	1.4	1.3	6.8	5.0	5.7	9.1
	World	1.4	1.2	1.2	1.4	1.1	1.1	2.3	0.9	6.9	1.8	2.2	3.0	2.1	1.7	6.9	4.8	6.3	9.0
	European	1.9	1.6	1.7	1.9	1.5	1.5	3.0	1.3	9.7	2.2	2.7	3.9	2.9	2.3	8.3	5.3	7.6	11.4
195	African	0.2	0.4	0.4	0.4	0.5	0.4	0.3	0.2	0.3	0.5	0.1	1.1	0.1	0.6	0.3	0.9	0.2	0.7
	World	0.2	0.5	0.4	0.4	0.5	0.5	0.4	0.3	0.4	0.6	0.1	1.3	0.0	0.6	0.4	0.6	0.2	0.6
	European	0.3	0.5	0.5	0.5	0.6	0.5	0.4	0.3	0.5	0.6	0.2	1.7	0.0	0.7	0.4	0.6	0.2	0.5
196	African	0.6	0.6	0.5	0.5	0.7	0.6	1.3	0.7	1.6	0.5	0.6	0.7	1.0	0.7	0.3	0.4	0.2	1.1
	World	0.7	0.7	0.6	0.5	0.7	0.7	1.6	1.2	2.0	0.5	0.6	0.7	1.2	0.9	0.4	0.4	0.2	0.9
	European	0.8	0.8	0.7	0.6	0.8	0.8	1.9	1.6	2.3	0.6	0.6	0.8	1.3	1.0	0.4	0.5	0.2	0.8
197	African	1.0	1.1	1.0	1.2	1.1	0.9	1.1	0.4	1.7	0.8	0.7	1.3	0.8	0.7	1.0	0.6	0.7	2.0
	World	1.3	1.3	1.2	1.4	1.3	1.0	1.4	0.5	1.7	0.8	0.9	1.6	0.9	0.9	1.1	0.7	0.5	2.4
	European	1.5	1.6	1.5	1.7	1.6	1.2	1.7	0.7	1.9	1.3	1.1	2.0	1.1	1.1	1.2	0.8	0.5	2.9
200	African	0.9	1.3	1.5	1.2	1.0	1.5	0.9	0.9	1.1	0.5	1.0	1.8	1.3	2.2	1.4	2.0	1.2	1.1
	World	1.3	1.8	2.0	1.7	1.5	2.1	1.3	1.4	1.3	0.8	1.6	2.8	1.6	3.4	2.4	3.6	1.8	2.3
	European	1.7	2.3	2.7	2.2	2.0	2.7	1.8	2.0	1.8	1.2	2.1	3.8	2.0	4.7	3.4	4.9	2.7	3.4
201	African	1.8	1.4	1.4	1.4	1.4	1.6	1.4	1.7	1.2	1.6	1.6	1.7	0.9	1.2	1.1	1.2	0.6	0.6
	World	1.8	1.4	1.4	1.5	1.4	1.5	1.3	2.0	1.2	1.5	1.7	1.9	1.0	1.5	1.5	1.2	0.8	1.3
	European	2.0	1.6	1.5	1.7	1.5	1.7	1.4	2.3	1.6	1.6	1.9	2.3	1.3	1.9	2.1	1.5	1.2	1.6
203	African	0.7	0.6	0.5	0.4	0.6	0.7	0.6		0.4	0.5	0.7	1.0	0.3	0.9	0.4	0.6	0.3	1.5
	World	1.3	1.1	0.9	0.8	1.1	1.2	1.0		0.9	1.0	1.3	1.9	0.6	1.7	0.9	1.3	0.6	3.3
	European	1.9	1.5	1.2	1.2	1.5	1.7	1.4		1.3	1.6	1.9	2.7	0.8	2.5	1.5	2.0	0.9	6.2
204	African	3.9	3.3	3.1	3.3	3.1	3.3	4.3	3.1	3.0	2.1	4.2	4.5	2.5	4.0	4.1	3.9	3.5	4.3
	World	5.4	4.2	3.9	4.2	4.1	4.0	5.5	4.2	4.2	2.6	5.7	6.2	3.2	5.6	5.1	5.6	4.4	5.3
	European	6.5	5.0	4.7	5.2	5.0	4.6	6.6	5.2	5.0	3.2	7.0	7.8	3.8	6.9	5.8	7.2	5.3	5.2
202,205	African	0.2	0.6	0.5	0.4	0.5	0.2	0.2	0.7*	0.1	0.6*	0.6	0.2	0.0	0.3	0.4	0.0	0.5	1.6
	World	0.2	0.6	0.6	0.5	0.6	0.3	0.2	1.1*	0.2	0.9*	0.9	0.3	0.0	0.5	0.6	0.0	0.7	2.2
	European	0.3	0.7	0.7	0.6	0.9	0.4	0.3	1.6*	0.3	1.3*	1.2	0.4	0.1	0.6	0.8	0.0	1.0	2.9
OTHER	African	4.9	2.5	2.7	1.8	2.7	2.4	5.0	4.3	1.6	4.0	4.9	3.5	3.3	2.9	3.6	4.7	2.5	5.1
	World	9.2	4.2	4.7	2.9	4.6	4.0	8.9	7.2	2.9	7.0	9.2	6.4	5.4	4.8	6.5	9.1	3.9	9.7
	European	14.0	6.0	6.8	4.2	6.6	5.7	13.9	10.6	4.1	10.0	14.1	9.2	7.8	6.8	9.7	13.2	5.9	15.0
140-205	African	141.1	124.1	120.7	117.4	116.0	111.6	117.8	135.1	140.8	106.7	105.7*	123.1	106.3	126.0*	137.3	161.6	110.1	172.7
	World	217.0	185.9	186.3	185.1	176.1	169.6	184.7	203.1	209.7	162.7	162.9*	188.9	163.0	189.3*	192.5	230.3	149.9	252.0
	European	307.1	254.4	260.3	261.4	242.3	233.0	259.9	281.3	289.4	225.2	226.4*	261.0	225.6	260.2*	260.8	312.4	203.8	338.1

* See notes to Tables 27, 29, 30, 33 and 34.

REFERENCES

ALI, M.Y. and MUIR, C.S. (1965). "Malignant renal neoplasms in Singapore : survey of incidence mortality and pathological features."
Brit. J. Urol., **36,** 463.

AMERICAN CANCER SOCIETY (1953). *Manual of tumor nomenclature and coding.* Prepared by a Subcommittee of the Statistics Committee, American Cancer Society, Philadelphia, Pa.

AMERICAN MEDICAL ASSOCIATION (1961). *Standard nomenclature of diseases and operations.* Edited by R.J. Plunkett and A.C. Hayden. American Medical Association, Chicago, Ill.

BAILARD, J.C. III, THOMAS, L.B., THOMSON, A.D., EISENBERG, H. and VICK, R.M. (1966). "Morphology and survival rates of cervical cancer in Connecticut and southwest England", in : *National Cancer Institute Monograph,* 19. National Cancer Institute, Bethesda, Md.

BASHFORD, E.F. (1905). "The statistical investigation of cancer". *Scientific Reports of the Imperial Cancer Research Fund No. 2 Part I.* Taylor and Francis, London.

BASHFORD, E.F. (1908). "The ethnological distribution of cancer". *Third scientific report of the Imperial Cancer Research Fund.* Taylor and Francis, London.

BJARNASON, O.(1963). *Uterine carcinoma in Iceland.* M.D. thesis, Reykjavik.

BRAS, G. and WATLER, D.C. (1965). "Neoplasms in Jamaica". *Brit. J. Cancer,* **19,** 681

CAMPBELL, P.C. (1963). "The Connecticut Tumor Registry today". *Connecticut Health Bulletin, Connecticut State Department of Health,* 77.

CANCER REGISTRY OF NORWAY (1961). *The incidence of cancer in Norway, 1953-58.* The Norwegian Cancer Society, Oslo.

CANCER REGISTRY OF NORWAY (1964). *The incidence of cancer in Norway, 1959-61.* The Norwegian Cancer Society, Oslo.

CASE, R.A.M. (1956). "Cohort analysis of cancer mortality in England and Wales, 1911-54, by site and sex". *Brit. J. prev. soc. Med.,* 10, 172.

CASEY, R.S. and PERRY, J.W. (1958). *Punched cards : their application to science and industry.* Reinhold, New York.

CLEMMESEN, J. (1955). "The Danish Cancer Registry, under the National Anti-Cancer League". *Dan. med. Bull,* 2, 124.

CLEMMESEN, J. (1965). *Statistical studies in the aetiology of malignant neoplasms : I Review and results, II Basic tables Denmark 1943-57.* Munksgaard, Copenhagen.

CORREA, P. and LLANOS, G. (1966). "Morbidity and mortality from cancer in Cali". *J. nat. cancer Inst.,* 36, 717.

CORREA, P. LLANOS, G. and AGUILERA, B. (1964). "Estudio sobre causes de muerte en Cali". *Antioguia med.,* 14, 359.

DAVIES, J.N.P. (1958a). "Results achieved by the Kampala cancer survey". *Acta Un. int. Cancr.,* 13, 887.

DAVIES, J. N. P. (1958b). "Collection of statistical data on cancer in Africa". *Acta Un. int. Cancr.*, 13, 905.

DAVIS, J. N. P. (1963). "Some aspects of the cancer situation in Uganda". *Proc. roy. Soc. Med.*, 56, 532.

DAVIS, J. N. P., ELMES, S., HUTT, M. S. R., MTIVALYE, L. A. R., OWOR, R. and SHAPER, L. (1964). "Cancer in an African community, 1897-1956". *Brit. med. J.*, 1, 259 and 356.

DAVIES, J. N. P., KNOWELDEN, J. and WILSON, B. A. (1966). "Incidence rates of Cancer in Kyadondo County, Uganda 1954-1960". *J. nat. cancer Inst.* (in press).

DAVIES, J. N. P. and WILSON, B. A. (1954). "Cancer in Kampala, 1952-1953". *E. Afr. med. J.*, 31, 395.

DAVIES, J. N. P., WILSON, B. A. and KNOWELDEN, J. (1958). "Cancer in Kampala : a cancer survey in an under-developed country". *Brit. med. J.*, 2, 431.

DAVIES, J. N. P., WILSON, B. A. and KNOWELDEN, J. (1962). "Cancer incidence of the African population of Kyadondo (Uganda)". *Lancet*, 2, 328.

DOLL, R. (1966). "World-wide distribution of gastro-intertinal cancer". *J. nat. cancer Inst.* (in press).

DUNGAL, N. (1950). "Lung cancer in Iceland". *Lancet*, 2, 245.

EDINGTON, G. M. and MACLEAN, C. M. U. (1965). "A cancer rate survey in Ibadan, Western Nigeria, 1960-63". *Brit. J. Cancer*, 19, 471.

FERBER, B., HANDY, V., GERHARDT, P. R. and SOLOMON, M. (1962). *Cancer in New York State, exclusive of New York City, 1941-1960 : a review of incidence, mortality, probability and survivorship.* Bureau of Cancer Control, New York State Department of Health, Albany, N. Y.

FLEGG, H. and LUTZ, W. (1959). "Report on an African demographic survey". *J. soc. Res.*, 10, 1.

GENERAL REGISTER OFFICE (1966a). *Code of surgical operations*, 1956, reprinted with corrections, 1966. General Register Office, H. M. S. O., London.

GENERAL REGISTER OFFICE (1966b). *Classification of occupations.* General Register Office, H. M. S. O., London.

GREENBERG, R. A. (1959). "The Connecticut Tumour Registry". *Connecticut Health Bulletin, Connecticut State Department of Health,* 73.

GRISWOLD, M. H., WILDER, C. S., CUTLER, S. J. and POLLACK, E. S. (1953). *Cancer in Connecticut, 1935-1951.* Connecticut State Department of Health Hartford, Conn.

GUTKIND, P. and SOUTHALL, A. W. (1956). *Townsmen in the making.* Institute of Social Research, Kampala.

HENDERSON, M. and CURWEN, M. P. (1961). "Cancer of lung in S. W. England". *Brit. J. Cancer*, 15, 19.

HIGGINSON, J. and OETTLE, A. G. (1957b). "The incidence of cancer in the South African Bantu" *Acta Un. int. Cancr.*, 13, 949.

HIGGINSON, J. and OETTLE, A. G. (1958a). "Cancer survey by S. A. I. M. R. among South African Bantu". *Acta Un. int. Cancr.*, 14, 531.

HIGGINSON, J. and OETTLE, A.G. (1958b). "Carcinoma of the oesophagus in the South African Bantu". *Acta Un. int. Cancr.*, **14**, 554.

HINGGINSON, J. and OETTLE, A.G. (1960). "Cancer incidence in the Bantu and "Cape Coloured" races of South Africa : report of a cancer survey in the Transvaal (1953-55)". *J. nat. Cancer. Inst.*, **24**, 589.

HINGGINSON, J. and OETTLE, A.G. (1966). "Cancer incidence in the South African Bantu : Johannesburg (1953-1955). Age-specific rates with direct standardization to a standard African population". *S. Afr. J. med. Sci.*, (in press).

HOFFMAN, F.L. (1915). *The mortality from cancer throughout the world.* Prudential Press, Newark, N.J.

HOGBEN, L. and CROSS, K.W. (1960). *Design of documents : a study of mechanical aids to field enquiries.* MaxDonald and Evans, London.

KNOWELDEN, J. and OETTLE, A.G. (1962). Cited by Davies, Wilson and Knowelden.

MACLEAN, C.M.U. (1965). "Tradition in transition : a health opinion survey in Ibadan, Nigeria". *Brit. J. soc. prev. Med.*, **19**, 192.

MEINSMA, L. (1963). *Vijfjaagsoverlevingscijfers na Kankerbehandeling* (survival rates after cancer treatment). H.J. Paris, Amsterdam.

MEINSMA, L. (1964). "Voeding en Kanker" *Voeding*, **25**, 357.

MEINSMA, L. (1965). *Resultaten behandeling kankerpatienten, 1956-1958* (Results of cancer treatment). Landelijke Organisatie voor de Kankerbestrijding, Amsterdam.

MUIR, C.S. (1964). "Demography and age-sex distribution of the necropsy population of multiracial Singapore" *Singapore med. J.*, **5**, 96.

MUIR, C.S. (1965). "The incidence of laryngeal cancer in Singapore". *J. Lar. Otol.*, **79**, 203.

MUIR, C.S. and SHANMUGARATNAM, K. (1965). "Incidence of uterine cancer in Singapore". *Israeli J. med. Sci.*, **1**, 214.

MUIR, C.S. and SHANMUGARATNAM, K. (1966). "Incidence of nasopharyngeal cancer in Singapore". *U.I.C.C. symposium on cancer of the nasopharynx.* Munksgaard, Copenhagen.

NEW ZEALAND DEPARTMENT OF HEALTH (1965). *Cancer data : deaths, 1964, and cases reported, 1963.* Medical Statistics Branch, Department of Health, Wellington.

OETTLE, A.G. (1957). "The incidence of mammary cancer in the Bantu". *Proc. Second Internat. Symp. on Mammary Cancer.*

OETTLE, A.G. (1960). "Cancer in the South African Bantu". *Cancer Progress,*

OETTLE, A.G. (1964). "Cancer in Africa, especially in regions south of the Sahara". *J. nat. Cancer Inst.*, **33**, 383.
and HINGGINSON, J. (1956). "The incidence of primary carcinoma of the liver in the Southern Bantu. Part II : Preliminary report on incidence". *J. nat. Cancer inst.*, **17**, 281.

PAYNE, P.M. (1961). "Cancer registration, planning and policy." *Postgraduate med. J.*, **37**, 350.

PAYNE, P.M. (1964). "Methods of cancer registration in S.E. England with special reference to the use of a medium sized electronic data processing system". In : *Atti dei colloqui sui rapporti tra fisica e medicina.* Arti grafiche saturnia, Trento.

PAYNE, P.M. (1965). "Cancer registration, its methods, problems and uses". In : *A decade of progress.* Cancer Institute, Madras.

PEDERSEN, E. and MAGNUS, K. (1959). *Cancer registration in Norway. The incidence of cancer in Norway, 1953-54.*The Norwegian Cancer Society, Oslo.

PRATES, M.D. and TORRES, F.O. (1959). "A cancer survey in Lourenço Marques". *J. nat. Cancer Inst.,* **35,** 729.

PRICE, C.H.G. (1962). "Incidence of osteogenic sarcoma in Southwest England and its relationship to Paget's disease of bone". *J. Bone Joint Surg.* **44B,** 366.

RAVNIHAR, B. (1960). "Eight years of cancer registration in Slovenia (Yugoslavia)". *Acta Un. Int. Cancr.* **16,** 1578.

RAVNIHAR, B. (1963). "The management of carcinoma of the lung". *Acta Un. int. Cancr.,* **19,** 1361.

RINGERTZ, N. , TÖRNBERG, B., SJÖSTRÖM, A. and SWENSON, D. (1962). *Cancer incidence in Sweden, 1959.* National Board of Health, the Cancer Registry, Stockholm.

RINGERTZ, N., TÖRNBERG, B., SJÖSTRÖM, A. and SWENSON, D. (1963). *Cancer incidence in Sweden, 1960.* National Board of Health, the Cancer Registry, Stockholm.

RINGERTZ, N., TÖRNBERG, B., SJÖSTRÖM, A. and SWENSON, D. (1965). *Cancer incidence in Sweden, 1961.* National Board of Health, the Cancer Registry, Stockholm.

SAXEN, E. and HAKAMA, M. (1964). "Cancer illness in Finland". *Ann. Med. exp. Biol. Fenn.,* **42,** Suppl. 2.

SEGI, M. (1960). *Cancer mortality for selected sites in 24 countries (1950-57).* Department of Public Health, Tohoku University School of Medicine, Sendai, Japan.

SEGI, M., FUKUSHIMA, I., FUJISAKU, S., KURIHARA, M., SAITO, S., ASANO, K. and NAGAIKE, H. (1957). "Cancer morbidity in Miyagi Prefecture Japan , and a comparison with morbidity in the United States". *J. nat. Cancer Inst.,* **18,** 373.

SEGI, M. and KURIHARA, M. (1962). *Cancer mortality for selected sites in 24 countries No. 2. (1958-1959).* Department of Public Health, Tohoku University School of Medicine, Sendai, Japan.

SEGI, M. and KURIHARA, M. (1963). *Trends in cancer mortality for selected sites in 24 countries (1950-59, graphic edition).* Department of Public Health, Tohoku University School of Medicine, Sendai, Japan.

SEGI, M. and KURIHARA, M. (1964). *Cancer mortality for selected sites in 24 countries No. 3 (1960-1961).* Department of Public Health, Tohoku University School of Medicine, Sendai, Japan.

SINGAPORE MINISTRY OF CULTURE (1966). *Singapore : facts and figures.* Government Printing Office, Singapore.

SNAEDAL, G. (1964). "Cancer of the breast". *Acta Chir.* Scand., Suppl. 338.

STEINITZ, R. (1963). *The Israel Cancer Registry : new cases of malignant neoplasms in 1960 and 1961.* Ministry of Health, Division of Chronic Diseases and Rehabilitation, Jerusalem.

STEINITZ, R. (1965). *The Israel Cancer Registry : malignant neoplasms in four-year period 1960-1963* Ministry of Health, Division of Chronic Diseases and Rehabilitation, Jerusalem.

STEINITZ, R. and TZUR, B. (1965). *Israel Cancer Registry, its data and data processing.* Ministry of Health, Division of Chronic Diseases and Rehabilitation in co-operation with the Israel Cancer Association, Jerusalem.

STOCKS, P. (1959). "Cancer registration and studies of incidence by surveys". *Bull. Wld Hlth Org.,* **20,** 697.

VELASQUEZ, G. (1965). "Needed research on morbity and health in Latin America". *The Milbank Memorial Fund Quarterly,* **43,** 354.

VICK, R.M. (1960). "A cancer records bureau". In : *British surgical progress.* Butterworth, London.

WATLER, D.C., BRAS, G., and McDONALD, H.G. (1959). "The incidence of malignant neoplasms in Jamaica". *W. Indian med. J.,* **8,** 249.

WORLD HEALTH ORGANIZATION (1950). "Report of the subcommittee on the registration of cases of cancer as well as their statistical presentation". In : "Report of the second session of the expert committee on health statistics", *Technical report series,* No. 25, World Health Organization, Geneva.

WORLD HEALTH ORGANIZATION (1952). "Second report of the subcommittee on the registration of cases of cancer as well as their statistical presentation". In : "Third report of the expert committee on health statistics". *Technical report series,* No. 53, World Health Organization, Geneva.

WORLD HEALTH ORGANIZATION (1957). *Manual of the international statistical classification of diseases, injuries and causes of death.* Seventh revision. World Health Organization, Geneva.

WORLD HEALTH ORGANIZATION (1959). "Third report of the subcommittee on cancer statistics". In : "Sixth report of the expert committee on health statistics". *Technical report series,* No. 164. World Health Organization, Geneva.

WORLD HEALTH ORGANIZATION (1962). "Cancer control; first report of an expert committee". *Technical report series,* No. 251. World Health Organization, Geneva.

WORLD HEALTH ORGANIZATION (1964). *The application of automatic data processing systems in health administration.* European Office, World Health Organization, Copenhagen.

WORLD HEALTH ORGANIZATION (1965a). *Epidemiological and Vital Statistics Reports,* 18, No. 12, World Health Organization, Geneva.

WORLD HEALTH ORGANIZATION (1965b). *World Health Statistics Annual,* 1962, Part I. World Health Organization, Geneva.

WORLD HEALTH ORGANIZATION (1966). "Cancer treatment; report of an expert committee". *Technical report series,* No. 322. World Health Organization, Geneva.

APPENDIX

No single index can be used to indicate the "reliability" of cancer incidence data, in the full sense of the word. Several indices have been used, but none do more than fill in a corner of the picture. The most commonly reported is the proportion of cases histologically confirmed. If registration is complete, this provides an indication of the extent to which patients with a clinical diagnosis of cancer are fully investigated; and it can be used to provide a firm estimate of a minimum incidence, which the true incidence certainly exceeds. It should be noted, however, that a high proportion will be recorded if the Registry draws its material principally from pathological departments and it may be obtained by a Registry which, by not obtaining the co-operation of hospital departments of medicine and surgery or of general practitioners, fails to record a large proportion of affected patients. The cases on which the Singapore rates in chapter IV are based, were, for example, 100 per cent histologically confirmed - simply because registration depended wholly on the receipts of a pathological report. Alternatively a low proportion does not necessarily mean that the corresponding incidence data are unreliable; it may merely be that the process of registration has not demanded histological information.

The proportion of cases known to be histologically confirmed at 14 of the co-operating registries are shown separately for each primary site in Appendix Tables 1 (for males) and 2 (for females). Definitions of the international list numbers are given in chapter III. Notes concerning minor modifications of the definitions, adopted in this report by the individual registries, are given in the description of the registries and in the footnotes to the relevant cancer incidence Tables in Chapter IV.

It should be noted that in the Connecticut and New York State material histological confirmation is taken to include all cases confirmed at autopsy; and that in the Israel material, it is taken to include cases confirmed at autopsy, if it is also stated that specimens were taken for microscopic examination. In the Israel material cases are also assumed to have been histologically confirmed if the patients were treated by radical surgery or if a specific histological diagnosis is given (unless there is reasonable doubt about whether a biopsy was performed).

Another useful index is the proportion of cases registered as a result of the receipt of information from death certificates. This, unfortunately, can be construed in different ways and comparison of the proportions reported by different registries is liable to be misleading unless the registries are consulted to make sure that the figures imply the same thing. Appendix Tables 3 and 4 show respectively for males and females the proportions of registrations dependent on death certification for each primary site at 8 of the co-operating registries.

The low figures for the Liverpool regional registry of England and Wales indicate the proportion of cases which were registered solely on the basis of death certification information. They exclude cases that were first notified from death certification, but which were subsequently confirmed by evidence obtained on inquiry to hospitals. The Icelandic data similarly are limited to cases notified from death certification, when inquiry showed that the patient had never entered hospital. In contrast, the Connecticut and New York State data include all cases first notified from death certification, so long as no evidence was subsequently obtained to show that the diagnoses were incorrect.

It should be noted, that even in Connecticut, where the cancer registry is highly organized and has been long established, information about some cases is still received first from death certificates. When the proportion first notified in this way is large it must be suspected that the figures for cancers in sites which normally have a high survival rate are substantially underestimated, whereas other figures (such as those for leukaemia, or cancer of the stomach or lung) may be almost complete. In the New Zealand registry (the figures for which are not given in the Appendix Tables) an attempt has been made to overcome this discrepancy by multiplying the recorded incidence rate for each site by a factor equal to the total number of deaths recorded for cancer of that site divided by the corresponding number of deaths in patients whose cancers had previously been registered.

APPENDIX TABLE 1

Percentage of cases confirmed histologically: male

INTER-NATIONAL LIST No.	REGISTRY													
	S. Africa Johannesburg (Bantu)	Uganda Kyadondo	Colombia Cali	Jamaica Kingston	Puerto Rico	U.S.A. Connecticut	U.S.A. N.Y. State	Israel	Japan Miyagi prefecture	ENGLAND and WALES Birmingham region	ENGLAND and WALES Liverpool region	Finland	Iceland	Netherlands 3 provinces
140		-	100	100	100	97	97	82	50	58	48	89	92	72
141		-	100	85	97	91	81	94	50	65	57	83	100	97
142		100	100	100	86	92	88	95	50	91	80	96	100	100
143-4	89	-	100	100	98	91	86	98	88	70	62	77	50	97
146		-	-	78	100	90	73	92	67	87	63	82	100	100
145,147-8		100	91	93	96	88	77	88	100	69	68		67	98
150	76	88	53	81	75	71	62	53	25	60	54	53	66	78
151	44	39	73	72	59	72	55	69	27	54	48	44	68	70
152	*	100	60	100	88	94	73	76	0	79	85	73	100	91
153	*	0	72	75	78	82	68	85	28	60	70	66	71	82
154	*	100	100	75	89	86	78	89	33	69	68	70	97	87
155.0	62	62	92	96	71	74	47	90	15	68	73	82	90	96
155.1		100	90	85	74	81	62	84		56	72			83
156	*	13	-	100	42	50	58	47	4	20	29	26	47	67
157	*	71	43	74	46	65	47	51	15	27	38	49	68	55
160	88	100	100	80	92	96	85	100	64	93	85	89	90	94
161	75	100	92	92	96	90	83	93	55	82	78	93	92	94
162-3	36	42	78	72	57	69	60	67	29	49	51	52	82	92
170	100	100	100	80	100	89	86	89	80	80	93	100	100	86
177	48	38	86	63	73	77	65	55	37	41	48	53	71	62
178	*	100	90	100	86	96	89	94	56	97	97	90	93	97
179	*	68	93	92	98	94	88	100	50	91	87	100	88	93
180	82	77	100	100	87	80	71	81	58	72	85	75	98	92
181		100	82	92	84	91	83	88	47	72	58	75	83	97
190	100	83	88	100	88	97	84	96	100	96	92	100	100	98
191	89	91	94	56	100	97	98	64	55	46	42	96	93	82
192	*	88	100	100	100	85	65	73	43	97	80	90	83	100
193	*	50	74	96	71	80	62	68	20	61	80	72	53	82
194	*	0	100	88	100	98	80	94	33	75	74	100	93	91
195	*	67	-	100	100	85	74	95	0	70	64	67	40	77
196	*	100	69	92	92	77	57	96	63	74	66	69	69	93
197	*	100	91	100	100	97	82	91	0	90	88	94	100	100
200		88	100	100	93	86	75	94	58	92	88	100	87	97
201		92	88	100	97	92	74	85	27	95	93	92	91	97
203	98	50	100	80	84	73	46	60	0	60	78	40	25	91
204		100	100	99	68	85	52	100	41	41	56	55	49	99
202,205		-	88	100	80	94	78	100	0	79	75	35	100	100
OTHER	*	18	67	57	71	71	66	54	16	59	50		55	73
140-205	*	73	84	79	80	82	71	74	29	56	56	61	74	83

* Not available.

APPENDIX TABLE 2

Percentage of cases
confirmed histologically: female

INTER-NATIONAL LIST No.	S. Africa Johannesburg (Bantu)	Uganda Kyadondo	Colombia Cali	Jamaica Kingston	Puerto Rico	U.S.A. Connecticut	U.S.A. N.Y. State	Israel	Japan Miyagi prefecture	ENGLAND and WALES Birmingham region	ENGLAND and WALES Liverpool region	Finland	Iceland	Netherlands 3 provinces
140		-	100	80	71	100	90	87	-	50	55	95	100	50
141		100	86	100	98	87	79	75	63	75	70	100	67	96
142	100	100	100	82	86	86	90	98	57	94	88	97	88	97
143-4		50	88	96	98	100	87	89	25	75	76	94	50	100
146		-	-	60	83	100	74	93	100	95	84	90	90	100
145,147-8		0	100	100	93	88	77	93	0	80	72		33	100
150	50	33	75	80	69	79	65	70	17	62	72	47	63	100
151	50	67	68	71	54	63	47	58	22	37	42	34	57	87
152	*	-	100	-	92	68	65	86	50	63	83	65	100	74
153	*	33	100	71	67	78	67	82	25	57	55	58	75	93
154	*	89	100	92	92	86	76	88	24	63	63	69	79	86
155.0	39	90	84	100	64	78	34	90	11	70	95	70	80	100
155.1		-	91	96	86	85	65	85		58	67			85
156	*	20	-	100	53	60	57	27	6	35	24	15	59	50
157	*	75	81	57	48	59	40	57	12	29	39	38	69	62
160	0	75	100	100	91	87	81	93	55	83	84	87	83	100
161	50	-	75	100	92	93	81	81	82	79	72	92	50	100
162-3	38	-	86	71	56	71	54	61	15	48	76	49	66	87
170	65	50	86	87	97	90	80	90	62	79	64	92	96	91
171	76	62	97	92	97	97	92	97	66	85	92	96	95	98
172	*	70	94	90	98	99	92	99	77	92	89	95	98	98
173	*	100	100	100	100	100	85	100	44	100	100	66	100	100
174	*		-	-	37	83	54	47	19	53	-		53	100
175	*	92	97	94	94	91	73	86	54	84	85	85	94	92
176	*	88	83	90	96	90	88	94	88	87	84	86	100	93
180	83	100	86	100	83	83	70	79	47	70	81	66	78	93
181		20	82	90	92	84	79	76	63	58	60	64	77	92
190	83	-	100	83	93	97	89	95	67	97	96	100	93	94
191	100	92	96	59	100	96	98	62	83	46	50	94	90	82
192	*	100	100	90	93	83	74	78	67	82	80	93	100	100
193	*	100	70	82	73	80	59	76	43	64	83	81	61	82
194	*	70	94	90	92	95	89	91	63	80	72	87	88	97
195	*	100	100	50	50	74	72	89	0	80	50	67	100	65
196	*	75	71	78	91	90	46	90	45	69	58	69	80	88
197	*	100	90	100	100	100	86	98	40	87	90	100	100	100
200		92	88	100	88	79	77	92	58	91	87	88	91	97
201		100	100	100	97	87	73	88	50	88	90	97	90	96
203	84	-	50	58	67	80	48	53	100	59	68	41	50	89
204		100	100	100	69	83	45	100	51	38	42	37	62	97
202,205		-	100	100	75	89	71	96	0	84	75	20	100	99
OTHER	*	17	69	60	60	67	60	49	46	55	52		69	73
140-205	*	72	90	85	86	86	76	78	37	67	65	69	80	90

* Not available.